GET CONNECTED

To Content Updates, Study Tools, and More!

Meet SIMON 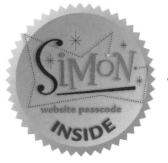 Your free online website companion

Introduction to Health Information Technology

sign on at:

http://www.harcourthealth.com/SIMON/Davis/introHIT/

what you'll receive:

Whether you're a student or an instructor, you'll find information just for you. Things like:
- Content Updates
- Links to Related Publications
- Author Information . . . and more

plus:

WebLinks

Hundreds of active websites relevant to Health Information Management. The WebLinks are continually updated, with new ones added as they develop. Simply tear along the perforated edges of the card and register with the listed passcode. Passcodes expire 18 months after initial registration.

If this book is used or if the section at the right has been removed, please go to the web address above to see options for gaining access to this book's web enhancements.

W.B. SAUNDERS COMPANY

DAVLACQYFEGG

Introduction to

Health Information Technology

Nadinia Davis, MBA, CIA, CPA, RHIA
Assistant Professor
Health Information Management
Kean University
Union, New Jersey

Melissa LaCour, RHIA
Program Director
Health Information Technology
Delgado Community College
New Orleans, Louisiana

Introduction to

Health Information Technology

W.B. SAUNDERS COMPANY
A Harcourt Health Sciences Company
Philadelphia   London   New York   St. Louis   Sydney   Toronto

W.B. SAUNDERS COMPANY
A Harcourt Health Sciences Company

The Curtis Center
Independence Square West
Philadelphia, Pennsylvania 19106

Library of Congress Cataloging-in-Publication Data

Davis, Nadinia
Introduction to health information technology / Nadinia Davis, Melissa LaCour.—1st ed.

p. ; cm.

Includes index.

ISBN 0–7216–8353–3

1. Medical informatics.   2. Medicine—Information technology.   3. Information resources manage-
ment.   I. LaCour, Melissa.   II. Title
 [DNLM: 1. Delivery of Health Care—organization & administration—United States.   2. Information
Management—organization & administration—United States.   W 84 AA1 D249i 2002]

R858 .D386 2002

362.1′068′4—dc21   2001049542

Editor-in-Chief: Andrew Allen
Acquisitions Editor: Maureen Pfeifer
Associate Developmental Editor: Rebecca Swisher
Manuscript Editor: Amy Norwitz
Production Manager: Pete Faber
Illustration Specialist: Lisa Lambert
Illustrator: Lisa Weischedel

INTRODUCTION TO HEALTH INFORMATION TECHNOLOGY   ISBN 0–7216–8353–3

Printed in the United States of America.

Last digit is the print number: 9   8   7   6   5   4   3   2   1

This book is dedicated to all of those individuals who have inspired me to enter the Health Information Management profession, to participate in the educational process, and to volunteer with the associations.

I would particularly like to thank Marion Gentul, RHIA, CCS, for her constant support and guidance. You were right—this is a very exciting profession!

Thanks to my colleagues at Kean University (formerly my instructors!), Natalie Sartori, MEd, RHIA, and Barbara Manger, MPA, RHIA, for their encouragement.

To Maureen Pfeifer, W.B. Saunders Acquisitions Editor, and all of the editorial and production staff who worked with us: thank you for your faith in us, and apologies for the missed deadlines!

To the reviewers: thank you for slogging through those horrible early drafts.

Finally, to my family: thank you for your patience and understanding through this process.

NADINIA DAVIS

This work is dedicated to my husband, Ricky: your love and support gave me strength! To my children, Brett and Beth: you are my greatest inspiration! To my parents, Bill and Ginger Brewer: your encouragement, love, and support give me courage! To my sister, Christy: thank you for always being there when I need you!

To Nadinia Davis: thanks for the friendship, memories, and guidance . . . this has been an exciting experience! To Bob Garrie: thanks for the connection!

A special thank-you to Maureen Pfeifer, Scott Weaver, Erin Nihill, Helaine Tobin, and the numerous W.B. Saunders editorial and support staff who have made this book a reality.

To Kim Mercadal, Christy Biggers, and Harold Gaspard: IT is finished!

And to the educators and mentors who have touched my life along the way: Bill and Nancy Lochmann; Stevan Nielsen; Helen Baxter, RHIA; Sandy McCall, RHIA; Mary Ann Torsch, RHIA: you have made a difference in my life.

MELISSA URSO LACOUR

INTRODUCTION

The purpose of this text is to introduce the reader to health information technology both as a work-based, task-oriented function and as a part of a larger profession of health information management. The book is organized such that the reader is taken from a broad view of the health care industry, to the basic elements of health information technology, through personal experience in a physician's office, and then on to the acute care and other environments and a variety of technical issues. The content progresses such that the individual will be functional in the particular topic discussed in each chapter and, upon mastery of those elements, will be able to understand the following chapters. The book is designed in this way to derive maximum benefit from the natural learning process. For example, if one were going to learn about health care, what better place to start than in a physician's office? In the current health care environment, in many ways a primary care physician is the link to all other aspects of the health care continuum. So we begin quite naturally with the physician office scenario and move into other areas.

This book is both a teaching text that can be used in a classroom and a self-study text that can be used independently. Although the text stands alone, it is best used in conjunction with the accompanying workbook. While the workbook does not contain additional didactic information, it does contain a wealth of exercises and self-study materials so that the student can reinforce the learning.

This book is designed to meet the needs of students at the beginning of their course of study in health information. It can easily fit into a one quarter– or one-semester course in introduction to health information technology or introduction to medical records science, both in degree programs and in certificate courses, such as coding and tumor registry. We believe that a complete integration of computer-based terminology and concepts is necessary to effectively address the basic issues of health information technology. We also believe that because health information technology is a competency-based program, the textbook should follow that competency basis as closely as possible. In addition, we believe that certain technology courses within an accredited program in health information technology, such as coding and statistics, are not appropriately addressed extensively in an introductory text. To those ends,

- We have integrated computer-based terminology and concepts, statistics, and legal and coding issues into the various chapters wherever they arise naturally. For example, the calculation of average length of stay arises from a discussion of facility types.

- Every chapter objective tracks a specific task competency that is pertinent to an introductory course.
- Each chapter builds on the previous chapters and encourages the application of key concepts at each level.
- Special health records are addressed only as elements of either an outpatient or inpatient record.

In order to understand what health information technology is, it helps to have a broader picture of health information management in general. Ever since physicians and other caregivers have been documenting their care of patients, they have had individuals working with them to help, at a minimum, store and retrieve that documentation. In the late nineteenth century and early twentieth century, the individuals who performed that function, most notably in hospitals, were the medical record librarians. (We like to imagine these people in the basement with the cobwebs and the dust mites, scurrying around trying to file and retrieve charts.)

The health information management profession has grown over the last 70 years as a result of health information management professionals', both individually and collectively, assuming increasing responsibilities as health care delivery has become a more complex industry. The field of health information management embraces a variety of individual functions and professional capacities, and a number of national and international professional organizations reflect the diversity of the profession in general. Notably, the American Health Information Management Association (AHIMA), based in Chicago, provides the national leadership for the broad-based management and technical aspects of health information management. AHIMA is an association of over 40,000 professionals, students, and associate members, all of whom have the common goal of ensuring quality health care through quality data.

Health information management today is so broad that its elements and the knowledge that individuals must acquire in order to successfully practice cannot be contained in one volume. This book was designed to start the process. It can be used as an introductory text in a health information management program. It can be used as the foundation text in a health information technology program. It can also be used by individuals who just wish to acquire some basic knowledge of health information technology and how it fits into the health care arena.

For whatever reason you are reading this text, remember that it is the beginning of the journey. The understanding of health information technology is not achieved by the end of this book. There are additional skills that must be obtained. One must acquire additional knowledge from other sources in order to be a successful practicing professional in this field. Also, the industry and the profession are changing constantly. We have no doubt that there will be elements in this book that will be outdated the moment it goes to press. However, that is the challenge of life-long learning.

We believe that health information technology is an exciting and rewarding career choice for students, and we have tried our best to infuse the narrative with that enthusiasm. We hope you enjoy using this text and would welcome any comments that you may have to improve it for our next edition.

ABOUT THE AUTHORS

Nadinia Davis

Nadinia Davis is an Assistant Professor of Health Information Management at Kean University in Union, New Jersey. She holds a bachelor's degree in political science from Villanova University in Pennsylvania and an MBA with a concentration in accounting from Fairleigh Dickinson University in New Jersey. Nadinia began her career working in a variety of administrative capacities and entered the financial services industry in 1980. Upon completing her master's degree, she joined the Corporate Audit Division of Merrill Lynch & Company. Nadinia rose to the position of Assistant Vice President there, at which point she decided to make a career change to health care, specifically health information management. She returned to school and obtained her post-baccalaureate certificate in health information management from Kean University. Nadinia has worked in a variety of capacities in acute care facilities. She has been a coding consultant and a director of medical records in a rehabilitation facility.

Nadinia has spent her entire career in health information management, lending her talents and expertise in a volunteer capacity to both the New Jersey Health Information Management Association and the American Health Information Management Association. In 1999, she received the NJHIMA Distinguished Member Award. In 2001, she completed a 3-year term on the Board of Directors of AHIMA.

Melissa LaCour

Melissa LaCour is the Program Director of the Health Information Technology department at Delgado Community College in New Orleans, Louisiana. Melissa holds a bachelor's degree in medical record administration from Louisiana Tech University. Melissa has held a variety of positions in health information management including manager of medical records at a rehabilitation center, release of information specialist in acute care, and assistant director and director of medical records in acute care. Melissa joined Delgado in August of 1996. She also volunteers her time with the Louisiana Health Information Management Association and the Greater New Orleans Health Information Management Association, of which she is a past president.

CONTENTS

UNIT ONE **CONTENT and STRUCTURE of HEALTH INFORMATION**

CHAPTER 1. **Health Care Delivery Systems** 2

Health Care Professionals 4

Physicians 4
Nurses 6
Allied Health Professionals 8

Patient Care Plan 8
Acute Care Facilities 10

Admission and Discharge 11
Length of Stay 12
Average Length of Stay 14

Ambulatory Care Facilities 15

Physician's Office 15
Group Practice 15
Clinic 16
Ambulatory Surgery 16
Radiology and Laboratory 16

Long-term Care Facilities 17
Behavioral Health Facilities 18

Drug and Alcohol Rehabilitation 19

Rehabilitation Facilities 19
Other Specialty Facilities 19

Adult Day Care 19
Respite Care 20
Hospice 20
Home Health Care 21

Comparison of Facilities 21

Facility Size 21
Ownership 23
Financial Status 23
Patient Population 23
Services 24

Continuum of Care 24

Childhood 24
Adult Care 25
Special Health Issues 25
Elder Care 25
Impact of Mergers and Acquisitions 25

Legal and Regulatory Environment 26

Federal 26
State 27
Local 28

Accreditation 28

Joint Commission on Accreditation of Healthcare Organizations . 29
Commission on Accreditation of Rehabilitation Facilities 30

Professional Standards 31

CHAPTER SUMMARY 33

REVIEW QUESTIONS 33

CHAPTER 2. Data Elements 36

Basic Concepts 38

Health 38
Data 38
Information 38
Health Data 39
Health Information 40

Overview of a Physician's Office Visit 42

Personnel 42
Clinical Flow 44
Services 45

Key Data Categories 45

Demographic Data 46
Socioeconomic Data 46
Financial Data 47
Clinical Data 48

Describing Data 50

Characters 50
Fields 51
Records 52
Files 53

Health Record 53

Health Information Management 53

Data Quality 54

Data Accuracy 55
Data Validity 55

Data Sets 55

CHAPTER SUMMARY 58

REVIEW QUESTIONS 58

CHAPTER 3. **Organization of Data Elements in a Health Record** 60

Organization of Data Elements 62

Integrated Record 62
Source-Oriented Record 63
Problem-Oriented Record 64
Computer-Based Record 65
Problem List 67

Clinical Flow of Data 68

Admissions 68
Initial Assessment 70
Plan of Care 70

Medical Evaluation Process 71

SOAP Strategy 72

Clinical Data 73

Physicians 73
Nurses 80
Operative Records 82
Laboratory Data 82
Radiology Data 83
Other Clinical Data 83

Data Collection Devices 83

Forms 84
Computer-Based Data Collection 88

Data Quality 90
Forms Control 91
Other Types of Records 92
Data Sets 93
Other Health Care Settings 93

CHAPTER SUMMARY 95

REVIEW QUESTIONS 95

CHAPTER 4. **Postdischarge Processing** 98

Data Quality 100

Timeliness 100
Completeness 100

Controls 101

Preventive Controls 101
Detective Controls 103
Corrective Controls 104
Correction of Errors 105

Postdischarge Processing 106

Identification of Records to Process 107
Assembly 109
Quantitative Analysis 110
Coding 115
Retrieval 118
Abstracting 118

Tracking Records While Processing 119

Batch by Days 119
Loose Sheets 119
Efficiency 120

Other Health Information Management Roles 120

CHAPTER SUMMARY 121

REVIEW QUESTIONS 121

UNIT TWO **STORAGE, USES, and REPORTING of HEALTH INFORMATION**

CHAPTER 5. **Storage of Health Information** 126

The Paper Explosion 128
Master Patient Index 129

Manual Master Patient Index 132
Computerized Master Patient Index 133
Retention of Master Patient Index 136

Filing 137

Computer Files 137
Physical Files 138
Identification of Physical Files 141
Filing Methods 150

Computer Indexing. 155
Record Retention 155
Filing Furniture. 158
File Rooms 162

Alternative Storage Methods. 165

Microfilm. 165
On-site Storage 168
Off-site Storage 168
Selection of Storage Method 169

Chart Locator Systems 169

Manual Systems. 170
Computerized Systems 172

Security of Health Information. 175

Disaster Planning 175
Security from Fire 176
Security from Water Damage 177
Security from Theft or Tampering 177
Destruction of Health Information. 179

CHAPTER SUMMARY. 181

REVIEW QUESTIONS 181

CHAPTER 6. **Uses of Health Information** 184

Health Information and Its Uses. 186

Improvement of Patient Care 186
Support and Collection of Reimbursement 187
Licensure, Accreditation, and Certification 188
Administration 190
Prevalence and Incidence of Mortality and Morbidity 190
National Policy and Legislation 191
Development of Community Awareness of Health Care Issues . . . 193
Litigation. 193
Education 194
Research 194
Managed Care 195
Marketing 196

The Quality of Health Care 197
Quality Management Theories 198

Deming 199
Juran 199
Crosby. 200

History and Evolution of Quality in Health Care 200

Medical Education. 201
Standardization and Accreditation. 202
Federal Government. 204

Monitoring the Quality of Health Information 205

Quality Assurance 206
Performance Improvement 208

Health Information in Quality Activities 212

Quantitative Analysis 213
Qualitative Analysis 213
Clinical Pathways (Patient Care Plans) 218
Utilization Management 219
Case Management 219
Risk Management 220

Organization and Presentation of Data 222

Meetings 222
Quality Improvement Tools 223

Health Care Facility Committees. 228

Medical Staff Committees 228
HIM Committee 229
Infection Control Committee. 229
Safety Committee. 230

CHAPTER SUMMARY. 232

REVIEW QUESTIONS 232

CHAPTER 7. **Retrieval and Reporting of Health Information** 234

Organized Collection of Data. 236

Primary and Secondary Data. 236
Data Set 238
Creation of a Database. 240

Data Review and Abstracting 242

Data Quality Check 246

Data Retrieval. 248

Retrieval of Aggregate Data. 248
Indices. 249
Identification of a Population. 251
Optimum Source of Data. 252

Reporting of Data 253

Reporting to Individual Departments 253
Reporting to Outside Agencies 253

Statistical Analysis of Patient Information 254

Analysis and Interpretation 254
Presentation 256

Routine Institutional Statistics. 256

Admissions 256
Discharges 256
Census. 259
Hospital Rates and Percentages 264

CHAPTER SUMMARY. 267

REVIEW QUESTIONS 267

UNIT THREE REIMBURSEMENT and LEGAL ISSUES

CHAPTER 8. **Confidentiality and Compliance** 272

Confidentiality 274

Definition. 274
Legal Foundation. 274
Scope 274

Access 277

Continuing Patient Care 277
Reimbursement 278
Litigation. 279
Access by Patient 281

Consent 285

Informed Consent. 285
Admission 285
Medical Procedures 285
Release of Information 287

Preparing a Record for Release 293

Validation and Tracking 293
Retrieval 294
Reproduction 294
Certification 294
Compensation 295
Distribution 295

Internal Requests for Information 296

Sensitive Records 297

Compliance   298

Licensure   298
Accreditation   299
Corporate Compliance   300
Professional Standards   301

CHAPTER SUMMARY   302

REVIEW QUESTIONS   303

CHAPTER 9. **Health Care Reimbursement**   306

Reimbursement   308

Types of Reimbursement   308
Comparison of Reimbursement Methods   310

Insurance   311

History   311
Assumption of Risk   312
Types of Insurance   313

Government Intervention   319

Medicare   320
Medicaid   320
Tax Equity and Fiscal Responsibility Act of 1982 (TEFRA)   321
Medicare Prospective Payment System   321

Prospective Payment Systems   322

Diagnosis Related Groups   322
Ambulatory Patient Classifications   324
Resource Utilization Groups   325
Other Prospective Payment Systems   325

Billing   326

Patient Accounts   326
Chargemaster   326
Charge Capture   327
Uniform Bill (UB-92)   328
HCFA-1500   328

Impact of Coding   332

Coding Quality   332
Chargemaster Review   333

CHAPTER SUMMARY   335

REVIEW QUESTIONS   335

UNIT FOUR **SUPERVISION and PROFESSIONAL DEVELOPMENT**

CHAPTER 10. **Human Resource Management** 340

Human Resources 342
Organization Charts 343

Facility Organization 344
Health Information Management Department Organization 347

Health Information Management Department Workflow . . . 349

Health Information Management Functions 349

Department Planning 354

Mission 355
Vision 356
Goals and Objectives 356

Prioritization of Department Functions 357
Evaluation of Department Operations and Services 358
Department Policies and Procedures 358

Policy and Procedure Review 362

Health Information Personnel 362

Job Analysis 362
Job Description 364

Employee Productivity 365

Manual Productivity Reports 368
Computerized Productivity Reports 369

Employee Evaluations 370

Poor Evaluations 371

Hiring Health Information Management Personnel 371

Advertisement 371
Application 373
Interviewing 378
Assessment 379

Fair Employment Practices 379
Department Equipment and Supplies 380

Supplies 381
Monitoring Use of Department Resources 383

Ergonomics 383

CHAPTER SUMMARY 386

REVIEW QUESTIONS 387

CHAPTER 11. **Training and Development** 390

Orientation. 392

Organization Orientation. 392
Health Information Management Department Orientation 395
Clinical Staff Orientation 396

Training 399

Assessment of Education Needs 399
Audience 400
Format 400
Environment 401
Calendar of Education 401

In-service Education 402
Educating the Public 403
Continuing Education 403
Communication. 405

Employee-to-Employee Communication 407
Health Information Management Department and Physicians . . . 407
Health Information Management Department and Outside
Agencies or Parties. 407
Written Communication 408
Electronic Communication 408

Department Meetings. 410

Agenda 410
Meeting 411
Minutes 413
Meeting Records 413

CHAPTER SUMMARY. 414

REVIEW QUESTIONS 414

APPENDICES

Managing Personal Workforce Readiness 418
Jonathan L. Butler

Glossary 441

Test Your HI-Q Suggested Answers 465

INDEX 485

CONTENT and STRUCTURE of HEALTH INFORMATION

1

Health Care Delivery Systems

Chapter Outline

Health Care Professionals
Physicians
Nurses
  Licensed Practical Nurse
  Registered Nurse
  Advanced Nursing Specialties
Allied Health Professionals

Patient Care Plan

Acute Care Facilities
Admission and Discharge
Length of Stay
Average Length of Stay

Ambulatory Care Facilities
Physician's Office
Group Practice
Clinic
Ambulatory Surgery
Radiology and Laboratory

Long-term Care Facilities

Behavioral Health Facilities
Drug and Alcohol Rehabilitation

Rehabilitation Facilities

Other Specialty Facilities
Adult Day Care
Respite Care
Hospice
Home Health Care

Comparison of Facilities
Facility Size
  Number of Beds
  Discharges
Ownership

Financial Status
Patient Population
Services

Continuum of Care
Childhood
Adult Care
Special Health Issues
Elder Care
Impact of Mergers and Acquisitions

Legal and Regulatory Environment
Federal
  Medicare
State
  Licensure
  Reporting
Local

Accreditation
Joint Commission on Accreditation of
  Healthcare Organizations
Commission on Accreditation of Rehabilitation Facilities

Professional Standards

Reference

Suggested Reading

Web Sites

Chapter Summary

Review Questions

Professional Profile

Application

By the end of this chapter, the student should be able to:

- Identify and describe the major medical specialties.

- Distinguish among nursing occupations.

- Identify and describe the major allied health professions and their principal occupational settings.

- Define ambulatory care.

- Distinguish between inpatients and outpatients.

- Calculate the length of stay for a patient, given the admission and discharge dates.

- Define acute care facility.

- Define rehabilitation facility.

- Define long-term care facility.

- Describe the differences among health care facilities.

- Describe government involvement in health care.

- Define accreditation.

- List major accreditation organizations and the facilities they accredit.

Vocabulary

accreditation

activities of daily living (ADLs)

acute care facility

allied health professionals

average length of stay

bed count

behavioral health facility

children's hospital

consultation

continuum of care

deemed status

diagnosis

ethics

home health care

hospice

hospital

inpatient

integrated delivery system

laboratory

length of stay

licensure

long-term care facility

mental health facility

nurse

outpatient

palliative care

physiatrist

physician

primary care physician

primary caregiver

procedure

psychiatrist

radiology

referral

rehabilitation facility

respite care

We begin our introduction to health information technology with an overview of the health care delivery system. You have probably experienced the need for health care at one time or another. You may know a lot about certain types of health care because of your own illness or the illness of a family member. The purpose of this chapter is to acquaint you with the basic structure and terminology of the health care industry.

Health Care Professionals

A wide variety of professionals work in health care. They vary from doctors and nurses to therapists and technicians to administrative personnel. Each of these professionals plays a vital role in the delivery of health care. In this chapter, we introduce you to some of them.

Physicians

A **physician** is a person who is licensed to practice medicine. To become licensed, a physician attends college, then medical school, and then serves a residency in his or her specialty. A *resident* performs professional duties under the supervision of a fully qualified physician. Residency can last from 4 to 8 years, depending on the specialty. The medical licensing examination can be taken after the first year of residency. The practice of medicine is regulated by each individual state, which administers the examination and issues the license.

A physician earns a degree as a Doctor of Medicine (MD) or a Doctor of Osteopathy (DO). MDs and DOs are trained in schools that focus on different philosophies of medical treatment and diagnosis. A medical doctor studies the allopathic philosophy, which is a scientific-based approach to medicine. An osteopathic doctor uses both allopathic philosophy and a manipulative approach to medicine. Both are eligible for licensing. As a general rule, both are eligible to practice medicine in hospitals; however, that is a decision of individual hospitals.

As an example of the educational background of a physician, consider the following: a physician who specializes in family or general practice (see Overview of a Physician's Office Visit in Chapter 2) has attended college for 4 years and medical school for another 3 years. After medical school, the graduate may take a licensure examination. Because the physician intends to become a general practitioner, he or she would then apply for a residency of 3 or more years in internal medicine or family practice.

Beyond licensing, physicians may pursue additional training and take an examination to become board certified. Board certification is developed and administered by the specialty board that sets standards of education for the physician's specialty. The American Board of Medical Specialties consists of 24 medical specialty boards. Among the 24 medical specialties, there are 42 subspecialties (Raffel and Raffel, 1994, p 151). For example, gastroenterology is a subspecialty of internal medicine. Another example of board certification is certification by a pediatrician (a physician who specializes in the treatment of children) from the American Academy of Pediatric Medicine. Board-certified physicians are fellows of their respective academies.

Physicians are generally classified by *medical specialty*. They can specialize in a particular disease or condition, a body or organ system, or a task. For example, an oncologist is a physician who diagnoses and treats cancers. An obstetrician takes care of pregnant women. A physician can be a gastroenterologist, specializing in diseases of the digestive system. A urologist specializes in diseases of the urinary system. There are several tasks that physicians perform that are considered specialties, even though many physicians may perform them to a certain extent. For example, a radiologist interprets x-rays and other types of examinations that generate film records of internal organs. A gastroenterologist may know how to read an x-ray, but it is not his or her specialty. Some specialties may focus further on the patient's age group. A pediatric oncologist deals with children's cancers. Table 1–1 lists some common medical specialties.

HIT Bit

If you have not yet studied medical terminology, here is a brief lesson. Medical terms consist of combining forms, prefixes, and suffixes. These parts are assembled to form words, which can easily be deciphered when you know the definitions of the parts. For example, we just used the word "oncologist." This word is assembled from the following parts:

onc/o = cancer
-logy = process of study
-ist = one who specializes

Therefore, an "oncologist" is "one who specializes in the study of cancer." The following are the word parts of some of the other specialties we mentioned.

gastr/o = stomach
enter/o = intestine
ped/i = children
iatr/o = treatment
-ic = pertaining to
oste/o = bone
pathy = process of disease

Can you decipher the words in Table 1–1 now that you know their parts?

Most individuals have a relationship with a general practitioner, also known as a family practitioner. He or she is the physician who coordinates care among the various specialists the individual may need. The general practitioner may identify

Table 1–1. Common Medical Specialties

Physician Specialty	Description
Allergist	Diagnoses and treats patients who have strong reactions to pollen, insect bites, food, medication, and other irritants
Anesthesiologist	Administers substances that cause loss of sensation, particularly during surgery
Cardiologist	Diagnoses and treats patients with diseases of the heart and blood vessels
Dermatologist	Diagnoses and treats patients with diseases of the skin
Family practitioner	Delivers primary health care for patients of all ages
Gastroenterologist	Diagnoses and treats patients with diseases of the digestive system
Gynecologist	Diagnoses and treats disorders of, and provides well care related to, the female reproductive system
Neonatologist	Diagnoses and treats diseases and abnormal conditions of newborns
Obstetrician	Cares for women before, during, and after delivery
Oncologist	Diagnoses and treats patients with cancer
Ophthalmologist	Diagnoses and treats patients with diseases of the eye
Orthopedist	Diagnoses and treats patients with diseases of the muscles and bones
Pathologist	Studies changes in cells, tissue, and organs in order to diagnose diseases and/or to determine possible treatments
Pediatrician	Delivers primary health care to children
Psychiatrist	Diagnoses and treats patients with disorders of the mind
Radiologist	Uses x-rays and other tools to diagnose and treat a variety of diseases

a suspicious skin problem and send the patient to a dermatologist for evaluation and treatment. The process of sending a patient to another physician in this manner is called a **referral.** The general practitioner referred the patient to a dermatologist to be diagnosed or treated. Alternatively, the general practitioner may have asked the dermatologist to evaluate the patient's condition and confirm the general practitioner's ideas and/or give recommendations for treating the patient. This process is called a **consultation.** A physician who coordinates the care of a patient, through referrals and consultations, is called a **primary care physician (PCP).** A general or family practitioner is most often the PCP for his or her patients. However, not all PCPs are family practitioners. For example, some women choose to use their gynecologists as their PCPs. A pediatrician is frequently the PCP for a child.

Nurses

A **nurse** is a clinical professional who has received post–secondary school training in caring for patients in a variety of health care settings. There are several levels of nursing education, each qualifying the nurse for different positions. Historically, most nurses graduated from a hospital-based certificate program. Another large percentage received their training through associate degree programs. A growing number of nurses have a bachelor's and/or master's of science degree in nursing. Today, almost all nurses are college educated at some level. Nurses, like doctors, take licensing examinations. Table 1–2 lists the various levels of nursing and their educational requirements.

TABLE 1–2. Levels of Nursing Practice	
Title	**General Description and Requirements**
Surgical Technician/Technologist (CST, if certified)	HOE program; associate degree; certification can be obtained from the Association of Surgical Technologists.
Nurse Assistant Geriatric Aide Home Health Care Assistant Certified Nurse Technician	High school graduate or equivalent (preferred); 6- to 18-mo HOE program; certification or registration required in all states for long-term care facilities, obtained by completing state-approved program.
Licensed Vocational Nurse Licensed Practical Nurse	High school graduate or equivalent; graduation from a 1- to 2-yr state-approved HOE practical/vocational nurse program; licensed by state of employment or by the National Federation of Licensed Practical Nurses.
Registered Nurse	Minimum high school graduation or equivalent; programs leading to registration are offered at the associate, bachelor's, and master's degree levels. Licensure in state of practice.
Nurse Practitioner	Registered nurse; complete an accredited course in nurse practitioner training.

HOE, Health Occupations Education.

Adapted from Simmers L: Diversified Health Occupations, 4th ed. ©1998. Reprinted with permission of Delmar, a division of Thomson Learning. Fax 800-730-2215.

LICENSED PRACTICAL NURSE

A *licensed practical nurse (LPN)* receives training at a technical or vocational school. The training consists of learning to care for patients' personal needs and other types of routine care. LPNs work under the direction of physicians and/or registered nurses.

REGISTERED NURSE

In addition to caring for patients' personal needs, a *registered nurse (RN)* administers medication and renders other care at the request of a physician. RNs particularly focus on assessing and meeting the patients' need for education regarding their illness. Registered nurses may specialize in caring for different types of patients. For example, a nurse may assist in the operating room or care for children or the elderly, each of which requires special skills and training. Registered nurses who want to move into management-level or teaching positions generally pursue a master's degree and sometimes a doctoral degree.

ADVANCED NURSING SPECIALTIES

In response to physician shortages and a desire by nurses for greater independence, several advanced specialties in nursing practice have developed, under the general title of *nurse practitioner (NP)*. Examples of these specialties are nurse midwives and nurse anesthetists. A nurse midwife focuses on the care of women during the period surrounding childbirth: pregnancy, labor, delivery, and after delivery. A nurse anesthetist is trained to administer anesthesia and to care for the patient during the delivery of anesthesia and recovery from the process.

Nurse practitioners have a master's degree and additional training and licensing beyond the RN.

Allied Health Professionals

Allied health (or health-related) **professionals** can be both clinical and nonclinical professionals who provide a variety of services to patients, generally at the request or under the direction of a physician or registered nurse. A *clinical professional* is one who provides health care services to a patient. *Nonclinical professionals* support the clinical staff and provide other types of services to a patient. Health-related professions include x-ray technicians, a variety of therapists, and health information management professionals. We discuss health information professionals in Chapter 2. Table 1–3 lists examples of health-related professions, their principal work environments, and their basic educational requirements.

HIT BIT

Physicians identify and treat illnesses. They can also help prevent illnesses through patient education and various types of inoculations. Nurses and professionals in other health-related disciplines help physicians prevent, identify, and treat illnesses. Identification of the illness is the **diagnosis**. A **procedure** is performed to help in the identification and treatment processes.

Diagnosis	Procedure	
	Diagnostic	*Therapeutic*
A disease or abnormal condition	*The evaluation or investigative steps taken to develop the diagnosis or monitor a disease or condition*	*The steps taken to alleviate or eliminate the cause or symptoms of a disease*
Examples:		
Appendicitis	Physical examination Blood test	Appendectomy
Cerebrovascular accident (stroke)	Physical examination Neurologic examination Computed tomography scan	Medication Physical therapy Occupational therapy Speech therapy Psychological counseling
Myocardial infarction (heart attack)	Physical examination Blood test Electrocardiogram	Medication Coronary artery bypass graft

Patient Care Plan

Developing a diagnosis is generally the responsibility of the physician. However, the treatment of the patient involves many different individuals, including the patient. The *patient care plan* may be as simple as instructions to "take two aspirin

TABLE 1–3. Examples of Health-Related Professions

Title	Description	Requirements
Certified Coding Specialist or Certified Coding Specialist/Physician-office based Health Unit Coordinator	Assigns, collects, and reports codes representing clinical data. Primarily employed in health care facilities. Transcribes physician's orders, prepares and compiles records during patient hospitalization. Primarily employed in acute care, long-term care, and clinics.	Certification by examination from the American Health Information Management Association. High school graduate or equivalent; community college; hospital training program; completion of a vocational education program in the area of ward clerk, unit secretary, or health unit coordinator. Certification available from the National Association of Health Unit Coordinators.
Occupational Therapist	Focuses on returning patient to maximum functioning in activities of daily living. Primarily employed in rehabilitation facilities, but may work in virtually any health care environment.	Bachelor's degree; licensure required in most states; certification (registration) can be obtained from the American Occupational Therapy Association.
Phlebotomist	Draws blood for donation and testing. Primarily employed in health care facilities and community blood banks.	High school graduate or equivalent. Ten- to twenty-hour certification program in a hospital, physician's office, or laboratory. Completion of a vocational education program as a phlebotomist.
Physical Therapist	Focuses on strength, gait, and range of motion training to return patients to maximum functioning in activities of daily living. Primarily employed in rehabilitation facilities, but may work in virtually any health care environment.	Bachelor's or master's degree; licensure by state of practice.
Registered Dietitian	Manages food services; evaluates nutritional needs, including planning menus and special diets and educating patients and family. Primarily employed in health care facilities.	Bachelor's degree; registration can be obtained from American Dietetic Association; licensure, certification, or registration required in many states.
Registered Health Information Technician	Provides administrative support targeting the collection, retention, and reporting of health information. Employed primarily in health care facilities, but may work in a variety of different settings, including insurance and pharmaceutical companies.	Associate degree from accredited HIT program; registration by examination from the American Health Information Management Association.
Registered Health Information Administrator	Provides administrative support targeting the collection, retention, and reporting of health information, including strategic planning, research, and systems analysis and acquisition. Employed primarily in health care facilities, but may work in a variety of different settings, including insurance and pharmaceutical companies.	Bachelor's degree from accredited HIA program; registration by examination from the American Health Information Management Association.
Respiratory Therapist	Delivers therapies related to breathing. Primarily employed in health care facilities.	Associate or bachelor's degree; licensure or certification required in most states; registration can be obtained from the National Board for Respiratory Care.

and drink plenty of fluids" or it may be a multiple-page document with delegation of responsibilities. For example, suppose a patient has been diagnosed with insulin-dependent diabetes mellitus (IDDM), a disease caused by chronic high blood glucose that can be controlled only with medication (i.e., insulin).

- A nurse may be responsible for educating the patient about medication regimens.
- A psychologist can help the patient deal with the stress of chronic illness.

- The patient's family will need to learn about IDDM and what to do in a crisis.
- If the patient is elderly and lives alone:
  - ❑ A home health care worker may be brought in to check the patient's blood sugar at home.
  - ❑ A nutritionist can provide the patient with education about proper diet.
  - ❑ The patient may need physical therapy for safe conditioning exercises.

The patient, of course, must be involved every step of the way. A well-documented patient care plan helps all members of the interdisciplinary care team work together to deliver the best possible care to the patient.

Acute Care Facilities

Now that you have an idea of "who's who" in health care, let's turn our attention to the facilities in which health professionals work. The first type of facility is the **acute care facility.** The typical patient in an acute care facility either is acutely ill or has some problem that requires the types of evaluation and treatment procedures that are available in the facility. The word "acute" means "sudden" or "severe." Applied to illnesses, it refers to a problem that generally arises swiftly and/or severely. In an acute care facility, patients are cared for as "inpatients." An **inpatient** typically remains in the facility overnight. Therefore, inpatients are patients whose evaluation and treatment result in admission to and discharge from the facility on different days.

The acute care facility may be thought of as a hospital. When we say that a patient is going to the hospital, we usually mean that he or she is going to an acute care facility. However, the term "hospital" has a broader definition. Fundamentally, a **hospital** provides room and board and services for patients to stay overnight. Diagnostic and therapeutic care are provided to patients as directed by physicians. Hospitals are licensed by the state in which they operate, and each state defines hospitals for these purposes. Some states include the requirement for an "organized medical staff" in their definition of a hospital. An acute care facility is, therefore, a type of hospital.

Typically, an acute care facility is also distinguished by its having an emergency department and surgical (operating) facilities. In other words, the facility is able to treat patients who need immediate medical care for serious injuries or illnesses. The facility is also able to provide services for surgical procedures, such as appendectomies and hip replacements.

Historically, acute care facilities have been *stand-alone* hospitals. Although they may have provided a variety of different services to the community, they did not have a formal business affiliation with other hospitals. In recent years as a result of economic pressures, hospitals are consolidating. Sometimes they merge, which means that two or more hospitals combine their resources. Other times, one hospital acquires (purchases) the other. The differences between a merger and an acquisition are primarily organizational and financial.

In recent years, partly as a cost-cutting measure and partly for increased customer service, acute care facilities have expanded into ambulatory care services. They have done this in three ways: ambulatory surgery, clinics, and ancillary services (see discussion under Ambulatory Care Facilities).

Admission and Discharge

Admission is the process that occurs when the patient is registered for evaluation and/or treatment in a facility. In most facilities, the admission process involves a variety of data collection activities (see Chapter 2). The *admission date* is defined as the actual calendar day that the patient is registered. Therefore, whether he or she arrives at 1:05 AM or 11:59 PM on January 5, the admission date is the same: January 5.

Discharge is the process that occurs when the patient leaves the facility. Discharge implies that the patient has previously been admitted to the facility. The *day of discharge* is defined as the actual calendar day that the patient leaves the facility. Note that a physician's order for a patient to leave the facility is required for a normal discharge. However, there are other events that also cause a discharge. A patient may die or may leave against medical advice (AMA). Both of these events are discharges on the calendar day on which they occur.

On average, patients in acute care stay less than 30 days. Actually, the average number of days that a patient spends in a given acute care facility depends on what types of patients are treated in the facility. Many acute care facilities have an average patient stay between 3 and 6 days, significantly less than 30 days.

TEST YOUR HI-Q

If a patient is admitted as an inpatient on Monday at 10 AM but dies on Monday at 3 PM, is that patient still considered an inpatient?

Length of Stay

The time that a patient spends in a facility is called the **length of stay (LOS).** Length of stay is the measurement, in days, of the time between admission and discharge. Figure 1–1 illustrates how to calculate a patient's length of stay. For example: A patient enters the facility on Monday, July 1, and is discharged on Thursday, July 4. The easiest way to calculate the length of stay is to subtract the dates. Four minus one is three; therefore, the length of stay is 3 days.

It is important to note that when counting the length of stay, *count the day of admission but not the day of discharge.* In the previous example, the patient is considered to have stayed in the hospital on 3 days: July 1, July 2, and July 3. On July 4 the patient is no longer there. This is a fairly easy calculation when the patient enters the facility and leaves the facility during the same month because we can just subtract the days in the month.

Length of stay is more difficult to determine if the patient enters and leaves the facility in different months. For example, if the patient enters the hospital in July and leaves in August, three calculations are required. Step 1: Calculate how many days the patient was there in July. Step 2: Calculate how many days the patient was there in August. Step 3: Add the two together. Figure 1–2 gives an example of this calculation. The patient is admitted on July 26 and discharged on August 6. Step 1: The patient is in the hospital in July for 6 days. Remember that we have to count the day of admission. Step 2: The stay in August is only 5 days, because we do not count the day of discharge. Step 3: Add the 6 days in July to the 5 days in August. The length of stay for this patient is 11 days.

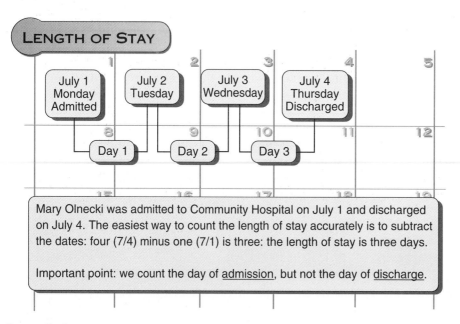

LENGTH OF STAY

| July 1 Monday Admitted | July 2 Tuesday | July 3 Wednesday | July 4 Thursday Discharged |

Day 1   Day 2   Day 3

Mary Olnecki was admitted to Community Hospital on July 1 and discharged on July 4. The easiest way to count the length of stay accurately is to subtract the dates: four (7/4) minus one (7/1) is three: the length of stay is three days.

Important point: we count the day of <u>admission</u>, but not the day of <u>discharge</u>.

Figure 1–1.

Calculation of length of stay within a calendar month.

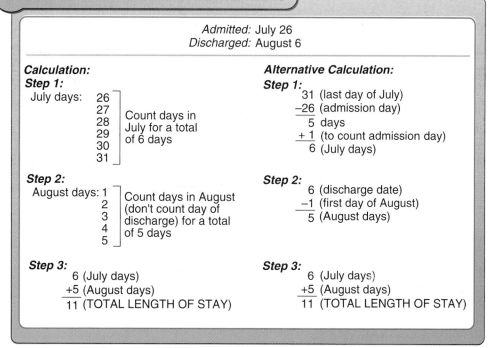

LENGTH OF STAY ACROSS MONTHS

Admitted: July 26
Discharged: August 6

Calculation:

Step 1:
July days: 26
27
28   Count days in
29   July for a total
30   of 6 days
31

Step 2:
August days: 1
2   Count days in August
3   (don't count day of
4   discharge) for a total
5   of 5 days

Step 3:
6 (July days)
+5 (August days)
11 (TOTAL LENGTH OF STAY)

Alternative Calculation:

Step 1:
31 (last day of July)
−26 (admission day)
5 days
+ 1 (to count admission day)
6 (July days)

Step 2:
6 (discharge date)
−1 (first day of August)
5 (August days)

Step 3:
6 (July days)
+5 (August days)
11 (TOTAL LENGTH OF STAY)

FIGURE 1–2.

Calculation of length of stay across calendar months.

If you want to do this arithmetically without actually listing the days in the month, you can subtract the days in July and add back one for the admission date and subtract the days in August and then add the July and August days (see Fig. 1–2). In a computerized environment, the computer very nicely calculates this type of information for you. However, it sometimes is necessary to calculate length of stay manually.

HIT BIT

To calculate length of stay from one month to the next, it is important to know how many days there are in a month. There are 4 months that have 30 days: April, June, September, and November. February has 28 days, except in leap years (every 4 years), when it has 29 days. All of the other months have 31 days.

If you have trouble remembering how many days there are in a particular month, try creating a mnemonic. Using the first letters of each of the 30-day months, create a silly sentence that will help you associate them. You will want to use April and June in the sentence, because there are other months that begin with those letters. For example: "April and June are Not Summer" or "April's Sister is Not June." As a child, you may have learned the jingle: "Thirty days hath September, April, June, and November; all the rest have 31, except February alone, which has 28 in time, and each leap year 29."

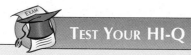

TEST YOUR HI-Q

A patient was admitted on March 14 and discharged on May 3. What was the length of stay?

Average Length of Stay

Length of stay is very important in defining the type of facility and in analyzing its patient population. **Average length of stay (ALOS)** is calculated by adding up the LOSs for a group of patients and dividing by the number of patients in the group. Figure 1–3 illustrates the ALOS of patients in an acute care facility using patients who were discharged in July as an example. In the example, the total length of stay of all the patients put together is 55 days. Fifty-five days divided by five patients gives the average number of days, 11 days. This type of an average is called the *arithmetic mean*.

ALOS refers to the arithmetic mean of all the patients' LOSs within a certain period of time. Usually we calculate ALOS monthly or annually or in some relevant time period. ALOS might also be calculated by medical specialty, and it can even be calculated in terms of a specific physician's practice. These calculations are useful in determining whether a physician or a particular medical specialty conforms to the average in a particular hospital or whether the physician or specialty is higher or lower in terms of LOS.

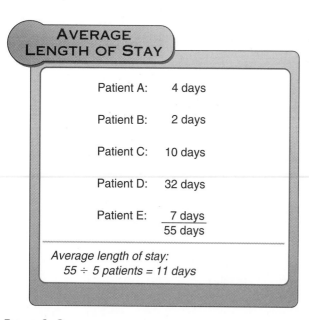

AVERAGE LENGTH OF STAY

Patient A:	4 days
Patient B:	2 days
Patient C:	10 days
Patient D:	32 days
Patient E:	7 days
	55 days

Average length of stay:
55 ÷ 5 patients = 11 days

FIGURE 1–3.

Sample calculation of average length of stay.

One of the characteristics of an acute care facility is that the ALOS of its patient population is less than 30 days. In reality, the ALOS of an acute care facility is significantly less than that, depending on what type of patients are treated there. For example, a hospital with a large number of mothers and their newborns, whose stay in the facility is generally 1 to 3 days, will tend to have a very low ALOS: perhaps only 4 or 5 days. On the other hand, a hospital with a large number of patients with serious trauma, burns, and transplants might have an ALOS closer to 12 or 13 days.

Ambulatory Care Facilities

As we discussed earlier, many hospitals are expanding to offer a variety of different services. For example, a patient at Smart Hospital may be an inpatient who is having an operation or may be an outpatient visiting a physician in the clinic. When discussing a health care facility, its services, and its patients, it is important to identify which patients are being discussed.

In an *ambulatory care facility,* patients are admitted and discharged on the same day. A patient whose evaluation and/or treatment is intended to occur within one calendar day is an ambulatory care patient, also known as an **outpatient.** The concepts of admission and discharge have little relevance in an ambulatory care facility, because both processes typically are intended to take place on the same day. An ambulatory care admission, then, is referred to as a *visit* or an *encounter.* If we want to count the number of patients who were admitted to a physician's office, for example, we would say that we were counting the number of visits or encounters. Visits and encounters may not be synonymous. When analyzing such activity for statistical purposes, it is very important to understand how such terms are defined and used within the facility.

Physician's Office

A *physician's office* is one type of ambulatory care facility. Most of us have been to a physician's office, so this is a good place to start our discussion. Most physicians maintain an office where patients can visit. There are many different types of physicians, as we shall see later in our discussion. Some physicians have offices attached to their homes; others have space in office buildings.

Group Practice

Sometimes, physicians share office space and personnel with other physicians. This helps to reduce the cost of maintaining an office. It also provides professional collaboration among physicians. This combination of physicians is called a *group practice.* Group practices may have only one type of physician, such as a group of family practitioners, or may comprise several different specialties, called a multispecialty group. An internist may be in practice with a pediatrician and a gynecologist, for example. One of the advantages of a group practice is that physicians can assist with each other's patients, to the extent that such assistance is permissible by the limitations of the individual physician's specialty.

Clinic

A *clinic* is a facility-based ambulatory care department that provides general or specialized services such as those provided in a physician's office. Clinics may be funded and/or established by charitable organizations, the government, or different types of health care facilities. For example, a community health center is a type of clinic that provides primary care in a specific geographic area. Originally, many of these centers were located in areas accessible to economically depressed populations. Many acute care facilities have developed clinics that resemble physicians' office services. A hospital may have clinics that serve particular patient populations, such as an infectious disease clinic or an orthopedic clinic. Clinics may also closely resemble multispecialty group practices. Large teaching facilities may have many clinics available. The clinic may be part of the physicians' general practice, the physicians may be employees of the parent facility, or they may donate their time.

Ambulatory Surgery

Ambulatory surgery is a service that lets patients come in, have a surgical procedure performed, and go home the same day. These are fairly low risk procedures from which full recovery is expected and for which the patients do not need intensive nursing care afterward. Examples include endoscopies, cataract surgery, certain biopsies, and some foot surgeries. This service is sometimes called "outpatient surgery," "same-day surgery," or "one-day surgery." Ambulatory surgery can either be hospital based or take place in a freestanding facility.

HIT BIT

"Ambulatory" literally means the "process of walking." So an ambulatory care patient is theoretically walking in and out. However, the name is a little misleading. Ambulatory care patients are not always ambulatory. "Ambulatory" also refers to a patient who is *able* to walk. However, patients in wheelchairs can visit physicians at the office. Some patients are driven to the physician's office in special vans that look like ambulances. Clearly, in neither case do the patients actually walk into the office, but they are ambulatory care patients.

Radiology and Laboratory

Acute care facilities offer a broad range of evaluation services, such as radiology and laboratory services. The **radiology** department performs and reviews x-rays. The **laboratory** analyzes body fluids, such as blood. These evaluation services are called *ancillary,* or *adjunct, services.* Many of these services are offered in free-standing facilities as well. Some freestanding services lease space in other health care facilities, such as acute care hospitals, so that it is not always obvious that the service is not part of the hospital.

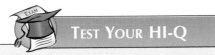

TEST YOUR HI-Q

The lines between inpatients and outpatients may become blurred given certain circumstances. An emergency department patient who is treated and released is clearly an outpatient. However, if the patient enters the emergency department at 11 PM and leaves at 4 AM, the patient clearly came on one day and left on the next. Is this patient an inpatient or an outpatient? Why? Additionally, some patients are kept in the hospital for *observation.* This is a special category of patients, neither outpatients nor inpatients, who may stay in the hospital for up to 24 hours without being admitted as an inpatient. Can you think of a reason why this category of patients was created?

Long-term Care Facilities

You may be more familiar with the term "nursing home." For many years, these were primarily facilities that took care of elderly patients who were ill or whose families could no longer care for them at home. Patients often moved into a nursing home and lived there until they died. Today, **long-term care facilities** treat a wide variety of patients who need more care than they would be able to get at home, but who do not generally need the intensity of care provided by an acute care facility. In addition, the philosophy of these facilities has changed so that the focus is less on making a home for the patient and more on maintaining his or her health and preparing the patient to go home, if possible.

By definition, a long-term care facility has an average length of stay in excess of 30 days. This is an important difference between acute care and long-term care. Because the ALOS is over 30 days, we know that a long-term care facility manages patients on an inpatient basis. In long-term care, we refer to those inpatients as *residents.*

There are other fundamental differences between long-term care facilities and acute care facilities. Although both care for inpatients, their focus and delivery are significantly different. Because long-term care patients are considered residents, there is a greater emphasis on comfort, activities of daily living, and recreational activities such as games and crafts. Group activities are common in order to facilitate residents' interaction and socialization.

Table 1–4 compares some of the services available in selected health care facilities.

TABLE 1–4. Comparison of On-site Services Provided in Health Care Facilities				
Service or Department	**Physician's Office**	**Acute Care**	**Long-term Care**	**Rehabilitation**
Nursing	Maybe	Yes	Yes	Yes
Medical staff	One, two, or many	Many; visit many patients daily	Many; visit patients as needed or defined	Many; visit many patients daily
Patient registration	Yes	Yes	Yes	Yes
Dietary	Not usually	Yes	Yes	Yes
Health information management	Not a separate function in small facilities	Yes	Not always a separate function	Usually
Patient accounts	Yes	Yes	Yes	Yes
Volunteers	Only in large facilities	Yes	Yes	Yes
Radiology	Maybe	Yes	Limited, if any	Usually
Laboratory	Maybe	Yes	Limited	Limited
Physical therapy	May be associated within group practice	Small department	Varies; may have small department	Large department
Occupational therapy	May be associated within group practice	Small department	Varies; may have small department	Large department
Emergency	Urgent	Yes	No	No
Surgery	Minor procedures	Yes	Minor procedures	Minor procedures
Pathology	No	Yes	No	No

Behavioral Health Facilities

Behavioral health facilities are defined by their patient population. Patients in **behavioral health facilities** either have or are being evaluated for psychiatric illnesses. These facilities may also be referred to as **mental health facilities** or psychiatric facilities. These facilities can be inpatient, outpatient, or both. Large behavioral health facilities may be administered by the state or county government. In addition, there are many small, private facilities. There is no standard in terms of ALOS. Outpatient services may be provided in stand-alone clinics or as part of an inpatient facility.

Although some patients in behavioral health facilities may have additional medical conditions that require treatment, the primary thrust of care is delivered by **psychiatrists** (physicians), psychologists (nonphysician specialists), and social services personnel. Particularly in an inpatient facility, there may also be on staff a physician known as an internist. The internist is responsible for treating patients for any medical conditions that they may have.

Drug and Alcohol Rehabilitation

Although treatment is referred to as rehabilitation, drug and alcohol abuse or dependence is considered a psychiatric condition. There are two phases of treatment: detoxification and rehabilitation. Detoxification refers to the treatment of a patient who is going through withdrawal of substances from his or her body. This withdrawal may take 3 to 4 days. Rehabilitation is the treatment of the patient by psychiatrists, psychologists, drug and alcohol counselors, and social workers, so that the patient learns how not to return to drugs and alcohol in the future. Although treatment varies, initial rehabilitation may take weeks or months, with continuing treatment throughout the patient's life.

Rehabilitation Facilities

The focus of *rehabilitation* is to return the patient to the maximum possible level of function in terms of **activities of daily living (ADLs)**. ADLs include self-care issues such as bathing and toileting as well as practical concerns such as ironing and cooking. This type of rehabilitation is referred to as physical medicine and rehabilitation. These facilities may be inpatient, outpatient, or both.

Rehabilitation facilities treat patients who have suffered a debilitating illness or trauma or who are recovering from certain types of surgery. For example, a patient may have survived a car accident but may have suffered a head trauma and other injuries that require extensive therapy. Patients who have had knee replacement surgery need therapy to learn to function with the prosthetic joint.

As with behavioral health patients, rehabilitation patients may have medical conditions that require treatment while they are in therapy. There is an internist on staff at inpatient facilities to treat these conditions. However, the thrust of treatment is the therapy. Rehabilitation therapy occurs under the direction of a **physiatrist,** a physician who specializes in physical medicine and rehabilitation. Physical therapists (PTs), occupational therapists (OTs), speech therapists, social services, and psychologists play large roles, to varying degrees, in the rehabilitation of individual patients.

Other Specialty Facilities

Other types of facilities are defined by medical specialty or by the types of patients that they treat. Some specific facilities are adult day care, respite care, home health care, and children's hospitals. Figure 1–4 shows examples of facility differences.

Adult Day Care

Adult day care is an outpatient facility that specializes in taking care of elderly or physically impaired adults. When the patient's family is caring for the individual at home, the **primary caregiver** may have to work full-time or part-time and

HEALTH CARE FACILITIES

Some facilities are defined by length of stay:

Ambulatory care facility: Patients are admitted and discharged on the same day

Acute care facility: Patients remain at least overnight and, on average, stay less than 30 days

Long-term care facility: Patients remain at least overnight (inpatient) and, on average, stay longer than 30 days

Other facilities are defined by the medical specialty or by the types of patients they treat:

Rehabilitation facility: Physical medicine, PT, and OT; may be inpatient or outpatient

Behavioral health facility: Psychiatric diagnosis; may be inpatient or outpatient

Children's hospital: Treats only children, usually 16 years old and younger; may be inpatient or outpatient

FIGURE 1–4.

Comparison of health care facilities by characteristics and patients. OT, occupational therapy, PT, physical therapy.

can't be home with the patient all day. The family member can take the patient to the adult day care facility. Adult day care provides activities, social interaction, some therapies, and some medical treatment. Medical treatment usually consists of ensuring that the patient takes the proper medication at the appropriate time.

Respite Care

Caring for a patient in the home can be a physically and emotionally draining experience for the primary caregiver. **Respite care** provides temporary relief for the primary caregiver. Respite care is not specifically a facility as much as it is a type of service. It may take place in a long-term care, rehabilitation, adult day care, or mental health facility. In some cases, it may be delivered in the home.

Hospice

A **hospice** provides palliative care for the terminally ill. **Palliative care** refers to making the patient comfortable in terms of easing pain and other discomforts. Hospice care can be delivered to the patient in an inpatient setting or in the home. A hospice also provides support groups and counseling for both the patient and his or her family and friends. Hospice services may continue for the survivors after the patient's death.

Home Health Care

As the name implies, **home health care** involves a variety of services provided to patients in the home. Services range from assistance with ADLs to physical therapy to intravenous drug therapy. Personnel providing these services also vary, from aides to therapists, to nurses and doctors.

HIT Bit

You may have noticed that many of the terms and phrases used in health care frequently are shortened to a few recognizable letters. An abbreviation made from the initial letters or parts of a term is called an *acronym.* Acronyms and other abbreviations shorten writing time and save space. However, acronyms can also cause confusion. AMA, for example, means "against medical advice." It is also the abbreviation for the American Medical Association and the American Management Association. There are also interdisciplinary issues with abbreviations. Dr. means "doctor" to a health care professional. To an accountant, it means "debit." Therefore, abbreviations should be used carefully. Health care facilities must define acceptable abbreviations and should enforce the restriction on the use of abbreviations to only those that have been approved.

Comparison of Facilities

We have talked about differences between types of facilities. What about facilities that are the same type, such as two acute care facilities? How do we compare them? No single description, statistical or otherwise, separates one hospital from another. In comparing hospitals, we look at many different characteristics together. Only then can we obtain a real understanding of the differences between them. In this section, we discuss ways of differentiating between like facilities and also mention a few more specific differences between types of facilities.

Facility Size

One way of distinguishing one facility from another is by the facility size. Frequently not only is a facility described as being acute care or long-term care or ambulatory care or rehabilitation, but it also is differentiated by number of beds or by number of discharges. The size of an ambulatory care facility is defined by the number of encounters or the number of visits. These concepts are detailed in the following sections.

NUMBER OF BEDS

In an inpatient facility, beds are set up for patients to occupy. There are two basic ways to view beds: licensed beds and bed count. *Licensed beds* are the number of beds that the state has approved the hospital to have. For now, think of licensed beds as the maximum number of beds allowed to the facility.

Facilities don't always need all of their licensed beds. For example, a facility may not have enough patients to fill all of the beds. It is very expensive to maintain the equipment and the staffing for an empty room. Facility administrators look at beds in terms of whether they are occupied. If the percentage of occupied beds is low over a period of time, then administrators may decide to close some of the beds. Therefore, a facility may equip and staff only as many beds as it needs for the forseeable future. This number of beds, which can be less than the number of licensed beds but not more, is called the bed count. **Bed count** is the number of beds that the facility actually has set up, equipped, and staffed, in other words, the beds that are ready to treat patients.

In comparing facilities, we often refer to the size of the facility in terms of its licensed beds. It is also useful to analyze a facility's licensed beds versus bed count over time. A seasonal or otherwise short-term closing of beds is not automatically a matter of concern and may, in fact, be an indication of sound administration. Long-term low bed count (as compared to licensed beds), on the other hand, may be an indication of serious problems. Over the last 10 years, many hospitals have been forced to close beds as a result of the payer-driven shift from acute care to ambulatory care. Because licensed beds are granted based on the needs of the community, long-term reduction of bed count may signal that the facility is no longer needed in its community.

DISCHARGES

Another measure of the size of a facility is the number of discharges in a period, usually expressed monthly or annually. Number of discharges is a measure of activity, as opposed to a measure of physical size. Although two acute care facilities may each have 250 beds, one of them may discharge 15,000 patients per year while the other discharges 25,000 patients per year. Higher numbers of discharges require larger numbers of administrative and other support staff.

Occupancy, the percentage of available beds that have been used over a period of time, is one explanation for the difference in the number of discharges. To calculate occupancy, divide the number of days that patients used hospital beds by the number of beds available. If the number of days that patients used hospital beds is 7000, and the number of beds available is 8000, then the occupancy rate is 62.5%. The number of beds available can be based on either bed count or licensed beds. A facility may use bed count internally to monitor the rate at which available beds are being used, but may use licensed beds to compare use over time because licensed beds are less likely to change.

LOS is another explanation for different discharge numbers. The longer a patient stays in the hospital, the fewer individual patients can be treated in that particular bed. Therefore, if a hospital has an ALOS of 6 days, it can treat half as many patients as a hospital with an ALOS of 3 days. For example, to calculate the ALOS of a 200-bed hospital that has 6000 "beds" or "days" available to treat patients in the month of June, multiply 200 beds times 30 days in June equals 6000. If the ALOS is 6 days, then the hospital is able to treat an estimated 1000 patients for 6 days (6000 divided by 6 equals 1000). If the ALOS is 3 days, then the hospital is able to treat an estimated 2000 patients—twice as many as the hospital with an ALOS of 6 days. That means twice as many admissions, twice as many discharges, and twice as much work for many of the administrative support staff who process these activities (see Chapter 4).

Ownership

Health care facilities may exist under many different types of ownership. Some facilities, such as physician group practices and radiology centers, are owned by individuals or groups of individuals. Facilities may be owned by corporations, government entities, or religious groups. Frequently, the ownership of the organization has an impact on both the operations and the services provided by the facility. For example, a facility owned by a religious organization may not allow abortions to be performed by their physicians. A government-owned facility may require supplies to be purchased from government-approved vendors.

Financial Status

Another way to distinguish institutions from each other is by their tax status: for-profit or not-for-profit. A for-profit, or proprietary, organization has owners. It can have few or many owners or shareholders. Ford Motor Company is an example of a for-profit organization with many shareholders. A not-for-profit institution operates solely for the good of the community and is considered to be owned by the community. It has no shareholders who have a vested interest in the economic viability of the organization.

The tax status of an organization has little or no impact on the day-to-day operations of the organization. The fundamental impact is on the distribution of net income. In a not-for-profit organization, net income must be reinvested in the organization or the community. In a for-profit organization, net income may, at the discretion of the board of directors, be distributed in whole or in part to the shareholders of the organization.

Patient Population

As we have already discussed, facilities may differ in terms of the types of patients that they treat. Rehabilitation facilities and mental health facilities treat patients with different types of problems. Many facilities specialize in treating only certain types of diseases. For example, Deborah Heart and Lung Center in New Jersey specializes in treating cardiac and respiratory problems. It would not accept a patient whose only problem is a broken leg. Another common type of specialty hospital is a **children's hospital.** The medical treatment of children requires smaller equipment as well as specialized equipment and clinical skills. A children's hospital would not normally accept a 35-year-old patient.

Services

Depending on the type of patients that they treat, facilities offer a variety of different services. These services are often organized into departments. For example, an acute care facility has an emergency department and a surgery department. It also offers radiology, laboratory, and pathology services. If an acute care facility offers physical therapy, it may be a small department. Often, therapy is provided at the patient's bedside. A rehabilitation facility does not have an emergency department, but it may have a room set aside for performing minor surgical procedures. It may have radiology and laboratory services, but it probably does not have a pathology department. Because physical therapy is a major component of rehabilitation, physical therapy is a large department. A large amount of space is available for treatment, including a variety of specialized equipment.

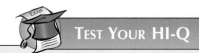

TEST YOUR HI-Q

Deluxe Hospital is a 460-bed facility with an average of 35 discharges per day. The ALOS is 6 days. Deluxe has an emergency department, several operating suites, and a wide variety of ancillary services. The most common reason for admission is childbirth, followed by heart and lung problems. What kind of a facility is Deluxe? What services might it provide?

Continuum of Care

With so many different caregivers working in such a variety of facilities, communication among them is essential. The coordination among caregivers to treat a patient is called the **continuum of care.** Continuum of care is a concept with two separate but related elements. First, it refers to communication among all the patient's care providers in a facility from his or her admission to discharge. As a patient moves from place to place in a facility, communication among all his or her caregivers ideally should be as smooth and coordinated as possible. Second, continuum of care refers to all of the patient's experiences from one facility to another, either throughout a particular illness or throughout the life of the patient. We illustrate the continuum of care from birth to death for a female patient in the subsequent text.

Childhood

The patient, Emily, is born in an acute care facility. As a child, Emily is treated by a pediatrician. The pediatrician is her primary care physician. She receives extensive well care: preventive vaccinations, checkups, and developmental assessments.

Adult Care

As Emily ages and grows into adulthood, she visits a general practitioner as her new primary care physician. The general practitioner would benefit from having the information about all of the patient's childhood diseases, immunizations, and problems that she has experienced previously. Emily would then see her primary care physician on a regular basis. As she becomes an adult, she also visits a gynecologist for regular examinations.

Special Health Issues

When Emily becomes pregnant, she is examined and followed by her obstetrician throughout the pregnancy and cesarean delivery. Later on in life, as she becomes older, other illnesses may arise. For example, the patient in her late 30s develops diabetes. Her primary care physician refers her to an endocrinologist for treatment of the diabetes. After Emily discovers a lump in her breast, she undergoes a mammography and is referred to a surgeon for a diagnosis. Then the patient enters an acute care facility to have a lumpectomy. Note that at this point in our example, Emily has had at least three admissions to an acute care facility and has visited at least three specialists in addition to her primary care physician. How confusing would it be if none of these physicians was aware of the treatment she had received from the others?

Elder Care

As an elderly woman, Emily falls and breaks her hip. She needs to have a hip replacement, and is treated by an orthopedic surgeon in an acute care facility for hip replacement surgery, after which she is transferred to a rehabilitation facility for a couple of weeks of rehabilitation to enable her to resume her activities of daily living. Eventually Emily becomes incapacitated and is unable to take care of herself. She develops Alzheimer's disease and is seen by a neurologist and a psychiatrist. Ultimately, she is be admitted into a nursing home for round-the-clock nursing care.

Throughout all of these encounters with various facilities and specialists, the previous history of Emily's encounters should follow her smoothly. The orthopedic surgeon will want to know her experiences under anesthesia when she had breast surgery, and about her reaction to anesthesia when her baby was born. This information should be available to subsequent surgeons.

Impact of Mergers and Acquisitions

As noted previously, hospital mergers have increased in recent years. Many health care organizations are doing this consolidation along the continuum of care. In other words, they are not just buying multiple acute care facilities, they are buying physician's office practices, rehabilitation facilities, and long-term care facilities as well as acute care facilities. Thus, they are able to provide patients with seamless coordination of care along this continuum. Such enterprises are referred to as **integrated delivery systems (IDSs).** There are many who see this as an efficient delivery of health care throughout the lifetime of a patient.

Legal and Regulatory Environment

In addition to the issues previously discussed, various facilities have different ways of operating or functioning. More often, the guidance or mandate under which activities are performed arises from legislation, regulation, and accreditation issues. In this section, we explain the legal environment of health care. Because this is frequently a topic of another entire text or course, our discussion is limited to the issues that bear directly on the activities of a health information technology professional. Federal, state, and local government all have an impact in varying degrees on health care institutions and delivery. Table 1–5 summarizes government impact on health care.

Federal

The federal government has a major impact on health care through regulatory activity. The federal legislature (Congress and the Senate) enacts laws, which the executive branch (the President) must then enforce. Enforcement arises from

TABLE 1–5. Federal Agencies Involved in Health Care		
Department	**Agency**	**Health-Related Functions**
Department of Health and Human Services	Food and Drug Administration	Ensures safety of foods, cosmetics, pharmaceuticals, biologic products, and medical devices
	Health Care Financing Administration	Oversees Medicare and the federal portion of Medicaid
	National Institutes of Health	Supports biomedical research
	Centers for Disease Control and Prevention	Provides a system of health surveillance to monitor and prevent outbreak of diseases
	Health Resources and Services Administration	Helps provide health resources for medically underserved populations
	Indian Health Service	Supports a network of health care facilities and providers to Native Americans, including Alaskans
Department of Defense	Military Health Services System	Maintains a network of health care providers and facilities for service personnel and their dependents
Department of Veterans Affairs	Veterans Affairs facilities	Maintains a network of facilities and services for armed services veterans and sometimes their dependents
Department of Labor	Occupational Safety and Health Administration	Regulates workplace health and safety

the delegation of executive responsibilities to various agencies. In terms of health care, the critical regulatory agency is the Health Care Financing Administration (HCFA), which administers Medicare and part of Medicaid.

MEDICARE

Medicare is an entitlement to health care benefits for persons of advanced age (over 65) or those with certain chronic illnesses (e.g., end-stage renal disease). Health care facilities are not automatically eligible for reimbursement from Medicare simply on the basis of treating a Medicare patient. To be eligible for reimbursement from Medicare, a health care facility must comply with Medicare's Conditions of Participation (COP). COP addresses the quality of providers, certain policies and procedures, and financial issues and is updated in the *Federal Register.* Another important area of federal regulation concerns release of information pertaining to patients with drug and alcohol diagnoses (discussed in Chapter 8).

State

The impact of state government on health care organizations varies from state to state. Here we discuss some of the most common involvements, licensure and reporting.

LICENSURE

In order to operate any health care facility, a license must be obtained from the state in which the facility will operate. The process of **licensure** varies among states. Often, the state's legislature passes a hospital licensing act or other similar law that requires hospitals to be licensed and delegates the authority to regulate that process to a state agency, possibly the state's Department of Health. The delegated agency then develops and administers the detailed regulations, which are part of the state's administrative code. The licensure regulations contain a great deal of useful information pertaining to the operations of a health care facility, including the minimum requirements for maintaining patient records. Some states' regulations are very detailed and specific as to the organization and structure of a facility, including such items as services to be provided, medical staff requirements, nursing requirements, committees, and sanitation. Licensure is specific to the type of health care facility being operated. The regulations governing acute care facilities differ somewhat from the regulations governing long-term care facilities, which are in turn different from regulations governing rehabilitation facilities.

It is fundamentally the responsibility of the board of directors or board of trustees of a facility to ensure compliance with each of the requirements of the license. The board delegates the day-to-day operations of the facility to management, through the chief executive officer or administrator of the hospital.

Many state agencies visit hospitals on a regular basis and review the hospital operations and the documentation for compliance with the license of the facility. Of particular note are long-term facilities, which tend to be scrutinized very closely. Many states defer their acute care facility reviews to alternative methods such as relying on the reviews of accrediting bodies, discussed subsequently.

REPORTING

There is a tremendous amount of reporting that occurs between health care facilities and state agencies. Typically, reporting includes information about general patient data, cancer, trauma, birth defects, and infectious disease. Additional reporting may result from health care workers' observation of inappropriate activities, such as child abuse, and health care workers have an obligation to report to the authorities certain types of suspected abuses. So the relationship between state government and health care facilities is extensive.

Local

Local government may also become involved in health care organizations, particularly in the aspect of zoning regulations. Because the facility is an important member of the local community, its activities may become deeply intertwined with those of the community.

Accreditation

So far, we've discussed federal statutes and regulations and the impact of licensure. Another issue that has a visible impact on the operation of a health care facility is voluntary accreditation. Whereas licensure is mandatory to operate a health care facility within a given state, accreditation is voluntary.

Accreditation begins with voluntary compliance with a set of standards that are developed by an independent organization. That organization then audits the facility to ensure compliance. A variety of accrediting bodies exist for different industries. Table 1–6 lists some health care accrediting bodies and the subjects of their activities.

HIT BIT

If you are studying health information management in a college that has an accredited health information management program, your program is accredited by the Commission on Accreditation of Allied Health Education Programs (CAAHEP), in cooperation with the Council on Accreditation of the American Health Information Management Association. CAAHEP also accredits a variety of different health programs (see Table 1–6). Also, the school as a whole may be accredited by a variety of different academic standard setting bodies.

TABLE 1–6. Accrediting Organizations in Health Care	
Accrediting Organization	**Facilities/Organizations Accredited**
Health Care Facilities	
Accreditation Association for Ambulatory Health Care	Ambulatory care facilities
American Osteopathic Association	Osteopathic hospitals
Joint Commission on Accreditation of Healthcare Organizations	Acute care, ambulatory care, behavioral health, long-term care, and rehabilitation facilities
Commission on Accreditation of Rehabilitation Facilities (CARF)	Rehabilitation facilities
National Committee for Quality Assurance (NCQA)	Managed care organizations
Community Health Accreditation Program (National League for Nursing)	Home and community-based health care organizations
Educational Programs	
Accreditation Council for Occupational Therapy Education	Occupational therapist and occupational therapy assistant programs
Liaison Committee of the Association of American Medical Colleges and the American Medical Association	Medical schools
Committee on the Accreditation of Allied Health Education Programs	Education programs for 18 specialties, including anesthesiologist assistant, athletic trainer, cardiovascular technologist, emergency medical technician-paramedic, health information administrator/technician, medical assistant, physician assistant, and respiratory therapist
National League for Nursing Accrediting Commission	Nursing schools
American Physical Therapy Association	Physical therapist and physical therapist assistant
Commission on Accreditation/Approval for Dietetics Education of the American Dietetic Association	Dietitian/nutritionist and dietetic technician programs

Joint Commission on Accreditation of Healthcare Organizations

Within the health care profession, the most important accrediting body is the Joint Commission on Accreditation of Healthcare Organizations (JCAHO). The JCAHO is an organization, located in Chicago, that sets standards for acute care facilities, ambulatory care networks, long-term care facilities, and rehabilitation facilities, as well as certain specialty facilities, such as hospice and home care.

The standards set by the JCAHO reflect optimum industry practice and in many ways define how the health care facility should operate in terms of patient care, the clinical flow of data, and documentation standards. Much of the activity of the JCAHO stems from the original 1913 American College of Surgeons (ACS) medical documentation standardization project. For many years after that project, ACS not only maintained the development of the standards of documentation for hospitals but also conducted the approval proceedings. In 1951, the ACS, along with the American Hospital Association, the American Medical Association, and the Canadian Medical Association, formed the Joint Commission on Accreditation of Hospitals, which took over that accrediting function. In 1987, the Joint Commission changed its name to reflect the variety of different organizations that were seeking accreditation.

The JCAHO has a tremendous impact on health care facilities for a number of reasons. First, accrediting surveys take place on a scheduled 3-year (maximum) cycle. So at least every 3 years, the facility is subject to an intensive review. The accreditation standards change to differing degrees annually, with interim changes as needed. Therefore, within the 3-year cycle of review, facilities need to be aware of the changes and to implement procedures to comply.

Second, a favorable accreditation status of a facility has an impact on its relationship with government entities. As was previously discussed, the Health Care Financing Administration, through Medicare, allows reimbursement from Medicare to those facilities that comply with Medicare's COP. This ordinarily entails a survey to ensure that the facility complies with COP. However, a facility that is accredited by the JCAHO is not normally required to be subject to the COP review. This is called **deemed status** because the facility is deemed to have complied with the COP. In addition, in some states JCAHO accreditation reduces or eliminates the need for state licensure surveys. So, in some cases, the voluntary accreditation by the JCAHO can alleviate two additional surveys—the state department of health and Medicare COP.

Finally, accreditation is also desirable for marketing purposes. As the public becomes more aware of quality issues in a facility, JCAHO accreditation becomes a symbol of quality to a certain extent.

Commission on Accreditation of Rehabilitation Facilities

Another important accrediting body is the Commission on Accreditation of Rehabilitation Facilities (CARF), also known as the Rehabilitation Accreditation Commission, which focuses on facilities that provide physical, mental, and occupational rehabilitation services. Accreditation of adult day care, assisted living, and employment and community services are also available. The JCAHO also accredits rehabilitation facilities, but it has slightly different requirements and standards, adapting acute care and ambulatory care requirements. In fact, many rehabilitation facilities may be accredited by both the JCAHO and CARF. The focus of the two reviews is slightly different, and rehabilitation facilities that are accredited by the JCAHO find themselves in something of a dilemma in complying with both sets of requirements. CARF requirements tend to be more prescriptive, and surveyors focus beyond physician/nurse documentation to emphasize documentation of occupational, physical, and other therapies. In recent years, JCAHO and CARF have collaborated to offer to facilities joint survey options. In this way, the surveys can be simultaneous and partially coordinated to reduce duplication of effort.

There are many organizations that accredit health care facilities and health care professional education programs. A partial list of these organizations and the facilities and institutions that they accredit is given in Table 1–6.

AHIMA CODE OF ETHICS

Preamble

This Code of Ethics sets forth ethical principles for the health information management profession. Members of this profession are responsible for maintaining and promoting ethical practices. This Code of Ethics, adopted by the American Health Information Management Association, shall be binding on health information management professionals who are members of the Association and all individuals who hold an AHIMA credential.

I. Health information management professionals respect the rights and dignity of all individuals.

II. Health information management professionals comply with all laws, regulations, and standards governing the practice of health information management.

III. Health information management professionals strive for professional excellence through self-assessment and continuing education.

IV. Health information management professionals truthfully and accurately represent their professional credentials, education, and experience.

V. Health information management professionals adhere to the vision, mission, and values of the Association.

VI. Health information management professionals promote and protect the confidentiality and security of health records and health information.

VII. Health information management professionals strive to provide accurate and timely information.

VIII. Health information management professionals promote high standards for health information management practice, education, and research.

IX. Health information management professionals act with integrity and avoid conflicts of interest in the performance of their professional and AHIMA responsibilities.

Revised and adopted by AHIMA House of Delegates, October 4, 1998.

Professional Standards

In addition to licensure and accreditation requirements, there is yet another level of requirements that must be followed in a health care organization. This last set of requirements is *professional standards*. On one hand, licensure and accrediting bodies take a general overview of the facility and tend not to specifically address the day-to-day activities of individual practitioners. Professional standards, on the other hand, are developed by the professional organizations that grant the credentials to the individuals who are performing health-related tasks.

In addition to professional standards that govern the behavior of a variety of health care professionals, many of those professionals are also licensed by the state in which they practice and come under those licensing regulations as well.

Specifically, physicians are licensed to practice medicine the same way that health care facilities are licensed to operate, and the requirements for licensure may vary from state to state.

Professional standards play an important role in determining the activities of health care professionals. Often, it is the professional standards of the individual practitioner that dictate the type and extent of documentation that is required in the performance of any type of therapy or evaluation of patients.

In the field of health information management, professional standards tend to revolve around issues of **ethics** and best practices. They also tend to target data quality, confidentiality, and access to health information. It is important in the practice of health information technology that we know and adhere to these professional standards. Professional standards in health information management are developed by the American Health Information Management Association (AHIMA) and take the form of an ethics statement as well as practice briefs and position papers, which are routinely published in the *Journal of the American Health Information Management Association*.

Reference

Raffel MW, Raffel NK: The U.S. Health System, Origins and Functions, 4th ed. Albany, NY, Delmar, 1994.

Suggested Reading

Peden AH: Comparative Records for Health Information Management. Albany, NY, Delmar, 1998.
Sultz, HA, Young KM: Health Care USA: Understanding Its Organization and Delivery, 2nd ed. Gaithersburg, Md: Aspen, 1999.

Web Sites

American Health Information Management Association: www.ahima.org
American Hospital Association: www.aha.org
Department of Health and Human Services: www.os.dhhs.gov
Department of Labor: www.dol.gov
National Library of Medicine: www.nlm.nih.gov
Veterans Administration: www.va.gov

CHAPTER SUMMARY

Health care is provided by a variety of different practitioners, including physicians, nurses, and therapists. Physicians may maintain their own offices as solo practitioners or work with other physicians in group practices. Physicians' offices are a type of ambulatory care facility. Other types of facilities are acute care, long-term care, and a variety of specialty facilities including rehabilitation facilities, mental health facilities, and children's hospitals. Facilities can be classified by length of stay, inpatient versus outpatient services, and financial status (i.e., for-profit or not-for-profit).

Government plays a role in the health care industry. Federal and state governments enact laws and enforce them through regulations. Health care facilities are licensed through the state, and there are a number of very specific reporting requirements. Another aspect of facility organization is accreditation status. Accreditation is very important for quality assurance and also for reimbursement. Lastly, professional standards play a role in determining the activities of a facility because each profession has its own standards of both care and documentation.

REVIEW QUESTIONS

1. List six medical specialties and describe what those professionals do. Research five medical specialties that were not listed in the text and discover what those professionals do.

2. Identify and describe five allied health professions and their principal occupational settings. Research four health-related professions that were not listed in the text and discover what those professionals do.

3. Distinguish between ambulatory care facilities and acute care facilities.

4. Distinguish between inpatients and outpatients.

5. List three services provided in acute care facilities that are not widely available in long-term care or rehabilitation facilities.

6. Describe government involvement in health care.

7. Distinguish between licensure and accreditation.

8. List major accreditation organizations and the types of facilities they accredit.

PROFESSIONAL PROFILE
Physician Office Liaison

My name is Melanie, and I have a very interesting position at a community hospital. I am a physician office liaison. I am responsible for helping the hospital maintain good relationships with the physicians on our staff. We are a small community hospital with 250 licensed beds. Our physicians are not employees of the hospital; they have privileges. This means that the hospital allows the physicians to admit their patients for treatment at the hospital. These physicians have private practices with their own offices and staff. It's my job to know them, to help with any problems they may have communicating with the hospital, and to coordinate the filing of their professional documentation.

I like my job, because I get to meet many really interesting people and I learn about their jobs as well. Even though I'm learning something new every day, I had to know a lot to get this job in the first place.

To be able to help a physician's office staff member, I have to know the various professionals who might work in an office and what they might do. It really helps that I know the difference between a medical assistant and a nurse practitioner. It's important that I know how a group practice works so that I can help the hospital keep track of which physicians can cover for each other.

The hospital collects statistics on physicians: how many patients they admit, what diagnoses they are treating, what procedures they are performing, and other information. I collaborate with other hospital departments to collect these reports and help present them at medical staff meetings. In order to do this, I have to know all the departments in the hospital and how they are related to each other. I also need to understand the reports.

One of my most important tasks is credentialing. When a physician applies for privileges, I do a background check, collect the licensing documentation, and prepare a presentation for the credentialing committee. Because privileges aren't permanent, I remind the physicians when they need to reapply and help gather the updated documentation. I need to understand the differences among the medical specialties and what board certification means.

Finally, I coordinate continuing education sessions for physicians and their office staff. My next project is to develop a newsletter of hospital and physician activities that I can e-mail to the physicians' offices.

How did I get this job? I'm a registered health information technician. I have an associate degree in health information technology (HIT) from my local community college. In the HIT program, I learned a lot about physicians, hospitals, and other health-related professions. The hospital was very happy to have a candidate for the job who already understood the system.

APPLICATION

An Ethical Dilemma

Vanessa is the supervisor of health information management at Community Hospital. She is a member of AHIMA and is studying to become a registered health information technician. Community Hospital has a new chief operating officer, Brad, who is new to the hospital and comes from another state. Brad is concerned that too many physicians are not completing their paperwork when patients are discharged. He would like Vanessa and her staff to send the paperwork out of the hospital to the physicians' offices for completion, because he thinks that the physicians would be more likely to do the work if it were on their desks. Vanessa knows that the state licensure regulations prohibit the removal of the paperwork from the hospital under normal circumstances.

Should Vanessa comply with Brad's request? Is compliance with Brad's request a violation of the AHIMA Code of Ethics?

2

Data Elements

Chapter Outline

Basic Concepts
Health
Data
Information
Health Data
Health Information

Overview of a Physician's Office Visit
Personnel
Clinical Flow
Services

Key Data Categories
Demographic Data
Socioeconomic Data
Financial Data
Clinical Data

Describing Data
Characters
Fields
Records
Files

Health Record

Health Information Management

Data Quality
Data Accuracy
Data Validity

Data Sets

Suggested Reading

Chapter Summary

Review Questions

Professional Profile

Application

In Chapter 1, we discussed various health care professionals and the settings in which they work. When health care providers are caring for patients, they listen to the patients and make observations. In this chapter, we narrow our focus to the physician's office and discuss the way health care providers gather their observations about patients. Because most of you have visited a physician at one time or another, your personal experience will help you relate to the chapter contents.

Basic Concepts

Before proceeding, we need to understand some basic terminology. Although these terms may be meaningful to you in other subjects, it is important that we define them in the context of health care.

Health

Because this book is about health information, we should certainly have an understanding of what *health* is. Health begins with the absence of *disease*. For the purposes of this discussion, let's consider a disease to be an abnormality caused by organic, environmental, or congenital problems. Therefore, a person with no diseases is considered "healthy." What if a person has no diseases, but is very emotionally upset over events in his or her life—is that person healthy? Not really. Long-term emotional upheaval can lead to a number of serious diseases. Therefore, emotional concerns detract from health. What about a child who does not get enough to eat but is currently free from disease? Is that child healthy? Won't that child eventually deteriorate into an unhealthy status over time? Of course. Therefore, health is a broader concept than merely the absence of disease. A person who is healthy is free of disease and is also free of outside physical, social, and any other problems that could lead to a disease condition.

Data

Health information starts with **data.** What are data? Data are units of knowledge. A unit of data is an item, idea, concept, or raw fact. We can collect data, yet not understand them. We can collect temperatures, blood pressures, or number of patients, but unless the items are structured or organized, they are only data— individual items of knowledge—and are not meaningful.

Information

In order to interpret data—to make sense of the facts and use them—we organize the items of data. Once they are organized, data become **information.** The terms "data" and "information" are often used synonymously, but they are not the same. "Get me the data" usually really means "get me useful information." Data are the units of knowledge, and information is data that we have organized

DATA VS. INFORMATION

DATA		*INFORMATION*	
Definition:	Individual units of knowledge	Definition:	Data with a frame of reference
Example:	Maria Gomez	Example:	Maria Gomez Temperature (oral) March 15, 1999
	104		1 PM 104°
	105		2 PM 105°
	104		3 PM 104°
	103		4 PM 103°
	102		5 PM 102°
	101		6 PM 101°
	100		7 PM 100°
	99		8 PM 99°

On the left, the data about Maria Gomez are not useful, because we do not have a frame of reference. Those same data, within the frame of reference of date and time, tell a story that is clinically significant.

FIGURE 2–1.

A list of data with a frame of reference becomes information.

(Fig. 2–1). On the left in Figure 2–1 is a list of data pertaining to Maria Gomez. We cannot tell what the data mean until we determine that they are her oral temperature, taken at 1-hour intervals. Then, the information becomes useful. The primary purpose of this book is to discuss data in the health care setting, how data are organized, stored, and retrieved, and how we can make information from data.

On the right in Figure 2–1, the temperatures are listed in chronologic order. With these few readings, it is easy to see that Maria's temperature is going down. If we took her temperature every hour for 5 days, we would have over 100 items of data, and even listing them in order would not be helpful. Therefore, the most useful information is often a picture, such as the graph shown in Figure 2–2. Here, we can see that Maria's temperature went up on day 2, but returned to normal and stayed there. The figure shows that the usefulness of information depends on its organization and presentation.

Health Data

Health data are items of knowledge about an individual patient or a group of patients. We can list all of a patient's diseases or list all of the patients who have a certain disease. In fact, our example of data in Figure 2–1 is really health data: We collected a series of temperatures from one patient.

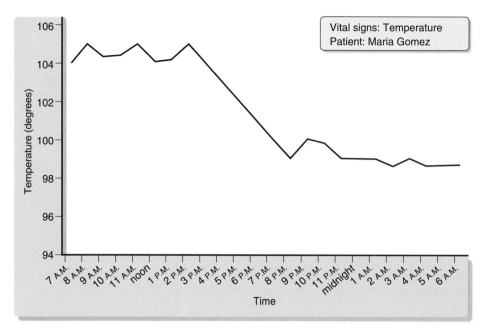

FIGURE 2–2.
The data presentation graph displays a large amount of data.

Similarly, we can obtain vast quantities of data on individual patients or groups of patients. Imagine that your local newspaper has just printed a list of 10,000 city residents and their diseases. Are these useful data? What could you do with these data? Unless you are prepared to perform some analytic procedures on it and organize it yourself, the list is not very informative. However, if the paper had printed the top 10 most common diseases of 10,000 residents, that's information you can use. This type of information is published frequently. For example, Figure 2–3 shows the top 10 causes of death in the United States in 1900 and 1997. Certainly, a list of the top 500 causes of death would not have been as useful.

Health Information

Health information is health data that have been organized. Health data related to 10,000 residents become health information when the data are organized in a way that is meaningful to the reader. Listing the top 10 diseases of your city's residents is useful health information. In Figure 2–1, the temperatures gathered become health information when we understand that those temperatures are for one patient at certain times of the day. This is information that physicians can use to make decisions. In Figure 2–3, the charts present interesting information that helps us to ask questions that lead to more information, and so on. The study of these types of health trends or patterns is called **epidemiology.**

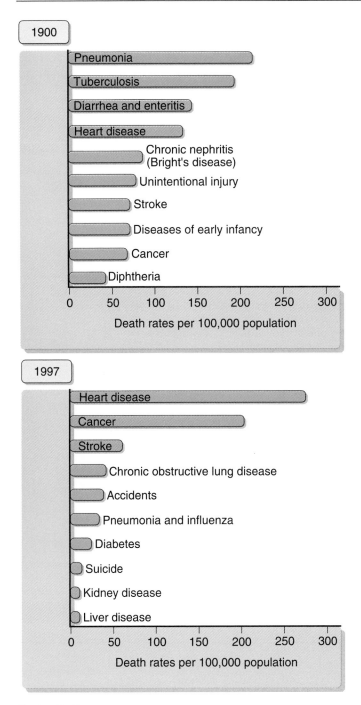

FIGURE 2-3.

The top ten causes of death in the United States: 1900 and 1997.
(Adapted from Grove RD, Hetzel AM: Vital Statistics Rates of the
United States, 1940–1960. Washington DC, US Government Printing
Office, 1968; and Hoyert DL, Koehanek KD, Murphy SI: Deaths: Final
Data for 1997. National Vital Stat Report 47, No. 19, June 30, 1999.)

Health information is a broad category: It may refer to the organized data that have been collected about an individual patient, or it can be the summary of information about that patient's entire experience with his or her physician. Health information can also be the aggregate information about all of the patients that a physician has seen. Further, we can take all of the physicians in a certain area and organize information about all of their patients and make broad statements about this array of information.

Health information, therefore, encompasses the organization of a limitless array of possible data items and combinations of data items. It can range from data about the care of an individual patient to the health trends of an entire nation.

HIT BIT

Is *data* a plural word or a singular word? "Datum" is the singular form of the Latin word and it represents one single item of knowledge. However, we rarely refer to one item of knowledge. Generally, we discuss a group of similar items, such as the temperatures listed in Figure 2–1, and we call the group "data". In this book you will notice that we use the plural form to refer to items of related data ("the *data are* significant"). Both ways are acceptable.

Overview of a Physician's Office Visit

Now that you have an understanding of some basic terminology, let's identify health data by hypothetically scheduling a visit to a physician's office to see how data are collected. Our visit will accomplish three objectives: identify the physician's office personnel, trace the clinical flow of a patient's data through the office, and list the data that are collected. Figure 2–4 shows the flow of activities in a typical physician's office. Obviously, different combinations of personnel and procedures are seen. Our visit is a general guide to the events so that you can understand the flow of information.

Personnel

After you have identified the physician you want to visit, you call the office for an appointment. You will probably not talk directly to the physician; very likely you will speak to someone who works with the physician. This may be any of a number of different allied health personnel. A *medical secretary* has a basic knowledge of office procedures, scheduling, filing, and billing. A *medical assistant* has all of that knowledge and some basic clinical knowledge, such as taking blood pressure and temperature. A *physician assistant* is a highly trained clinical assistant who can take the medical history and assist the physician in treating patients. A *nurse* is a highly trained clinician who can collect a variety of information and assist in treating patients. A *nurse practitioner* is a nurse with extensive additional

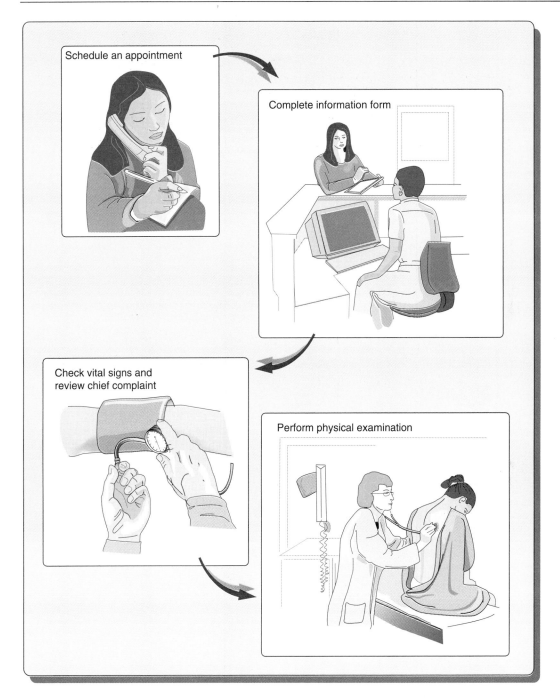

FIGURE 2–4.
Flow of activities in a physician's office.

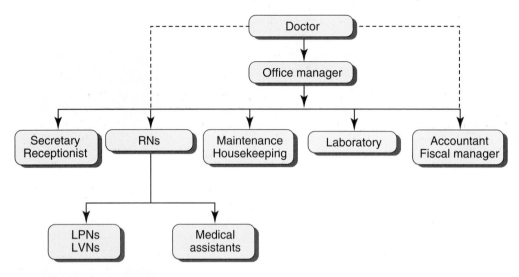

FIGURE 2–5.
Sample of employees in a physician's office. (From Simmers L: Diversified Health Occupations, 4th ed. ©1998. Reprinted with permission of Delmar, a division of Thomson Learning. Fax 800-730-2215.)

training. Nurse practitioners often work in areas in which there are not enough physicians. Figure 2–5 shows some employees common in a physician's office.

Clinical Flow

Our physician's office has a number of different personnel and employs a receptionist to handle telephone calls and appointments. When you called for an appointment, the receptionist asked for your name and telephone number and inquired whether you were a current patient. It is very important to know if the patient is a current patient, because a new patient takes more of the staff's time to collect data. The receptionist also asked why you wanted to see the physician. This is another aid to scheduling. A regular patient coming in for a flu shot takes far less of the physician's time than a new patient who complains of stomach pains. As we see in Chapter 9, identification of a new versus an established patient is also important for billing physician services.

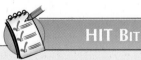

HIT BIT

Some physicians rely solely on appointments for scheduling office time. Other physicians employ open-access techniques. In **open access,** some appointments are made, but time is allowed for patients who call for a same-day appointment. Scheduling appointments requires knowledge of time budgeting, and implementation of open-access methods needs a firm understanding of the demand for time in relation to the number of patients per doctor.

When you get to the office, the receptionist asks you to fill out some forms. On these forms, you provide personal information: your name and address, your past medical history, and who is responsible for paying the doctor's bill. The receptionist or a medical secretary may then enter some or all of this information into the computer. As a new patient, a folder is labeled with your name and used to hold the form you completed as well as any other papers containing information about you that may be needed. If you were not a new patient, your existing folder would have been retrieved. This folder of information is also called the patient's *record*. Historically, the folder has been the only record; however, there is an increasing emphasis on keeping the data in the computer instead of on paper. You also sign forms that authorize the physician to treat you. Chapter 8 discusses this authorization and other types of consents and releases.

Once the record-keeping processes are completed, a medical assistant or nurse takes your temperature, blood pressure, height, and weight, data that develop a profile of information about you and your visit. Because this is your first visit, this profile is called your **baseline:** the information against which all future visits will be compared.

Eventually, the physician sees you, examines you, and develops an opinion about your disease or condition. Perhaps the physician recommends tests to determine the extent of disease or to help determine the diagnosis. If your diagnosis is clear, the physician prescribes treatment at this visit. Before you leave the physician's office, you either remit payment for the visit or sign a release for the insurance company.

Services

As we discussed in Chapter 1, a physician's office is only one type of ambulatory care setting. Although other ambulatory care settings provide different services than does a physician's office, the basic clinical flow of events is similar. For example, another type of facility is an ambulatory surgery center. In addition to the events described previously, an actual surgical procedure takes place. There is also time and a place set aside for the patient to recover from the surgery.

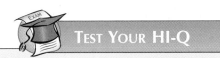

TEST YOUR HI-Q

What other services are provided in an ambulatory care setting? Describe the events that take place in other ambulatory care settings. How does the process differ from the one described in Figure 2–4? What other personnel are involved?

Key Data Categories

Let's think about what happens in a physician's office in the context of the data that are being collected about the patient. In our overview of a physician's office visit, we mentioned a number of questions that the physician's office personnel routinely asked. Let's organize these questions into meaningful categories.

Demographic Data

The first thing the physician would want to know is the patient's name and address. The physician needs the patient's name and address to develop a relationship with the patient and, perhaps, to send him or her correspondence, follow-up notices, or a bill. Other data that are needed include the home phone number, place of employment, work telephone number, and social security number. These data are needed when the physician has to contact the patient and also to distinguish one patient from another. This type of data about a patient is called **demographic data.** Because most of the data in this category pertain to locating and identifying the patient, this type of data is also called **indicative data.** Figure 2–6 shows a list of indicative data.

Socioeconomic Data

Another type of data about a patient that a physician collects is **socioeconomic data.** These personal data include the patient's marital status, education, and personal habits. Many students ask why we care about a patient's socioeconomic situation. One of the reasons that socioeconomic data are important is that the diagnosis of many illnesses, and sometimes their treatment, depends on an understanding by the doctor of the patient's personal situation. A list of socioeconomic data is presented in Figure 2–7.

Obviously, an asthma patient who smokes will be advised by his or her physician to quit smoking. This is an example of a personal habit that may be directly related to a disease condition. In addition, the socioeconomic, or personal life, of a patient sometimes dictates whether the patient will be compliant with medication or even whether he or she is able to obtain treatment. For example, if an elderly patient has just had a hip replacement, sending that patient home to a

INDICATIVE DATA

Definition: Data that help the user to contact the patient or to distinguish one patient from another

Name
Address
Home telephone number
Work telephone number
Social Security number
Birth date

FIGURE 2–6.

Sample indicative data.

SOCIOECONOMIC DATA

Definition: Personal data that give the user clues about potential problems and assistance in planning care

Marital status
Profession
Occupation
Employer
Religion
Sexual orientation
Personal habits
Race
Ethnicity

FIGURE 2-7.
Sample socioeconomic data.

third-story, walk-up apartment is going to be counterproductive to therapy. It will be very difficult for the elderly patient to get in and out of the house and certainly very difficult for him or her to get to therapy, particularly if there is no caregiver at home. Therefore, understanding a patient's personal life and living situation is very important in planning how to care for the patient.

Sometimes, the knowledge that a patient travels widely on business can lead a physician to suspect an illness that he or she would not consider if the patient never traveled. This patient's travels in certain areas of the world could have caused exposure to parasites not prevalent in his or her native area. The patient's complaint of gastrointestinal disturbances would lead the physician to suspect a parasite, whereas ordinarily he or she would consider only bacterial or viral causes.

Financial Data

When being treated in a health care facility, you should expect at some point that an invoice will be generated for the services and either you or your insurance company will be remitting payment. The physician requests information about the party responsible for paying the bill. This information comprises the **financial data.** As you can tell from the description, financial data relate to the payment of the bill for services rendered.

To understand the requirements of financial data, we need to define a few terms. A **payer** is the person or organization that is paying the bill. A payer is frequently an insurance company. It may also be a government agency, such as Medicare or Medicaid. Many patients have more than one payer. The primary payer is approached first for payment. A secondary payer is approached for any amount that the primary payer did not remit. For example, many elderly patients who are covered by Medicare have supplemental or secondary insurance with a different payer, such as Blue Cross Blue Shield Association. The physician first sends the bill to Medicare. Any amount that Medicare does not pay is then billed to Blue Cross Blue Shield Association.

Ultimately, the patient is responsible for payment of services that he or she received. If the patient is a dependent, a person other than the patient may be ultimately responsible for the bill. This person is called the **guarantor.** For example, if a child goes to the physician's office for treatment, the child, as a dependent, cannot be held responsible for the invoice. Therefore, the parent is responsible for payment and is the guarantor. Figure 2–8 lists financial data required by a health care facility.

Clinical Data

Clinical data are probably the easiest to understand and relate to the health care field. **Clinical data** are all of the data that are been recorded about the patient's health, including diagnoses and procedures. The following example illustrates clinical data.

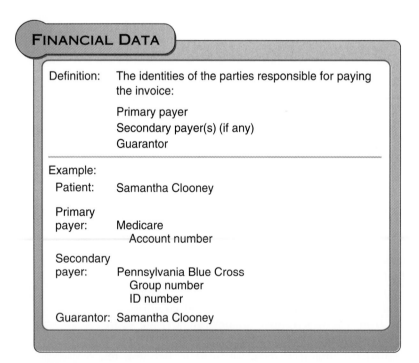

FINANCIAL DATA

Definition:	The identities of the parties responsible for paying the invoice:
	Primary payer
	Secondary payer(s) (if any)
	Guarantor

Example:
Patient: Samantha Clooney

Primary
payer: Medicare
            Account number

Secondary
payer: Pennsylvania Blue Cross
            Group number
            ID number

Guarantor: Samantha Clooney

FIGURE 2–8.
Sample financial data.

CLINICAL DATA

Definition: Data specific to the patient's diagnosis and treatment

Diagnosis
Temperature
Blood pressure
Laboratory reports
X-ray reports
Medications
Surgical procedures

FIGURE 2–9.

Sample clinical data.

Imagine that you are a patient going to the physician's office for pain in the abdomen. The physician knows that pain in the abdomen can be caused by a variety of conditions. The pain is merely a **symptom,** a description of what the patient feels or is experiencing. Other symptoms may include nausea, dizziness, and headache. The physician may order a number of tests and performs a physical examination to determine which of those conditions is responsible for the abdominal pain. Some of these tests include x-rays and blood tests. Ultimately, the physician may conclude that the abdominal pain is caused by an inflamed appendix, or appendicitis. Appendicitis is the diagnosis, and the blood test and physical examination are the procedures. The physician records both the examination and the results of the tests in the patient's record. Clinical data comprise the bulk of any patient's record. All of the previous data that we have discussed—demographic, socioeconomic, and financial—can usually be contained in one or two pages in the front of a patient's health record. The rest of the record is the clinical data. Figure 2–9 lists examples of clinical data.

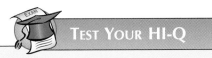

TEST YOUR HI-Q

Think about a disease with which you are familiar and create a list of all the data elements that you think a physician and allied health personnel in a physician's office would generate for the disease. You can make up the data, but make the list as complete as you can. This exercise will give you an idea of how complex health information is, even at the physician's office level.

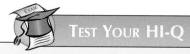

TEST YOUR HI-Q

Can you give two examples in your personal life of data and two examples of information? Think of two examples of how health data differ from health information.

Describing Data

Now that we have discussed data theoretically, let's explore data from a practical standpoint. We collect data for a reason and store the data for later use. It's a little like grocery shopping. We buy food that we need now and store it in the proper place for later use. Similarly, we collect the data that we think we need and store these data in the proper places for when we need them.

Whether we are collecting data to be stored on paper or in a computer, the data must be organized in such a way that we can understand them and retrieve the records later. The first step in collecting the data is determining what data are needed. Earlier in this chapter we started to explain the process of collecting data as it relates to health care by defining the types of data that we need.

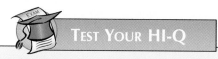

TEST YOUR HI-Q

List and describe the four key data categories and what they contain.

To take the analogy of grocery shopping further: Just as food comes in appropriate containers, data also come in packages. Data are collected and stored in logical segments. Individual data items are collected and packaged into useful bundles, according to the category of data. Think about your hypothetical visit to a physician's office. What data did the physician need? How were the data obtained? Data are collected piece by piece in logical segments. The logical segments are called *characters, fields, records,* and *files.*

Characters

A **character** is a letter, a single-digit number, or a symbol. "A" is a character, as well as "3" and "&." A character is the smallest unit of data that we can collect. Characters are the building blocks of data. When we put characters together, we make words and larger numbers and other types of written communication. The physician needs to know what characters to combine to make the words that are the patient's name, for example. Placing the characters in the correct order is important so that we collect the correct data.

HIT BIT

In this chapter we have been discussing data that are represented by written communication. These data can be collected and stored in a computer. In a computer, the smallest segment of data is a *bit*. A bit is the computer's electronic differentiation between two choices: on and off. Strings of bits in specific combinations of on/off patterns make *bytes,* which are represented on the computer screen as *characters.*

Fields

A **field** is a series of related characters that have a specific relationship to each other. Usually a field is a word, a group of related words, or a specific type of number. The number 07036 could be a field containing a zip code. Therefore, the field "zip code" contains five characters: 0, 7, 0, 3, and 6. Other typical fields that create a logical data segment are first name, last name, social security number, and telephone number.

Fields are defined by the type of data they contain. A field containing nothing but characters would be an *alphabetic* field. For example, a field for first name would be an alphabetic field (abbreviated "alpha"). A field containing only numbers would be a *numeric* field. A field for dollars is an example of a numeric field. A fields can also be a combination of alphabetic and numeric characters; this is called an *alphanumeric* field. A field for street address is an alphanumeric field.

Fields are generally given logical names to identify them. Figure 2–10 illustrates data fields and definitions. The listing of fields is one component of creating a **data dictionary.**

DATA DICTIONARY

Name	Definition	Size	Type	Example
FNAME	Patient's first name	15 Characters	Alphabetic	Jane
LNAME	Patient's last name	15 Characters	Alphabetic	Jones
HTEL	Patient's home telephone number	12 Characters	Alphanumeric	973-555-3331
TEMP	Patient's temperature	5 Characters	Numeric	98.6

Here is a simple example of part of a basic data dictionary. Can you see why the telephone number is not 10 numeric characters? Why is the temperature 5 characters?

FIGURE 2–10.

Common fields of data, including definitions.

Records

In the same way that characters combine to make fields, fields combine to make records. So, if we take a number of fields that have some logical connection to each other and group them together, we have created a **record.** A very simple example of fields that combine to make a record is an entry in a telephone address book. You can accumulate characters and create fields that are very familiar, such as first name, last name, street address, state, and city. Similarly, a physician keeps track of patients using groups of fields that combine to make a record of the patient's demographic data. A simple example of how fields combine to make a record is shown in Figure 2–11. Whether the data are collected on paper or in a computer, the size of the field must be considered in order to ensure uniformity in recording and retrieving the data.

DESCRIBING DATA

Name	Definition	Size	Type	Example
FNAME	Patient's first name	15 Characters	Alphabetic	Marion
LNAME	Patient's last name	15 Characters	Alphabetic	Smith
ADDRESS	Patient's home street address	25 Characters	Alphanumeric	23 Pine Street
CITY	City associated with ADDRESS	15 Characters	Alphabetic	Anywhere
STATE	State associated with ADDRESS	15 Characters	Alphabetic	IOWA
ZIP	Postal zip code associated with ADDRESS	5 Characters	Alphanumeric	31898
Telephone	Patient's home telephone number	14 Characters	Alphanumeric	(319) 555-1234

This record has seven fields:

Marion   Smith

23 Pine Street

Anywhere   Iowa   31898

(319) 555-1234

Each field is underlined to illustrate the number of characters allowed in the field, compared with the number that this record required. Is there a more efficient way to capture STATE? The telephone number is captured differently than the example in Figure 2-10. Can you see why? Can you think of a third way to capture it?

FIGURE 2–11.

Address book example of how fields combine to make a record.

Files

Obviously, creating a record of a patient's name and address is really just the beginning of the data that a physician collects on a patient. The physician collects numerous records of different types of data, and this group of related records is called a **file.** In Figure 2–12, the entire telephone address book is a file made up of individual records. Files can be large or small, depending on the number of records they contain. A patient's entire health history can be contained in one file, depending on how it is organized. An "electronic patient record" is developed by linking the data records collected about each patient. The special terminology and skills to accomplish this are beyond the scope of this text.

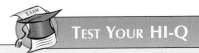

TEST YOUR HI-Q

Create a file of five records that contain name, address, and telephone number. Begin by defining the fields in data dictionary format and then show how you would represent these fields if you were trying to explain them to someone else.

Health Record

All of the data that have been collected about an individual patient are called a **health record** or **medical record.** *Medical record* is the term that has been used historically in the United States. Elsewhere, medical record may refer to the patient's record of a specific visit or group of visits to a health care facility, but "health record" refers to the patient's lifelong medical history. There is a noticeable shift in the United States to calling a patient's collective data a *health record.* For the sake of clarity, we refer to a patient's information as the health record, whether it refers to a single visit or the patient's collective experience.

The patient's "health record" is not the same as the term "record" used as a data element description. The health record historically has referred to the physical collection of papers on which patient information is recorded. As we move into a computer-based environment, we have continued to refer to the cumulative patient data as a "record," even though that terminology is not strictly accurate in a computerized setting.

Health Information Management

Health information management (HIM) is the profession that describes the sources and uses of health information and collects, stores, retrieves, and reports it. Health information management encompasses all of the tasks, jobs, titles, and organizations involved in the administration of health information. Health information management professionals are individuals who, by their activities or by their titles, are in a management capacity in terms of that administrative support.

DESCRIBING DATA

	Telephone Address Book	
Character:	A	A single letter, digit, or symbol.
Field:	Marion	A related string of characters. This field has six characters.
Record:	**Marion** Smith 23 Pine Street Anywhere, Iowa 31898 (319) 555-1234	A related group of fields. This record has seven fields (the street and number are considered one field).
File:	**Harry** Jones 76 Elm Street Anywhere, Iowa 31898 (319) 555-4321 **Samuel** Davis 98 Sycamore Terrace Anywhere, Iowa 31898 (319) 555-4567 **Jake** Schoner 65 Spruce Run Anywhere, Iowa 31898 (319) 555-2727 **Marion** Smith 23 Pine Street Anywhere, Iowa 31898 (319) 555-1234	A related group of records. This file has four records.

FIGURE 2–12.

Address book example of how records combine to make a file.

One area in the broad field of health information management is **health information technology (HIT).** Health information technology focuses on the day-to-day activities of health information management. Because this is an introductory text, we are primarily concerned with the health information technology activities and daily functions that support the collecting, storing, retrieving, and reporting of health information.

There are literally hundreds of different jobs with many different titles that health information management professionals perform throughout the world. Throughout this text, we present specific job descriptions and job titles that will assist you in planning your career in health information technology.

Data Quality

Have you ever heard the expression "garbage in, garbage out"? This expression is a humorous reflection on data quality in a computer environment. In other words, if the information you enter into the computer is wrong, then all you will get out of the computer is wrong information. Therefore, it is extremely important to ensure that your information is correct before you enter it. The same rule applies to data collected on paper. If your data on the paper record are incorrectly recorded, then you will retrieve incorrect data when you review it. This leads us to two of the key principles of data quality: **data accuracy** and **data validity.**

Data Accuracy

To be useful, the data have to be *accurate.* Think about how irritating it is for you to receive a telephone call when someone has dialed the wrong number. Sometimes a person writes the wrong number in his or her telephone address book. The data recorded are inaccurate. They are not correct. Receiving misdirected telephone calls is merely an annoyance. Receiving someone else's medication could be fatal. So the data must be accurate in order to be useful. If data are not accurate, then wrong impressions and knowledge are being conveyed to the user of the data.

Data Validity

Whether data are recorded on paper or electronically, their recording is subject to human error. Data must be *valid* in order to be useful. Validity pertains to the data's conformity with an expected range of values. For example, "ABCDE" is not a valid U.S. Postal Service zip code. Currently, zip codes in the United States contain only numbers. Similarly, 287° Fahrenheit is not a valid temperature for living human beings. A computer can be instructed to check specific fields for validity and alert the user to a potential data collection error.

HIT Bits

When creating fields in a computer, it is sometimes useful to tell the computer that a number is really alphanumeric. For example, if a zip-code field is labeled "numeric," most computer systems will drop the leading zeros. Zip code 07036 then becomes 7036 both on the screen and when printed out. This is not desirable if you are printing labels for mailing envelopes. Mail addressed this way would most certainly be delayed. Social security numbers are another tricky field to define. Again, a field containing a social security number should be defined as alphanumeric in order to preserve the zeros.

Data Sets

With a basic understanding of the concept of data—where it comes from, what types of things are collected, and why it is needed—we also need to know how the data are going to be used. All of the health data available can be volumi-

UNIFORM AMBULATORY CARE DATA SET

Section I: Patient Data Items
1. Personal identification (including name and facility reference number)
2. Residence
3. Date of birth
4. Sex
5. Race and ethnicity
6. Living arrangements and marital status (optional)

Section II: Provider Data Items
1. Provider identification
2. Location or address
3. Profession

Section III: Encounter Data Items
1. Date, place or site, and address of encounter
2. Patient's reason for encounter (optional — problem, diagnosis, or assessment)
3. Services
4. Disposition
5. Patient's expected sources of payment
6. Total charges

FIGURE 2–13.
Sections I, II, and III from the Uniform Ambulatory Care Data Set. (Redrawn from Abdelhak M, Grostick S, Hanken MA, Jacobs E: Health Information: Management of a Strategic Resource, 2nd ed. Philadelphia, WB Saunders, 2001, pp 108–110.)

nous and confusing. Individual physicians use the data to help treat individual patients and to improve the quality of their services. Health care consumers may use the data to select a physician or a treatment. In addition, insurance companies and government agencies may also want health data to pay patients' bills or track health trends. We discuss the uses of health data in Chapter 6. For most types of health care delivery, there is a minimum set of data that must be collected and reported on each patient. In ambulatory care, this minimum is called the **Uniform Ambulatory Care Data Set (UACDS).** The UACDS was developed in 1989 by committees working under the auspices of the Department of Health and Human Services.

Minimum data sets are easy to understand if you think about the key data elements you want to know about a patient, and then think about what someone else would want to know about the health care given to the patient. Figure 2–13 lists the elements of the UACDS.

Suggested Reading

Abdelhak M, Grostick S, Hanken MA, Jacobs E: Health Information: Management of a Strategic Resource, 2nd ed. Philadelphia, WB Saunders, 2001.

Johns M: Information Management. Albany, NY, Delmar, 1996.

Koch G: Basic Allied Health Statistics and Analysis, 2nd ed. Albany, NY, Delmar, 1999.

Kuzma JW: Basic Statistics for the Health Sciences, 3rd ed. Mountain View, Calif, Mayfield, 1998.

Osborn CE: Statistical Applications for Health Information Management. Gaithersburg, Md, Aspen, 2000.

CHAPTER SUMMARY

In this chapter we discussed some basic concepts of data. We learned the difference between data and information. We defined health, health data, and health information. A physician's office is one type of ambulatory care facility. It can be staffed by a variety of personnel, including receptionist, medical secretary, medical assistant, nurse, physician assistant, and nurse practitioner. In a physician's office, data are collected in these specific categories: demographic data, socio-economic data, financial data, and clinical data. Health records are the patient's collective health information, and they include ambulatory visits as well as inpatient stays in a facility, covering the health care the patient has received over a lifetime. Health information management professionals are concerned with the collection, storage, retrieval, and reporting of health information. Health information technology is one area of the health information management profession.

Data are collected in logical segments called characters, fields, records, and files. A patient's entire health history could be combined in one file, depending on how it is organized. One of the useful aspects of collecting data is that it can be analyzed in a variety of different ways, including by patient, physician, facility, or even country.

REVIEW QUESTIONS

1. Explain the difference between data and information.

2. Describe a patient's first visit to a physician. What data are collected? Who collects that data?

3. List and describe the responsibilities of the health care personnel who might work in a physician's office.

4. Distinguish among fields, records, and files.

5. For each of the elements of the Uniform Ambulatory Care Data Set, describe how you might define the field in a data dictionary.

PROFESSIONAL PROFILE
Patient Registration Specialist

My name is Michael, and I am a patient registration specialist at a large medical group practice. My primary responsibility is to register patients when they come into the facility to see a physician or a nurse practitioner. We keep all of our patient registration information in the computer, so I don't have to pull any files to update patient information. We get a lot of walk-ins in addition to patients with appointments, so our office is very busy.

When a patient is registering, I have to make sure that I enter the patient's demographic data correctly. I also must record the financial data so that the office can get paid! In addition to recording the data, I call the patient's insurance company to verify coverage. Every day, I call the patients who have appointments the next day to confirm their appointments. Sometimes they forgot and they really appreciate the reminder.

I started out as a receptionist here when I graduated from high school. I liked the environment and the people, so I enrolled in college to study health information technology. I'm about halfway through the program now and I was promoted to this position last month. I haven't decided what I want to do when I graduate, but there are a lot of opportunities here, working in the health information management department and in patient accounts.

APPLICATION

Creating a Data Dictionary

You are a health information professional working for Dr. Heath in his private practice. Dr. Heath has a large practice with several ancillary services attached. He and his partner see 50 patients a day in the practice, many of whom receive diagnostic procedures on-site. The diagnostic areas that Dr. Heath has are x-ray, electrocardiography, and laboratory. He is concerned because a number of patients have complained that in each area of care, the health personnel seem to ask the same questions. This is annoying and redundant. He is thinking of computerizing his data collection to streamline the data collection process. Before he does, he wants to make sure he understands the clinical flow of data in the facility. Dr. Heath seeks your advice and assistance in resolving his problem. What do you recommend? How would you go about implementing your recommendation?

3

Organization of Data Elements in a Health Record

Chapter Outline

Organization of Data Elements
Integrated Record
Source-Oriented Record
Problem-Oriented Record
Computer-Based Record
  Advantages and Disadvantages
Problem List

Clinical Flow of Data
Admissions
Initial Assessment
Plan of Care

Medical Evaluation Process
SOAP Strategy

Clinical Data
Physicians
  History
  Physical Examination
  Orders
  Progress Notes
  Consultations
  Discharge Summary
Nurses
  Nursing Assessment
  Notes
  Vital Signs
  Medication Administration
Operative Records
  Operative Report
  Anesthesia Report

Laboratory Data
Radiology Data
Other Clinical Data

Data Collection Devices
Forms
  Content
  Format
  Other Considerations
Computer-Based Data Collection

Data Quality

Forms Control

Other Types of Records

Data Sets

Other Health Care Settings

References

Suggested Reading

Chapter Summary

Review Questions

Professional Profile

Application

In the last chapter, we defined and explored data in terms of their components and structure, and we discussed the data that are collected in a physician's office. In this chapter, we discuss a number of different concepts related to data and also explore more data quality concepts. In addition, we describe the details of how data are organized in a health record—both data components and the record as a whole. We also compare physician's office records with health records in an acute care facility. Last, we discuss the development of data collection devices in paper-based and computer-based forms.

Organization of Data Elements

In Chapter 2, we discussed data theoretically. Our example of a telephone address book involved defining data in a certain useful format. We determined that data collected in a physician's office can be similarly defined. Although we defined a health record and discussed health data, we did not discuss how the data are compiled into a patient's health record. When we collect items of data we record them so that we remember them and can retrieve them later. Data can be recorded on paper or in electronic format, such as a computer. In Chapter 5, we discuss the intricacies of storing health data in both formats. In this chapter, we explore how health data are collected and recorded.

The primary purpose of recording data is communication, which is necessary for a variety of reasons. For example, the medical assistant may take a patient's vital signs for the physician's reference. The physician records patient data so he or she can measure the patient's progress at a later date. Therefore, recording health data is an important way for health care professionals to communicate and facilitate patient care. In Chapter 6 we discuss other uses for recording health data.

Integrated Record

When we record an item of data for the purpose of keeping track of it for later use, we can organize it many different ways. For example, the data can be organized in date order. The first piece of data is recorded with its date, and each subsequent piece of data is organized sequentially after the preceding piece of data. This method of recording data is particularly useful when we need to know when events happen in relation to each other. This method of recording data in date order is called a **date-oriented, sequential,** or **integrated record.** From the physician's office example in Chapter 2, it is obvious that organization of the data in date order is fairly useful and efficient for collecting data sequentially from each episode of care. Figure 3–1 illustrates the chronologic organization of data. In a paper record, it is easier to place the most recent pages on top, and therefore an integrated paper record may be organized in reverse chronologic order, but this is still considered an integrated record (Fig. 3–2).

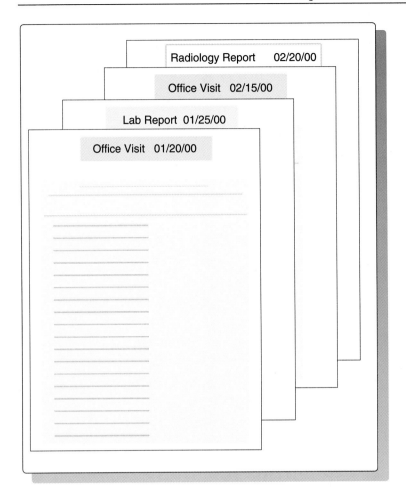

FIGURE 3–1.
Integrated record.

Source-Oriented Record

Besides the date-oriented organization of data, we can organize data by source. In other words, all of the data we get from the physician can be grouped together, all of the data we get from the nurse can be grouped together, and all of the information we get from the laboratory can be grouped together. This method of organizing data produces a **source-oriented record.** Organizing data by source is useful when there are many items of data coming from different sources. For example, a patient who is in the hospital for many days may require numerous laboratory and blood tests, and many pages of physician and nursing notes are compiled. If all of these pieces of data are organized in date order, we would have to know exactly what date something occurred in order to find the

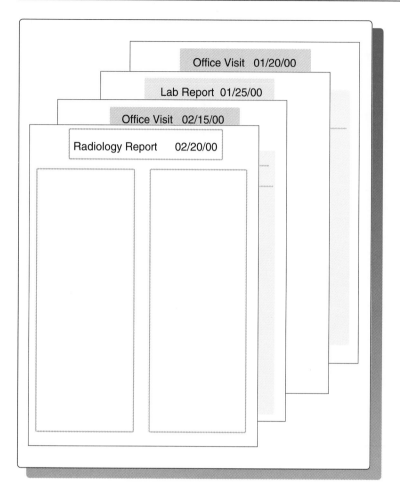

FIGURE 3–2.
Integrated record in reverse chronologic order.

data for it. Further, it would be very difficult to compare laboratory results from one date to the next. Consequently, in records that have numerous items from each type of source, the records tend to be organized in a source-oriented manner. Figure 3–3 illustrates a source-oriented record. Notice that within each source, the data are organized in chronologic order to facilitate finding specific items.

Problem-Oriented Record

The data can also be organized by the patient's diagnosis, or problem. For instance, all of the data on a patient's appendicitis and appendectomy can be organized together. Similarly, all of the data that pertain to the patient's congestive heart failure can be organized together. Such a method greatly facilitates the

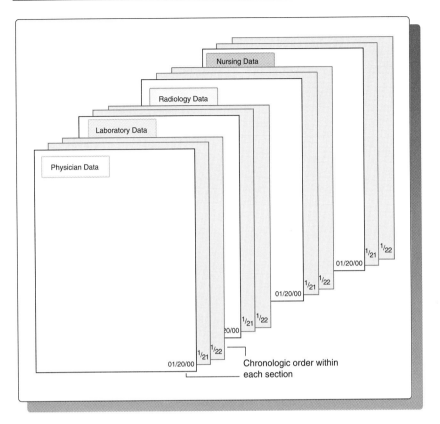

FIGURE 3–3.
Source-oriented record.

monitoring of individual patient conditions. This method of organizing data produces a **problem-oriented record** and is useful when the patient has several major chronic conditions that may be addressed at different times. For example, if a patient has congestive heart failure, diabetes, and hypertension, the patient might not be treated for all three simultaneously. Therefore, the records for each of the conditions may be kept separately. Problems that have been resolved are easily flagged, and current problems are more easily referenced. Figure 3–4 illustrates a simple problem-oriented record.

Computer-Based Record

In a computer-based record, data are collected in fields and records that are linked together in such a manner that the data can be referenced, displayed, or reported in any of the ways previously mentioned. This versatility is one of the major advantages of a computer-based record. The data are linked by reference numbers (e.g., medical record or billing number [see Chapter 5]) so that all data about the patient are accessible. A complete discussion of a relational data-

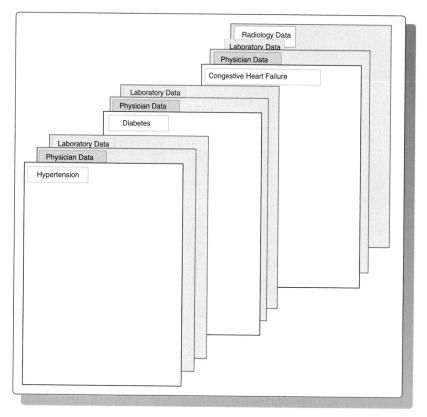

FIGURE 3–4.
Problem-oriented record.

base is beyond the scope of this text, but in Figure 3–5 we can see how computer records might be designed to link patient data together.

ADVANTAGES AND DISADVANTAGES

Each one of these methods of organizing data elements has its own advantages and disadvantages. The integrated record is simple to file, but subsequent retrieval and comparison of data are more difficult. The source-oriented record is more complicated to file, but retrieval and comparison of source data are facilitated. The problem-oriented record lends itself best to the long-term management of chronic illnesses; however, filing is complicated and duplication of data may be necessary so that laboratory reports related to different problems are included in all relevant sections. All of these methods are essentially paper-based organization systems. A well-designed computer-based system can solve filing and retrieval inefficiencies; however, cost and resistance to technology have been his-

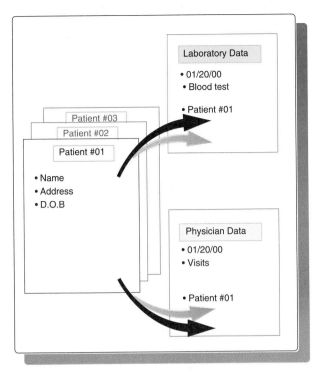

FIGURE 3–5.
Computer-based record.

torical barriers to universal implementation of computer systems. These barriers are crumbling, however, and many facilities are at or near full implementation of computer-based records.

It should be noted that the method of organizing a record is not patient specific. In other words, all patients' records are recorded in the same way. The method of organization is determined by its overall suitability to the particular environment and the needs that it satisfies.

Problem List

After several visits to an ambulatory care facility, a list of the patient's problems (diagnoses or complaints) is compiled. This problem list facilitates management of the patient's care and improves communication among caregivers. In a problem-oriented record, this list becomes an index to the record as well as a historical summary of patient care management. Therefore, the problem list is an integral part of a problem-oriented record. A simple problem list is shown in Figure 3–6.

PROBLEM LIST

Date	Problem #	Description	Date of Initial Diagnosis	Current Treatment	Comments
01/20/00	1	Hypertension	11/27/97	Diet	Follow-up 01/01
02/15/00	2	Sprain/right ankle	02/15/00	Wrap and rest Tylenol 1000 mg as needed	
03/15/00	2	Sprain/right ankle	02/15/00	None	Resolved

FIGURE 3–6.

Illustration of a problem list.

Clinical Flow of Data

In Chapter 2, you made a visit to a physician's office. After making an appointment, you came to the office, gave a history, reported financial information, met with the doctor, perhaps had some tests done, paid the bill, and left with a prescription. Let's turn our attention now to what happens in a hospital, and identify how the data flow in two types of facility are similar. For the moment, we will call the hospital an acute care facility.

Admissions

When a patient goes into the hospital, sometimes it is unexpected and he or she is taken to the emergency department. At other times the patient's visit is expected. In an expected visit, the patient has an "appointment," that is, the patient's physician (or someone in the physician's office) calls and arranges for admission. The patient may be admitted for diagnostic testing or for surgery; a woman may be coming in to give birth. The physician, or someone from the physician's office, calls in advance in much the same way that a patient calls a physician's office and makes an appointment. Thus, in a hospital, there is often an entire department whose function is similar to the registration clerk or receptionist in a physician's office. The patient registration department (also called the admissions department or patient access) is responsible for ensuring the timely and accurate admission of patients. Individuals who perform the clerical function of completing the paperwork may be called admitting clerks, registrars, or patient registration specialists. In a small hospital the admissions department may consist of only one person; however in a larger facility, a number of health care professionals are trained to register the patient into the hospital.

When the patient arrives at the admissions reception area, he or she supplies the same information given in a physician's office. First the admissions person asks the patient for proof of identity and then requests demographic and financial data, and some socioeconomic data. These data are kept together on a form known as a **face sheet** or an **admission record** (Table 3–1). It is important to file this form at the beginning of every record so that the patient is clearly identified to everyone who records or accesses data in it. Face sheet data are collected and recorded in the admissions department.

TEST YOUR HI-Q

The initial data collection for a patient begins to build the hospital's data set on that patient. In Chapter 2, we discussed the Uniform Ambulatory Care Data Set required in a physician's office. Each type of facility has its own particular data set that must be considered when planning data collection strategies. While you are reading this chapter, make a list of the items that you think would be appropriate to include in the data set required in an acute care facility—the Uniform Hospital Discharge Data Set (UHDDS).

TABLE 3–1. Sample Data Included in an Admission Record

Data Element	Explanation
Patient's identification number	Number assigned by the facility to this patient
Patient's billing number	Number assigned by the facility to this visit
Admission date	Calendar day: month, day, and year
Discharge date	Calendar day: month, day, and year
Patient's name	Full name, including any titles (MD, PhD)
Patient's address	Address of usual residence
Sex	Male or female
Marital status	Married, single, divorced, separated
Race and ethnicity	Must choose from choices given on the admissions form
Religion	Optional
Occupational	General occupation (e.g., teacher, lawyer)
Current employment	Specific job (e.g., professor, district attorney)
Employer	Company name
Insurance	Insurance company name and address
Insurance identification numbers	Insurance company group and individual identification numbers
Additional insurance	Some patients are insured by multiple companies. All information from all insurers should be collected
Guarantor	Individual or organization who is responsible for paying the bill, if the insurance company declines payment
Attending physician	Name of the attending physician; may also include the physician's identification number
Admitting diagnosis	Reason the patient is being admitted

These are typical items that are included in an admission record. Remember that the admission record contains the demographic, financial, and some socioeconomic data. What is missing from this list?

The "open-access" side of acute care facilities is the emergency department. Patients arriving in the emergency department are usually treated as ambulatory care patients. Sometimes the condition of the patient warrants admission to the hospital. In this case, the emergency department contacts the patient registration department to arrange admission. Patient information already collected is transferred to the patient registration department, and an inpatient stay is initiated. Because the patient is not likely to be in a condition to physically proceed to the patient registration department, data collection often takes place at the patient's bedside or with the assistance of family members.

Initial Assessment

After being formally admitted, the patient is taken to the appropriate treatment area. Sometimes this area is the nursing unit, and sometimes it is the preoperative area, where the patient is prepared immediately for surgery. In the treatment area, the patient is assessed by nursing staff in much the same way that a patient in a physician's office is assessed by a medical assistant or a nurse in the physician's office. In addition to the nursing assessment, the physician completes an assessment of the patient. An important part of the initial assessment is the preliminary diagnosis.

Plan of Care

Based on the initial assessments, a plan of care is developed for the patient. The initial plan may consist of tests and other diagnostic procedures. If the diagnosis has already been established, therapeutic procedures, such as surgery, may take place. All procedures, whether diagnostic or therapeutic, are undertaken only on the direct order of the physician.

TABLE 3–2. Comparison of Ambulatory Versus Inpatient Activities		
	Ambulatory Care (Physician's Office)	**Hospital (Acute Care)**
How to choose	Referral, advertisement, or investigation	Choices limited to facilities in which physician has privileges
Initiate contact	Call for an appointment; walk-in, if permitted	Emergency department or physician arranges admission
Collection of demographic and financial data	Receptionist, medical secretary	Patient registration or admissions department
Initial assessment	Vital signs and chief complaint recorded by nurse or medical assistant	Nursing assessment, physician takes history and physical examination
Plan of care	Prescriptions, instructions, diagnostic tests, and therapeutic procedures performed on an ambulatory basis	Medication administration, instructions, and diagnostic tests performed on an inpatient basis

Data Element	Explanation
TABLE 3–3. Data Required for a Consultation	
Patient's name	See Table 3–1
Patient's identification number	See Table 3–1
Physician's order	Required before the consultation is performed (see Table 3–7)
Date of request	Date that the attending physician requests the consultation
Specialty being consulted	Cardiology, podiatry, gastroenterology, etc.
Reason for consultation	Brief explanation of why the consultant's opinion is being sought
Authentication	Authentication of physician requesting consultation
Date of evaluation	When consultant saw patient
Consultant's opinion	Diagnosis or recommendations; may be an entire report, similar to an H&P (see Tables 3–5 and 3–6)
Report date	Date that consultant prepares report of the opinion
Authentication	Authentication of consultant

As you can see, an inpatient stay has similarities to an ambulatory visit. The primary differences are length of stay and volume of patient data collected. Table 3–2 compares an ambulatory care visit with an acute care, inpatient stay. The physician always coordinates the care of the patient. The degree of collaboration with other disciplines in developing the plan of care depends on the diagnosis and the health care setting. Rehabilitation facilities, for example, are characterized by highly interdisciplinary care plans. This is because therapies play the largest role in patient care, and the physician relies on feedback from rehabilitation therapists to direct further treatment. Care plan meetings take place on a regular basis and include patients and families. In acute care, the interdisciplinary activity is often not as formal or routine.

Physicians collaborate with each other by asking for advice; this is called a **consultation.** The **attending physician,** who is responsible for the patient's overall care, requests a consultation, citing the specialty information needed and the specific reason for the consultation. The **consultant** evaluates the patient and responds to the request with specific diagnostic and/or therapeutic opinions and recommendations. Table 3–3 lists the data required for a consultation. In addition, the nursing staff advises physicians of changes in the patient's status or problems that may arise.

Although each patient is treated individually, the process of treating a patient is based on standards of medical practice. Nursing practice has evolved its own standards of practice and has historically been diligent in documenting and providing evidence for that practice.

Medical Evaluation Process

A logical thought process supports the medical evaluation process, or development of a medical diagnosis. Data are collected in one of four specific categories: the patient's subjective view, the physician's objective view, the physician's opinion, and the care plan. In conducting the evaluation, the physician collects as much data as are necessary to develop a medical diagnosis. Initially, the data may support several different diagnoses. The physician continues to collect data until a specific diagnosis can be determined. For example, chest pain and shortness of breath can be symptoms of many diagnoses, including myocardial infarction, congestive heart failure, and pneumonia. The physician examines the patient and orders sufficient tests to conclude which diagnosis (or diagnoses) applies in each individual case.

SOAP Strategy

The physician begins the medical evaluation process by asking the patient about the medical problem and the symptoms he or she is experiencing. The patient's description of the problem, in his or her own words, is the **subjective** portion of the evaluation process. For example, the patient may have stomach pain. The patient may describe this as "abdominal pain," "pain in the belly," or "pain in the stomach." The physician's task is to narrow the patient's description through questioning. For instance, the patient can be assisted to identify the pain as a sharp, stabbing pain in the lower right portion of the abdomen. The physician also asks when the pain began, whether it is continuous or intermittent, and whether there are any other symptoms.

Once the physician has obtained and recorded the patient's subjective point of view about the medical problem, the physician needs to look at the patient objectively. In other words, he or she conducts a physical examination and explores where the stomach pain may be located. The patient says his or her stomach hurts, but the physician records that the patient has "tenderness on palpation in the right lower quadrant." Tenderness on palpation in the right lower quadrant is a classic indication of appendicitis. Other possible diagnoses include ovarian cyst and a variety of intestinal disorders, such as diverticulosis. The physician's **objective** notation is the specific anatomic location of the pain and the results of any laboratory tests that the physician ordered. The physician orders tests to confirm a likely diagnosis or to **rule out,** or eliminate, a possible diagnosis. In our examples, the physician is looking for an elevation of the white blood cell count that indicates the presence of an infection. Additional tests, such as an abdominal ultrasound, might be ordered, if the blood test results are negative or inconclusive.

Once the physician has obtained the patient's subjective view and has conducted an objective medical evaluation, he or she develops an **assessment.** The assessment is a description of what the physician thinks is wrong with the patient: the diagnosis or possible diagnoses. In the example, let us say that the physician has determined that the patient has appendicitis.

Once the physician has assessed what is wrong with the patient, he or she writes a **plan of treatment.** The plan may be for treatment or for further evaluation, particularly if the assessment includes several possible diagnoses.

This method of recording observations or clinical evaluations is called the **SOAP format:** *S*ubjective, *O*bjective, *A*ssessment, and *P*lan. Although physicians may not always follow this format exactly, they record their thoughts in this general manner. Table 3–4 lists the elements of a medical evaluation. Other clinical

TABLE 3–4. Medical Evaluation Strategy: The SOAP Format	
Data Element	**Explanation**
Subjective	The patient's report of symptoms or problems
Objective	The physician's observations, including evaluation of diagnostic test results
Assessment	The physician's opinion as to the diagnosis or possible diagnoses
Plan	Treatment or further diagnostic evaluation

personnel also record their observations, but not necessarily in the SOAP format. Many nursing evaluations are recorded by use of graphs or on preprinted forms. Graphs or preprinted forms are also used for clinical evaluations in physical therapy, respiratory therapy, and anesthesia records; also some operative records, and many maternity and neonatal records use preprinted or graphical forms.

Clinical Data

The volume and variety of clinical data that can be collected in an inpatient setting is enormous. Physicians, nurses, therapists, and numerous ancillary and administrative departments contribute notes, reports, and documentation of events. In this section, we discuss the major data elements that each of these professionals contribute. Data elements are gathered in logical groups, or collections, based on the nature of the data being collected. Figure 3–7 shows the contributors of health data and the collections of data that they contribute.

Physicians

When the patient is admitted, the physician conducts a medical evaluation. This evaluation begins with the subjective history, the objective physical examination, the assessment of a preliminary diagnosis or diagnoses, and a plan of care, for which orders are recorded. Medical decision making is a complex activity that depends on the number of possible diagnoses, the volume and complexity of diagnostic data that must be reviewed, and the severity of the patient's condition. This complexity is reflected in the physician's documentation. Figure 3–8 illustrates the components of medical decision making, and in the subsequent text each of these components of physician data is discussed.

HISTORY

A **history** is taken from the data that the patient reports to the physician regarding the patient's health. This data collection results generally in a dictated and typed report. In an ambulatory care setting, the history can be very short and focused. In an inpatient setting, however, the history is significantly more comprehensive. The history consists of the chief complaint, the history of the present

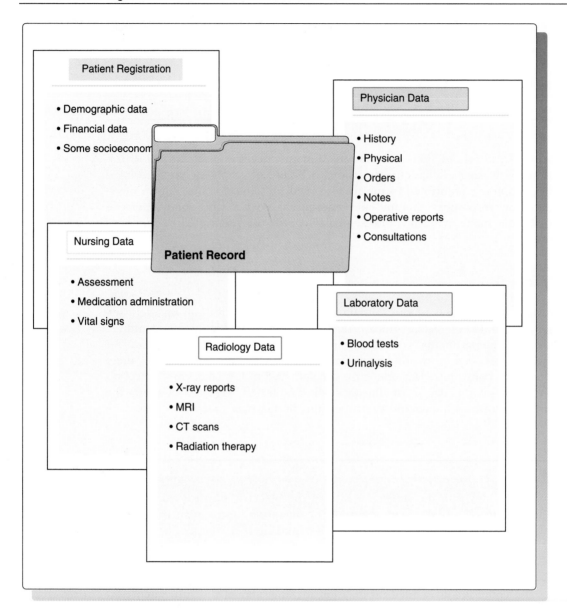

FIGURE 3–7.
Sample data elements in a health record, by source.

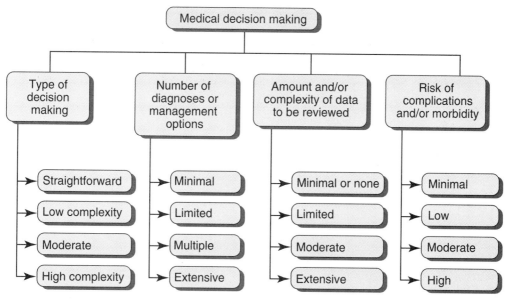

FIGURE 3–8.

Flowchart of medical decision making. (From Andress AA: Saunders Manual of Medical Office Management. Philadelphia, WB Saunders, 1996, p 96.)

complaint, a description of relevant previous illnesses and procedures, and a review of the relevant organs or body systems. The history is characterized by its complexity. The complexity of the history is directly related to the amount of data that the physician needs to evaluate the patient's problem.

For example, if a patient visits the physician's office because of a splinter in his or her finger, a simple, or problem-focused, history is directed toward the presenting problem, and very little else is discussed or observed. The history would probably contain nothing more than the events surrounding the occurrence of the splinter and possibly an inquiry as to whether the patient had received a tetanus vaccination in the past 10 years.

Sometimes, even in a fairly straightforward situation, the complexity of the issue may expand fairly rapidly. For example, the finger may appear to be infected. Perhaps a blood test needs to be taken. Perhaps there was a fall involved and there may be a suspected head trauma or fracture involved. The complexity of the history expands as the number of body systems are involved and the potential threat to life of the patient becomes more evident.

A patient admitted into an acute care facility, particularly when the underlying illness is still under investigation, requires more substantive evaluation. In that case, the physician collects a comprehensive history. The physician inquires more deeply into the patient's entire medical history and asks pointed questions about the patient's status with respect to more body systems. Table 3–5 lists the data elements that are collected in a history.

TABLE 3-5. Data Elements in a History	
Data Element	**Explanation**
Chief complaint	The reason for the encounter, usually as expressed by the patient
History of present illness	The patient's report of the events, circumstances, and other details surrounding the chief complaint
Review of systems	The patient's responses to the physician's questions regarding pertinent body systems, including Constitutional symptoms Eyes Ears, nose, mouth, and throat Cardiovascular Respiratory Gastrointestinal Genitourinary Musculoskeletal Integumentary Neurologic Psychiatric Endocrine Hematologic/lymphatic Allergic/immunologic
Past, family, and/or social history	Including the patient's prior illnesses and operations, socioeconomic concerns, and important family illnesses

All histories contain, at a minimum, the chief complaint and the history of present illness. The history can have four levels of complexity.

Level of History	History of Present Illness	Review of Systems	Personal, Family, and/or Social History
Problem focused	Brief	N/A	N/A
Expanded problem focused	Brief	Problem pertinent	N/A
Detailed	Extended	Extended	Pertinent
Comprehensive	Extended	Complete	Complete

Data from the American Medical Association. Adapted from Buck CJ: Step-by-Step Medical Coding, 3rd ed. Philadelphia, WB Saunders, 2000, pp 33–37.

PHYSICAL EXAMINATION

Once the appropriate history data are collected, the physician performs the objective portion of the evaluation: the **physical examination.** Like the history, the physical examination takes the form of a dictated and transcribed report. The physical examination (or more briefly, the *physical*) includes the physician's examination and observations of every pertinent body system. We say "pertinent" because the physical generally follows the same level of complexity as the history. For example, the patient with a splinter described earlier may require only an examination of the finger. In the absence of infection or other trauma, a problem-focused physical examination is appropriate. Also, it is not appropriate for the physician to perform a comprehensive physical examination on the splinter patient in the absence of any history indicating its necessity. In many cases, gynecologic and/or rectal examinations are frequently omitted, sometimes at the patient's request, and also when there is no suspicion of related abnormalities or disorders. The physical examination ends with the physician's assessment, also called the impression, and the initial plan of treatment. Table 3–6 lists data elements that are collected in a physical.

Sometimes the history and physical data are collected and reported together, as if they were one larger report, and it is referred to as the history & physical (H&P). Note that the H&P follows the medical evaluation process previously described. The subjective data (the patient's history) are followed by the objective data (the physical), and then the assessment and the plan of care are recorded.

The data collected in these two reports are critical for patient management; therefore, specific rules direct the completion of this data collection activity. For example, in an acute care facility, the Joint Commission on the Accreditation of Healthcare Organizations (JCAHO) requires that the history and physical be present in the record within 24 hours of admission, or before any surgical procedure takes place. The physician collecting and recording the data must **authenticate** the data. Authentication can be, for example, a signature on a dictated and typed report, a signature at the bottom of a handwritten note, or a password entered into a computer.

In an ambulatory care facility, the H&P may be the only data recorded at the time of the encounter, particularly if the patient's problem is minor. In an inpatient setting, the H&P is performed only on admission. In a residence setting, such as a long-term-care facility, the H&P must be updated periodically so that it represents the patient's current status. Health information management professionals must know the regulatory and accreditation requirements of this and any other data collection activity that occurs in facilities in which they are employed.

TABLE 3–6. Data Elements in a Physical Examination

Level of Examination	Body Area(s)/Organ System(s)*
Problem focused	Affected BA and OS
Expanded problem focused	Affected BA and other BA/OS
Detailed	Extensive affected BA/OS
Comprehensive	Complete BA and complete OS

*Body Areas and Organ Systems

Organ systems	Body areas
Eyes	Head
Ears, nose, mouth, and throat	Neck
Respiratory	Chest
Cardiovascular	Abdomen
Genitourinary	Genitalia, groin, buttocks
Hematologic/lymphatic/immunologic	Back
Musculoskeletal	Extremities
Skin	
Neurologic	General
Psychiatric	Constitutional (vital signs, general appearance)
Gastrointestinal	

Data from the American Medical Association. Adapted from Buck CJ: Step-by-Step Medical Coding, 3rd ed. Philadelphia, WB Saunders, 2000, pp 38–39.

ORDERS

While the patient is in the facility, the physician makes decisions about the patient's **treatment,** including directing any further diagnostic testing. For example, an appendectomy patient may have entered the hospital prediagnosed with appendicitis. The plan of treatment includes the appendectomy. Other patients enter the hospital with vague or multiple symptoms, and the physician is not entirely sure which one of several possible conditions the patient actually has. In the SOAP note example discussed earlier, we showed that right lower quadrant abdominal pain could have a number of different **etiologies,** or causes, and all of them are examined while the patient is in the hospital.

The doctor's instructions for laboratory tests, radiology examinations, consultations, and medication are all contained in a separate data collection called **physician's (doctor's) orders.** There are many different ways of recording physician's orders in a patient's record, varying from handwritten instructions on a piece of paper to direct entry into a computer. No tests or treatment can take place without the physician's order. Orders must be dated and authenticated by the physician. Nursing staff execute (put into effect) the orders by notifying the appropriate department or outside agency of the order. For example, medications may be requested from the hospital pharmacy, radiology tests may be arranged, or a consultant may be contacted. The nurse who executes the order authenticates and dates the activity.

Although each patient is treated individually, there are many conditions for which a predetermined plan of care is appropriate. This predetermined plan may include a specific series of blood tests, x-rays, and urinalysis. It may also consist of a set of preoperative or pretherapy activities. Such predetermined plans are called **standing orders.** Direction to put a set of standing orders into effect comes from the physician, who is still required to authenticate and date the orders.

Orders may be directly entered by the physician or dictated to a registered nurse, who then enters the orders. Orders that are dictated to a registered nurse are called *verbal orders*. Verbal orders that are dictated over the telephone are called *telephone orders*. Verbal and telephone orders are sometimes necessary in emergencies and when the physician is unable to be present at the hospital at the time the orders are required. Verbal and telephone orders must be authenticated by the physician, although they can be executed immediately. In an ambulatory care setting, orders may not be formally set apart from other data collections and may be incorporated in the end of the H&P or progress notes (see later). Nevertheless, the data elements of the physician's orders as described previously are present. Table 3–7 lists the data contained in an order.

PROGRESS NOTES

While the patient is being treated, the physician makes continuing observations and updates the assessment and plan. These **progress notes** are important evidence of the care that the patient has received and serve to document the physi-

TABLE 3–7. Data Contained in a Physician's Order

Data Required for an Order Personally Entered by the Physician

Data Element	Explanation
Patient's name	See Table 3–1
Patient's identification number	See Table 3–1
Order date	Date the order is rendered
Time	Time the order is rendered
Order	Medication, test, therapy, consultation, or other action directed by the physician
Physician's authentication	Physician's signature or password
Executor's authentication	Signature or password of party effecting the order
Execution date	Date the order was effected
Execution time	Time the order was effected

An important element of a physician's order is the time that it is rendered. The interpretation of the requirement to authenticate verbal orders as soon as possible is often "within 24 hours." Implicitly, this requires a date and time attached to both the order and the authentication. If the physician personally makes the order, then the date and time of both are the same. If it is a verbal order, then the nurse taking the order must record the date and time, and the physician would date and time the subsequent authentication. In a paper-based system, the time of the order is often omitted. However, in a computer-based order entry system, the time can be automatically affixed by the computer.

Data Required for a Verbal Order

Data Element	Explanation
Patient's name	See Table 3–1
Patient's identification number	See Table 3–1
Order date	Date the order is received
Time	Time the order is received
Nurse's authentication	Signature or password of party receiving the order
Order	Medication, test, therapy, consultation, or other action directed by the physician
Physician's authentication	Physician's signature or password
Physician's authentication date	Date the order is authenticated
Physician's authentication time	Time the physician authenticated the order
Executor's authentication	Signature or password of party effecting the order
Execution date	Date the order was effected
Execution time	Time the order was effected

cian's activities and evaluation process. Notes are often documented in the SOAP format: some physicians even write the SOAP acronym on the note. In an ambulatory care setting, progress notes may follow the H&P directly in the patient's medical record, or they may be omitted if all of the encounter data are included in the H&P. However, in an inpatient setting, progress notes become critical because days, weeks, or months may elapse from the time of the H&P taken at admission to the time of the patient's discharge. Notes must be authenticated and dated. In a facility in which physician residents are training, the resident may collect and record the data for the note. In many situations, and always for unlicensed residents, the resident's note must also be authenticated, or **countersigned,** by the attending physician.

CONSULTATIONS

Sometimes when a patient is in a hospital, the attending physician needs to call in an expert in a particular field. For example, if the appendectomy patient in our example also has chronic obstructive pulmonary disease, emphysema, asthma, or other severe respiratory problem, the attending physician may want to call in a pulmonary specialist to evaluate the patient's status prior to surgery. Some typical consultations that may be performed in an inpatient setting include an endocrinology consultation if the patient has diabetes mellitus; a podiatry consultation if the patient has overgrown toenails or onychomycosis; or a cardiology consultation if the patient has some sort of heart condition; and, as mentioned, a pulmonary specialist is consulted if the patient has respiratory concerns. Another typical type of consultation would be a psychiatric consultation if the patient suffers from depression or other behavioral health issues. Table 3–3 lists the data required in a consultation.

DISCHARGE SUMMARY

In an inpatient setting, a **discharge summary** of the patient's care is prepared by the attending physician or his or her designee. This summary includes a brief history of the problem, the discharge diagnosis and any other significant findings, a list of treatments and procedures performed, the patient's condition on discharge, and any instructions given to the patient or patient's caregiver. As with other data, the discharge summary must be authenticated and dated. The recording of the discharge summary often takes the form of a dictated and typed report.

Nurses

While the patient is in the hospital, the professionals who perform most of the patient's care, particularly in acute care and long-term care facilities, are the nurses and their ancillary staff. Nurses collect and record their own set of data about a patient. As with physician data, nursing data also require authentication and a signature.

NURSING ASSESSMENT

Nurses perform an assessment of the patient when the patient first enters the facility. The purpose of the **nursing assessment** is not to diagnose the patient's illness—that is the responsibility of the physician—but to diagnose the patient's care needs. The assessment includes determining the patient's understanding of his or her condition and whether the patient has any particular concerns or needs that are going to have an impact on the nursing care. The nursing assessment includes an evaluation of the condition of the patient's skin, learning needs, and ability to perform self-care.

TABLE 3–8. Data Required for a Nurse's Progress Note	
Data Element	**Explanation**
Patient's name	See Table 3–1
Patient's identification number	See Table 3–1
Date	Date of the note
Time	Time of the note
Note	Nurse's comments, observations, and documentation of activities
Nurse's authentication	Nurse's signature or password

Notes should be written as soon as possible after the activity has occurred. Thus, the date and time of the note coincide with the date and time of the occurrence. If a note is written after the fact, the date and time of the occurrence must be separately noted.

In a paper-based system, the note field is generally a large, alphanumeric field in which the author can comment freely. In a computer-based system, this field may be replaced with a series of fields from which the nurse can compose comments from predetermined menus, in addition to a free field for unique remarks. The actual content of the note is governed by nursing professional standards and facility requirements.

NOTES

Nurses also have to fill out **nursing progress notes.** In each shift the nurse writes down particular events or particular interactions with the patient. Patient complaints, and any activities of the nursing staff to solve those complaints, are noted. The elements of a nursing progress note are given in Table 3–8.

VITAL SIGNS

Nurses are also responsible for observing and recording the patient's vital signs while he or she is in the health care facility. Vital signs include temperature, blood pressure, pulse, and respiration. Frequently, vital signs are recorded in a graphical format, which can easily be referenced while the patient is in the facility. In Chapter 2 we showed that displaying a patient's temperature in a graph or picture facilitates review of the data (see Fig. 2–2). In a computer-based record, the data are also entered into a field that can then be linked to previous data collections to produce a report that is a graphical representation of the cumulative data over time. Other data that nurses collect in graph format include fluid intake and output and mechanical ventilation readings.

MEDICATION ADMINISTRATION

One of the most important nursing data collections is administration of **medications.** The name of the medication, dosage, date and time of administration, method of administration, and the nurse who administered it are important data elements.

Operative Records

The data elements that we have discussed are very common and occur in one form or another in almost all inpatient health records. However, physicians and nurses may collect and record other data in the health record, notably in the case of surgical procedures. The patient who has a surgical procedure requires two sets of data: the operative data and the anesthesia data.

OPERATIVE REPORT

The operative report is recorded as an operative note in the progress notes as well as a detailed, usually dictated and typed, **operative report.** The operative report lists the preoperative and postoperative diagnosis, the **surgeon** and surgical assistants, the procedures performed, and a detailed description of the **operation,** including the patient's condition and any blood loss. The operative report should be completed immediately following the procedure. As for all physician activities, the operative report is authenticated and dated. Additional data, such as instrument counts, are collected and recorded by nursing staff, separate from the operative report.

ANESTHESIA REPORT

The anesthesiologist performs preoperative and postoperative evaluations of the patient's condition. These may be documented in the progress notes or on a specially designed data collection device. During the procedure, a graphical representation of the patient's status is recorded continuously.

Laboratory Data

In an inpatient setting, the physician frequently orders routine laboratory tests, such as a complete blood count (CBC) and a urinalysis (UA). The CBC has many uses, as does the UA, and they may be ordered for specific diagnostic purposes. However, when these laboratory tests are performed at the time of the patient's admission, they help to identify preexisting infectious conditions. Infections identified after 72 hours of hospitalization are considered to be attributable to the facility: these are called nosocomial infections. **Laboratory tests** are performed only when ordered by the physician. The results of the tests are included in the health record. Laboratory results include both patient-specific data and data comparing the patient's test results against normative ranges of data.

In an ambulatory care setting, a single set of laboratory tests may be ordered. In an inpatient setting, the number of laboratory tests may increase dramatically. For some conditions, daily blood tests are appropriate. Therefore, multiple data fields recording the results of multiple tests are needed. Once again, the usefulness of a computer-based record is evident. Once the test result data are collected, a computer can display them in whole or in part as well as graphically.

Radiology Data

Radiology tests generate two sets of data: the original diagnostic image and the interpretation. The original diagnostic image is usually retained separately from the patient's record, which includes only the interpretation of the images. For example, a chest x-ray produces a large film, which is retained in special envelopes or files, usually in the radiology department. The radiologist's interpretation of the image on the film, another data collection that often takes the form of a dictated and typed report, becomes part of the patient's record.

Other Clinical Data

The previous discussion of clinical data includes only the basic data elements common to most patients. Depending on the diagnosis and the clinical setting, many other data elements are collected. For example, maternity patients are monitored for contractions, fetal activity, and stress during labor. Specific delivery data, such as number of previous births, types of deliveries, and conditions of the newborns, are collected. Assessment and therapy data are collected on rehabilitation patients. Data collection, as evident from this discussion, is rarely the collection of a single data field but is more often a record of several data fields collected repeatedly over time. At this point, let's turn our attention to how the data are collected.

Data Collection Devices

While the patient is in the hospital, an entire team of clinical personnel is collecting and recording data about everything that happens to the patient. The volume of data collected about a patient, and the way it is organized in a record, is the primary difference between the data compiled in a physician's office record and the data collected in an inpatient facility. If you recall, the physician's office data that we discussed in Chapter 2 was fairly brief for each encounter. Even a patient with multiple complications going to a physician's office will have a fairly brief record until he or she has visited many times. In a hospital, however, sometimes even the smallest procedures generate enormous volumes of data. Paper forms and computer screens are the primary **data collection devices** for health data.

Forms

In a paper-based record, most of the data are collected in a standard format that is devised by the individual facility. With some exceptions, notably obstetric patients and neonates, the forms in one hospital do not look the same as those in another hospital. The purposes of the forms are numerous:

1. A form reminds the user of which data have to be collected.
2. A form provides a structure for capturing that data so that the reader knows where to look to get the data he or she seeks.
3. The forms ensure that complete data are collected according to the clinical guidelines of the facility and of the profession and according to regulation.

Paper forms are frequently created by committees of the people who use them. Sometimes, there is an oversight committee, simply called the forms committee or documentation committee. This committee may be charged with ensuring that forms are created only when necessary, that duplicate forms are not created, and that the forms conform to hospital guidelines.

The demographic, financial, and some of the socioeconomic data that are collected in the patient registration record usually fit on one paper form, the admission record or face sheet, although it may take several computer screens to capture these data. Even facilities that collect the clinical data on paper tend to have computerized patient registration data.

CONTENT

Many considerations go into the development of a health data form. To illustrate this, let's develop one together. Suppose we decide to create a form for a physician's order. At the outset, we need creativity because as we proceed in the development of the form, we will find that we have to ensure that the form satisfies every user's needs. What data are needed on a physician's order form? (see Table 3–7 if you don't remember). The purpose of this form is to record the physician's instructions to nurses, therapists, consultants, and radiologists and to record anything else the physician decides must be done to care for the patient. The form must be flexible enough to record the hundreds of different medications, therapies, and instructions that a physician might give. On a paper form, these data are recorded by the physician, who writes the orders in his or her own handwriting. The purpose of the form is the most important consideration in its creation. The form for a physician's order has the very important purpose of communication of the patient's care to all of the health care team.

If a physician wants to tell a nurse to administer penicillin to a patient, then the nurse needs to know

- To which patient to give the medication
- The patient's medical record number to make sure that she or he gives the medication to the right patient (two people can have the same name)
- The exact medication
- The exact dosage
- The specific route of administration (e.g., oral or intravenous [via a needle into the bloodstream])
- When the order was given
- Who gave the order

Based on the purpose of the form and what information needs to be conveyed, how would you create a form that is able to capture this information? Generally, the patient's name and medical record number are recorded in the top right-hand corner of every page. Patient identification data must be on every page so that the data can be matched to the correct patient. The patient data most often go in the right-hand corner of the page because most records, particularly when the patient is still in the hospital, are kept in three-ring binders like a book. Having the patient's name and medical record number in the top right-hand corner makes the record very easy to check and avoids misfiling.

In addition to having the patient's identification on the form, we also need to include some information identifying the particular form. Typically included are the name of the facility, the title of the form, and any special instructions about the form. The top left-hand corner of the page is a handy place to put the name of the hospital and possibly its location (which is very useful if the hospital has many facilities), and the title of the form.

FORMAT

How many physician's orders can be put on one page of a paper record? Shall we put separate blocks for each order, or shall we create a form that has a lot of lines so that the physician can write as many different things as he or she wants for each order? This is a matter of personal preference. Frequently, you will see forms with the orders in blocks so that each block contains only one set of orders, and you will also see other order sheets that are a page of blank lines so that the physician can write free-form.

A major consideration in constructing a form is the size of the fields that will be included. Remember our discussion of data dictionaries in Chapter 2? On a paper form, the size of the field in characters must be accommodated, as well as the space needed to hand-write the data.

We must also consider the size of the form on the page. How close to the edge of the page can the form be printed? Will holes be punched in the form? If so, where will they be and how much space should be allowed? Figure 3–9 shows a form's design template.

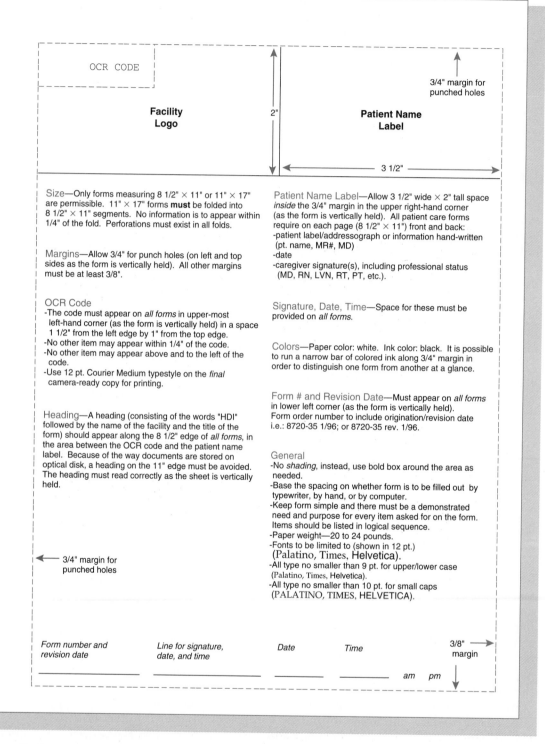

OCR CODE

**Facility
Logo**

2"

**Patient Name
Label**

3/4" margin for
punched holes

3 1/2"

Size—Only forms measuring 8 1/2" × 11" or 11" × 17" are permissible. 11" × 17" forms **must** be folded into 8 1/2" × 11" segments. No information is to appear within 1/4" of the fold. Perforations must exist in all folds.

Margins—Allow 3/4" for punch holes (on left and top sides as the form is vertically held). All other margins must be at least 3/8".

OCR Code
-The code must appear on *all forms* in upper-most left-hand corner (as the form is vertically held) in a space 1 1/2" from the left edge by 1" from the top edge.
-No other item may appear within 1/4" of the code.
-No other item may appear above and to the left of the code.
-Use 12 pt. Courier Medium typestyle on the *final* camera-ready copy for printing.

Heading—A heading (consisting of the words "HDI" followed by the name of the facility and the title of the form) should appear along the 8 1/2" edge of *all forms*, in the area between the OCR code and the patient name label. Because of the way documents are stored on optical disk, a heading on the 11" edge must be avoided. The heading must read correctly as the sheet is vertically held.

3/4" margin for
punched holes

Patient Name Label—Allow 3 1/2" wide × 2" tall space *inside* the 3/4" margin in the upper right-hand corner (as the form is vertically held). All patient care forms require on each page (8 1/2" × 11") front and back:
-patient label/addressograph or information hand-written (pt. name, MR#, MD)
-date
-caregiver signature(s), including professional status (MD, RN, LVN, RT, PT, etc.).

Signature, Date, Time—Space for these must be provided on *all forms*.

Colors—Paper color: white. Ink color: black. It is possible to run a narrow bar of colored ink along 3/4" margin in order to distinguish one form from another at a glance.

Form # and Revision Date—Must appear on *all forms* in lower left corner (as the form is vertically held). Form order number to include origination/revision date i.e.: 8720-35 1/96; or 8720-35 rev. 1/96.

General
-No *shading*, instead, use bold box around the area as needed.
-Base the spacing on whether form is to be filled out by typewriter, by hand, or by computer.
-Keep form simple and there must be a demonstrated need and purpose for every item asked for on the form. Items should be listed in logical sequence.
-Paper weight—20 to 24 pounds.
-Fonts to be limited to (shown in 12 pt.) (Palatino, Times, Helvetica).
-All type no smaller than 9 pt. for upper/lower case (Palatino, Times, Helvetica).
-All type no smaller than 10 pt. for small caps (PALATINO, TIMES, HELVETICA).

Form number and revision date

Line for signature, date, and time

Date

Time

3/8"
margin

am   *pm*

FIGURE 3–9.

Forms design template. (From Abdelhak M, Grostick S, Hanken MA, Jacobs E: Health Information, Management of a Strategic Resource, 2nd ed. Philadelphia, WB Saunders, 2001, p 19.)

Compliance with licensure and accreditation standards is another consideration. If the JCAHO requires that physician's orders must be authenticated, then we should facilitate that process on the form. There are two concepts we need to understand when we discuss authentication. The first concept is *authorship:* the author of an order is the person who wrote it. The second concept is *authentication:* the author's mark or signature. On a paper record, that mark or signature takes the form of the person's formal signature or, alternatively, his or her initials. Consequently, when we are designing the form, we need to make sure there is a place for the author's authentication. It also makes sense and may be a regulatory requirement to include a space so that the physician can record the date and time of the orders. This becomes important because there are many instances, from a clinical perspective, in which the time between the writing of the order and the execution of the order is crucial.

Now let us think some more about what else we need on the form. The physician's orders are written to communicate instructions to other health care providers. In a paper record the physician's orders are maintained in the nursing unit near the patient. The orders are not directly accessible to the radiology department, laboratory department, pharmacy, and the like. Someone has to take the orders and communicate them to the correct party. The nursing staff are usually charged with that responsibility. Therefore, our form must contain an area for the nursing staff to indicate that they have read and executed the order. In the case of medication, the medication needs to be ordered from the pharmacy, and then the medication has to be administered to the patient. Figure 3–10 shows a completed physician's order on a form that leaves separate blanks for each order.

OTHER CONSIDERATIONS

There are many other considerations in creating a form. So far, we have focused on what data need to be recorded on the form. In a paper record, we also need to consider a number of other issues.

- How heavy should the paper be? Should it be heavy card stock or copy machine weight?
- Should the form be one part, two parts, or more?
- If it is a multipart form, should there be carbon paper between the pages or should it be NCR (no carbon required) paper?
- What color paper should the form be printed on? White is best for photocopying, but would another color help the users of the form?

These are considerations that the forms committee reviews to ensure that the form conforms to the institution's guidelines. Designing forms was once a difficult and time-consuming process because forms needed to be developed with a pencil and paper, given to a printer, printed, and then returned to the organization. Today, we can develop forms using word processing software and reproduce them on a photocopy machine. Nevertheless, the large volume of forms re-

| Community Hospital City, State | Frank Bright ID #354792 |

DOCTOR'S ORDERS

Date 1/20/00	CBC c̄ diff	Date 1-20-00
Time 1 20 pm	UA exr	Time 1 30 pm
Date 1/21/00	KEFLEX 500mg	Date
Time 8 30 AM		Time
Date		Date
Time		Time
Date		Date
Time		Time

FIGURE 3–10.

Sample completed order form.

quired and the unique characteristics of some of the forms still often require the assistance of professional printers.

Computer-Based Data Collection

Paper-based forms are the traditional way of recording health data, and the skills that we have learned creating paper-based forms can be transferred to the creation of computer-based forms. Even when you are recording data into a computer, you're still recording it on a form—the computer screen; it just looks different. To create a computer-based form we have to have a name for the form. This is input at the top of the computer screen. The patient's name and medical record number are carried forward onto every screen after the data have been entered. Computerized data capture facilitates the improvement of data quality. In a computer-based record we don't have to "allow room" for entering data: we can allow exactly enough room for the particular data field. We also have the opportunity to program the computer to check the data for validity. In other respects, many of the same data collection considerations occur when developing a computer-based data record as for a paper-based record.

One consideration that becomes more important in computer data entry than in paper-record data collection is the sequence of data capture. On a paper-based form, the data can be entered in any order. Although the paper-based form may be designed to capture data in a logical sequence, as identified by the designers, there is no disadvantage inherent in recording items at the bottom of the form before recording items at the top if the data collector chooses to do so. In a computer-based data collection device, however, data collection may continue over several screen "pages." Flipping back and forth among the pages is confusing and time-consuming and may lead to errors and omissions. Although the computer can be programmed to check for incomplete data fields, this adds more wasted time, if the omission was caused by inefficient data capture. Consequently, computer-based data collection screens should collect data in the most efficient sequential order.

Let us talk about how the forms, within the context of a computer program, actually improve the data collection. First of all, we discussed that on a paper-based form, the patient's name and identification number go in the top right-hand corner, which is done manually: someone has to write it in, stamp it in, or affix a label in the corner. On a computer screen, the patient's name and medical record number are collected in other ways. The data enterer can type it in. Alternatively, the patient's name and identification number may be in a directory, from which the data enterer selects the patient's name and identification number and has it transferred to the form. In both paper and electronic form design, the element of human error is still a component of form completion.

If our physician's order form is completed in the computer, the data can be obtained in an expanded number of ways. For example, instead of a physician's actually typing or writing out the name of the drug, the dosage, and the route of administration, this information can be included in pop-up windows from a menu-driven pharmacy directory. This is particularly helpful, because the only elements included in the list are items that are definitely on the facility's approved drug list. In this particular instance, the use of a menu-driven computer-based data collection system significantly reduces the error that might occur if a physician ordered a nonapproved drug. Such a situation can easily happen if the physician has privileges at a variety of different hospitals, because approved drug lists in various hospitals are not necessarily identical. Further, the order entry can be linked to the pharmacy, generating the medication request without nursing intermediation. In addition, the order entry system can be linked to health data that we have already collected about the patient, such as sex, height, weight, age, and diagnosis. Then, if a physician ordered a drug at an excessive dosage for a newborn, for instance, a computer system could automatically generate a warning statement that the drug dosage was inappropriate. This would alert the physician that he or she had made an error, before any harm was done.

TABLE 3–9. Data Dictionary with Range of Valid Values					
Name	**Definition**	**Size**	**Type**	**Example**	**Valid Range**
Day	Day of the month	2 characters	Numeric	15	1–31
Month	Month of the year	2 characters	Numeric	08	1–12
Temperature	Patient's temperature	5 characters	Numeric	98.6	85–110

These are simple data elements that may appear in a patient health record. Although validity checks may include the size of the field, the range of values is also an important evaluation tool to check to prevent data entry errors. Can you see a problem with the valid range of values for Day? How can you fix the problem?

When determining a valid range of values for clinical measures, it is important to include a wide enough range so that extreme value can be entered; however, because some extreme values are not compatible with life, be careful to place reasonable limits on the values. Excessively wide ranges are not necessarily helpful in ensuring accurate data entry.

Data Quality

In Chapter 2 we mentioned data validity as a measure of data quality. Only valid data entered within a legitimate range of values for the type of data should be collected. For example, if you are collecting social security numbers, then the computer is looking for a nine-digit field. (Alternatively, you may choose to collect it as three fields of three, two, and four characters, respectively.) If someone tries to enter a social security number with 11 digits, that is not a valid entry. The range of valid entries is an element of the data dictionary. Table 3–9 illustrates a data dictionary with this additional element.

One problem with paper records is that clinicians may write an order but forget to sign it, so the order is not authenticated. In a computer system, authenti-

TABLE 3–10. Data Collection Device Design Issues	
Issue	**Considerations**
Identification of user needs	Not limited to the collectors of the data; also consider subsequent users of both the device and the data it contains.
Purpose of the data collection device	Both data collection and controls should be ensured for quality.
Selection of the appropriate data items and sequencing of data collection activities	Data items collected should fulfill the purpose of the device, without unnecessary fields. Consideration of the order in which data is collected is important.
Understanding the technology used	Not just paper vs. computer: How is the paper used, how is the computer used, what input devices are available and how will they be used?
Use of standard terminology and abbreviations as well as development of a standard format	Consistency in language and format helps to improve communication among users.
Appropriate instructions	Instructions on the form help to ensure consistency.
Simplicity	The simpler the device, the easier it will be to use.

Adapted from Abdelhak M, Grostick S, Hanken MA, Jacobs E: Health Information: Management of a Strategic Resource, 2nd ed. Philadelphia, WB Saunders, 2001, p 164.

cation is captured by a key word, or code, that the physician enters when he or she has completed the order. There are a number of different methods of capturing authentication data. We call these methods electronic signatures. An electronic signature does not capture the person's actual signature into the computer. Rather, it is the computer recognition of a unique code that only the author has in his or her possession. The computer can be programmed to reject orders that do not contain an appropriate authentication. The program would look for both the existence of the authentication (for data completeness), and the correct authentication (for data validity). Table 3–10 summarizes forms design issues.

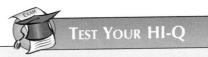

TEST YOUR HI-Q

Should the "correct" authentication be limited to the attending physician?

Forms Control

In a paper-based system, forms are used selectively depending on the type of patient record and the department using them. Someone in the hospital, frequently the director of the health information management department, needs to keep track of all approved forms. In reality, forms get passed around, photocopied, and shuffled from department to department. If a form is not used frequently, it often is lost to easy retrieval. When the form is needed but not readily available, the health care provider creates a new form even though the old form still exists. Therefore, a master forms file should be created and maintained. The master forms file contains every form used by the hospital and can be organized in any way that the hospital finds useful. One very efficient way to save a master forms file is to keep forms in the order of the departments that use them, for example, alphabetically by department name. Another way to maintain a master forms file is to give each form a numeric assignment and then save the forms in numeric order. In either case, the creation of an index and table of contents for the master forms file is necessary. The index is at the front of the file, and the title of each form and its individual number are listed in the table of contents. The responsibility for ensuring that forms are not duplicated and that each form conforms to the institution's needs is usually the responsibility of the forms committee, as previously mentioned.

The forms committee is an institutionwide committee that has the responsibility of reviewing all forms. Therefore, it is important that representatives of the major clinical services are included. For example, there should be a representative from nursing, physician staff (probably several representatives of different physician groups if there are numerous services in the facility), laboratory, and radiology; also, there should be a representative from health information management. Health information management frequently is in charge of the master forms file, and a health information professional should participate on the forms committee. In a computer-based environment, the forms are created and displayed on computer screens. The development of or addition to a computer system should be under the direction of a systems development team. However, only the clinicians and other health practitioners are truly aware of the data that need to be collected and how the data should be organized. The data dictionary then becomes critical in the developmental process. The data fields that are collected; who has access to them; and whether those with access can print, change, or view the data become increasingly important considerations. Existing institutional committees become involved in this development according to institution policies. Often, groups are formed for these new roles. In any event, health information management personnel should be as directly involved in these new groups as they were in the old.

Other Types of Records

The clinical flow of data is similar in every type of health care setting. We have primarily been discussing ambulatory or physician's office settings and inpatient visits in an acute care hospital. Other types of health care facilities require special records. For example, a patient can go into a hospital, have surgery, and leave on the same day; this is called same-day surgery. In those cases, the data collection is frequently compressed, so that the history and physical, some anesthesia information, and some procedural information (e.g., the operative report) are compressed into shorter documents because of the simplicity of the procedure.

These special records differ from the ones that we have already discussed because of the type of data that are collected. A classic example is obstetric and neonatal data. When a woman is pregnant and visits a physician for prenatal care, much data are collected on her progress and the progress of the fetus. Shortly before the woman is due to give birth, the data are transferred to the hospital in which she intends to deliver. The data become incorporated into the inpatient record.

Sometimes patients are gravely ill when they enter the hospital and are sent to special nursing care units called intensive care units. A patient with a serious heart problem might be cared for in a coronary care unit. Because of the intensity of nursing care in critical care units, nurses prefers to use graphical forms, which provide a great deal of visual data at a glance. In a paper record, this may consist of heavy stock foldout graphs, which can be as large as $8\frac{1}{2} \times 14$ inches or $8\frac{1}{2} \times 17$ inches. They indicate 24 hours of care. Vital signs are plotted on graphs that illustrate how the patient is being cared for and the patient's progress. Some of these forms are difficult to photocopy; however, they greatly facilitate recording patient data.

Data Sets

Earlier in this chapter, we asked you to think of a list of data elements for an acute care facility that would correspond to the **Uniform Hospital Discharge Data Set.** Here are the major elements of the UHDDS (Abdelhak et al, 2001, pp 113–114):

(handwritten note: UACDS, Marital status, provider: Location, address, profession, services, date of encounter)

(handwritten: Both)

1. Patient's identification number
2. Date of birth
3. Sex
4. Race and ethnicity
5. Residence
6. Health care facility identification number
7. Admission date
8. Type of admission
9. Discharge date
10. Attending physician's identification number
11. Surgeon's identification number
12. Principal diagnosis
13. Other diagnoses *or assmt*
14. Qualifier for other diagnoses
15. External cause-of-injury code
16. Birth weight of neonate
17. Other procedures and the date(s) of the procedure(s)
18. Disposition of the patient at discharge
19. Expected source of payment
20. Total charges

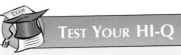

TEST YOUR HI-Q

From our discussion of data in this chapter, can you identify the sources of each of the elements of the UHDDS?

Other Health Care Settings

At this point, you should have a clear idea of what occurs in a physician's office and what goes on in an acute care facility, including how data are collected and by whom. We have touched briefly on the special data requirements of certain diagnoses and other health care facilities. The most important thing to remember is that the skills and the knowledge that you have acquired so far in this text are applicable to any health care delivery setting. Demographic, financial, socioeconomic, and clinical data are always collected in inpatient or resident settings. The volume and types of physician data, nursing data, and data from therapy, social services, and psychology vary, depending on the diagnosis and the setting. Health information management professionals who are employed in special health care settings need to become familiar with the unique data requirements of those settings.

Reference

Abdelhak M, Grostick S, Hanken MA, Jacobs E: Health Information: Management of a Strategic Resource, 2nd ed. Philadelphia, WB Saunders, 2001.

Suggested Reading

Andress AA: Manual of Medical Office Management. Philadelphia, WB Saunders, 1996.
Moisio MA, Moisio EW: Understanding Laboratory and Diagnostic Tests. Albany, NY, Delmar, 1998.
Skurka MA: Health Information Management: Principles and Organization for Health Record Services. rev ed. Chicago, American Hospital Publishing, 1998.

CHAPTER SUMMARY

In this chapter we discussed the clinical flow of data through an acute care visit. We compared the clinical flow of a patient's data in an acute care facility to the flow of the patient's data in an ambulatory care setting and illustrated the similarities and differences. We also discussed the various types of clinical data that are collected from physicians, nurses, laboratory, and radiology. We learned how to create a form and discussed the considerations in design of a paper form versus a computer-based input screen. We also discussed in more detail the data quality concepts of data validity and data completeness.

REVIEW QUESTIONS

1. Explain the SOAP strategy of medical evaluation.

2. List and explain the elements of an admission record.

3. Identify the appropriate source of the following data:
   a. Patient's name and address.
   b. Patient's latest blood test results.
   c. Patient's ability to explain his or her condition.
   d. Patient/family education activities.
   e. Plan of treatment on a specific day.
   f. Whether the patient had a consultation during the inpatient stay.

4. List and describe the data elements of the following:
   a. History
   b. Physical
   c. Medication administration

5. Develop a paper-based data capture device to record medication administration.

6. Compare and contrast the considerations in developing paper-based versus computer-based data collection devices.

7. Compare and contrast the elements of the Uniform Hospital Discharge Data Set to the elements of the Uniform Ambulatory Care Data Set.

PROFESSIONAL PROFILE
Transcriptionist

My name is Nicole, and I am a transcriptionist. I work for a large firm that performs transcription services for a lot of different facilities. I could work at home, if I wanted to, but I like going into the office. I work in a nice cubicle, which is in a room full of similar cubicles. My responsibility is to listen to what the physician dictated and to type exactly what the physician says. I learned transcription and took classes such as medical terminology and anatomy and physiology in the health-related professions program at my high school. I worked in a physician's office for a while and took some additional courses at my local community college.

My job isn't just typing. In order to transcribe accurately, I have to understand what the physician is saying and what it means. That means that I need to understand and use medical terminology correctly. I need to know the requirements of the various medical reports, such as the H&P and the discharge summary, so that I transcribe them in the right format. I also need to know the regulatory requirements pertaining to the reports. For example, I know that the H&P is more urgent than the discharge summary, so I always transcribe the H&P report first.

Some people think that my job will go away when computers can understand and transcribe human language quickly and accurately. I certainly won't need to type as much, but my skills will become more important in reviewing the clinical reports for completeness, accuracy, and other data quality issues. I'm looking forward to that. To better prepare myself for that function, I am studying to become a registered health information technician.

APPLICATION

Does Computerization Reduce the Use of Paper?

The computerization of a function is frequently referred to as a "paperless" environment. This is an interesting term. "Paperless" implies that no paper is used at all in the process. However, let's take a look at what happens when we computerize a patient's record. If we put the admissions data on a computer-based admissions form, and our health record is still largely paper-based, then we still print the admissions record on paper to include in the paper record. Many facilities that have a computer-based admissions record still print out the record for the benefit of those using the paper record.

The physician reports a history and physical that can be dictated into a computer; the transcriptionist can listen to the dictation on the computer and transcribe it into the computer using a word processing program. What happens to the history and physical then? It gets printed out as a paper record. In a computer-based environment, a transcription does not routinely get printed out, but you will find that many individuals print it out anyway to review in the convenience of their office. Even though we have not discussed computer security or the confidentiality of health records (see Chapter 8), this should already be raising red flags in your mind about whether this is an appropriate activity.

Think about the order entry system. The computer-based order entry system facilitates the entry of the order by the physician. However, when it is received in the pharmacy, the order is often printed out by the pharmacist while he or she is filling the order. More paper may be generated when a prescription is transferred to the nursing station for the patient. More paper is again generated if the order is printed out to be filed in paper format in the health record. This excessive generation of paper often occurs when a facility is in a transition from a paper-based record system to a computer-based system. However, with just this simple example, you can see that computerization of a patient record does not necessarily reduce paper immediately. How would you stop the excessive printing of data that can be viewed on the computer?

4
Postdischarge Processing

Chapter Outline

Data Quality
Timeliness
Completeness

Controls
Preventive Controls
Detective Controls
Corrective Controls
Correction of Errors

Postdischarge Processing
Identification of Records to Process
Assembly
Quantitative Analysis
   Elements of the Record
   Record Completion
   Deficiency System
Coding
   Nomenclature and Classification
   Inpatient Coding
Retrieval
Abstracting

Tracking Records While Processing
Batch by Days
Loose Sheets
Efficiency

Other Health Information Management Roles

Suggested Reading

Chapter Summary

Review Questions

Professional Profile

Application

CHAPTER OBJECTIVES

By the end of this chapter, the student should be able to:

- List and explain the elements of data quality.

- List, explain, and give examples of the three types of controls.

- Explain the flow of postdischarge processing of health information.

- List and explain the major functions of a health information management department.

- Explain the principles and process flow of an incomplete record system.

- Compare and contrast paper-based versus computer-based processing.

Vocabulary

abstracting

analysis

assembly

audit trail

classification

coding

completeness

concurrent analysis

concurrent coding

corrective controls

countersignature

CPT-4

data entry

deficiencies

deficiency system (incomplete system)

delinquent

detective controls

discharge register (discharge list)

DSM-IV

error report (exception report)

ICD-9-CM

ICD-10

ICD-O

loose sheets

nomenclature

postdischarge processing

preventive controls

quantitative analysis

retention

timeliness

universal chart order

We have spent the last two chapters discussing the elements of data, clinical data flow, and the organization of patient encounter data on paper- and computer-based forms in an ambulatory care facility and in an acute care, inpatient facility. In this chapter, we conclude the discussion of data ele-ments and introduce you to the controls that ensure that our data are accurate. To illustrate data control measures, we describe the role of health information management (HIM) professionals in postdischarge processing of patient data.

Data Quality

Whether the data are recorded by hand or entered into a computer, the process of recording data is called **data entry.** In health care, a patient's life can depend on the correctness of the data entered. Consequently, we are very concerned with the overall quality of the data that are recorded. We have already discussed the concepts of data accuracy and validity (see Chapters 1 and 2). In this chapter we add the concepts of data timeliness and completeness.

Timeliness

Timeliness refers to the recording of data in a reasonable amount of time, preferably concurrently with the time it is being collected. Numerous regulations, both on the licensure level from government and on the accrediting level from voluntary agencies, address the issue of when specific data need to be recorded. We have already discussed some of these regulations. For example, an operative report must be documented immediately after the operation. A history and physical (H&P) must be completed within 24 hours of admission or before a surgical procedure. Timeliness applies to many other activities, as we shall see in subsequent chapters.

Timeliness is important, particularly from the health care facility's point of view, because the patient's health record is part of the normal business records of the facility (see Litigation in Chapter 8). Therefore, data that are being entered into the health record must be recorded as concurrently as possible with the events that the data describe. For example, if a nurse is monitoring a patient at 3:00 PM, then the note that he or she records in the medical record must be written very shortly thereafter. Writing that same note at 9:00 PM, 6 hours after the actual observation, can impair the quality of the recorded note. Can the nurse really remember, 6 hours later, exactly what happened with the patient? Can a physician really remember, weeks later, exactly what happened on an operating table? Because this element is so important, a significant amount of time and energy is spent facilitating the timely completion of health records.

Completeness

Completeness refers to data's being collected or recorded in their entirety. A recording of vital signs that is missing the time and date is incomplete. A comprehensive physical examination that is missing mention of the condition of the

TABLE 4–1. Elements of Data Quality		
Element	**Description**	**Example of Errors**
Accuracy	Data are correct.	The patient's pulse is 76. The nurse recorded 67. That data entry was inaccurate.
Validity	Data fall within predetermined values or parameters.	99 degrees is a valid body temperature for humans; 990 degrees is not.
Timeliness	Data are recorded within a predetermined period.	Operative reports must be recorded immediately following surgery.
Completeness	Data exist in their entirety.	Date, time, or authentication missing from a record renders it incomplete.

This is a partial list of the elements of data quality. We will continue to identify data quality elements as we discuss different aspects of health information management.

patient's skin is incomplete. A progress note that is not authenticated is incomplete. Table 4–1 summarizes the data quality concepts that we have discussed so far. Good data are complete; therefore to ensure that good data are collected, we need to develop and implement data controls.

Controls

As you can see from our previous discussion of collecting data, there are many opportunities for errors to occur. We all know that humans make mistakes. Errors can occur in the simple act of hand-writing the data. If an individual's handwriting cannot be read by another health professional, then how can those data be considered valid or accurate? If only the person who wrote the data can decipher the writing, then the data are useless to others. If a nurse records a temperature of 98.6°F without the decimal point (986°F), the temperature recorded is not valid. Finally, if a physician does not dictate an operative report until a month after the operation was performed, how can that operative report truly reflect what actually occurred on that specific day? The patient's record is incomplete until the report is added to the record, and the report fails the test of timeliness.

One way that data can be protected so that they are accurate, valid, timely, and complete is through the development and implementation of controls over the collection, recording, and reporting of the data. We are discussing collection and recording of data in this chapter. Reporting of data is discussed in Chapter 7. There are three types of controls over the collection and recording of data: preventive, detective, and corrective (Table 4–2).

Preventive Controls

Preventive controls are designed to ensure that data errors do not occur in the first place. The best example of a preventive control is a computer validity check. For example, let's say you wanted to write a date into the computer and you indicated that the date is July 45, 2000 (i.e., 07/45/2000). If the computer

TABLE 4–2. Processing Controls		
Control	**Description**	**Example**
Preventive	Helps to ensure that an error does not occur	Computer-based validity check during data entry; examination of patient identification prior to medication administration
Detective	Helps to discover errors that have been made	Quantitative analysis, e.g., error report
Corrective	Correction of errors that have been discovered, including investigation of the source of the error for future prevention	Incomplete record processing

is programmed to prevent you from entering invalid dates, it might send you a message saying, "You have entered an invalid date—please re-enter." It might even make a loud sound or block the character "4" from being typed in the first position of the day field. This type of preventive control double-checks data validity and proves that the computer is extremely useful for data collection.

A noncomputer-based example of preventive controls are the procedural checks required in a nursing unit to ensure that patients receive the appropriate medication. For example, the nurse checks the patient's identification band before giving the medication to ensure that the medication is being given to the correct patient. The development of well-designed preprinted forms to collect data also helps to ensure that data collection is complete. These are just two examples of preventive controls that are routinely in place in a health care facility.

Preventive controls can be expensive and cumbersome to develop and implement. Therefore, the cost of a preventive control must always be balanced against its expected benefits. It is relatively easy to justify checking medications, orders, and patient identification, because the benefit to the patient is apparent. It is not quite as easy to justify developing a control to prevent the entry of an incorrect patient religion or ethnicity.

One simple way to prevent invalid data entries is with the use of multiple-choice questions on a printed form or computer screen. All of the valid choices are listed, so that the recorder merely chooses the correct one for the particular patient (Fig. 4–1). This method also prompts the user to complete the form. However, this method does not prevent inaccurate or untimely entries. As you can see, comprehensive preventive controls may be quite complex.

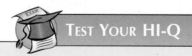

TEST YOUR HI-Q

When creating a paper form for new patients to complete at registration in a physician's office, what preventive control could be implemented to ensure that the patient lists all significant childhood illnesses?

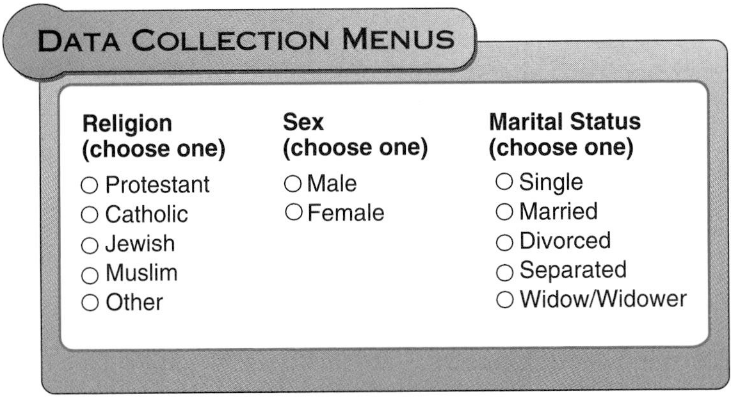

DATA COLLECTION MENUS

Religion
(choose one)
○ Protestant
○ Catholic
○ Jewish
○ Muslim
○ Other

Sex
(choose one)
○ Male
○ Female

Marital Status
(choose one)
○ Single
○ Married
○ Divorced
○ Separated
○ Widow/Widower

FIGURE 4–1.
Data collection menus improve data quality.

Detective Controls

Detective controls are developed and implemented to ensure that errors in data are discovered. Whereas a preventive control is designed to help prevent the person recording the data from making the mistake in the first place, a detective control is in place to find the data error after it is entered. In the previous date example, a computer-based detective control might be programmed to print out a list of entries that the computer recognizes as problematic. Such a printout is called an **error report** or **exception report.** Error reports are also generated when the computer or other system encounters a problem with its normal processing. For example, a fax machine can be programmed to print an error report describing the reason a fax transmission was not completed. In the previous medication administration example, a detective control could verify the medication ordered against the medication received to ensure that the order was filled correctly.

Detective controls are critical in a paper-based environment. Because there is no practical way to completely prevent erroneous data entry in a paper-based environment, the process of looking for errors is necessary. For example, nursing medication records may be reviewed on a regular basis to ensure that medication administration notes are properly entered. Also, if a physician fails to dictate an operative report on a timely basis, a control must be in place to detect the missing operative report. We discuss the process of implementing detective controls later in this chapter.

Detective controls are frequently the easiest and most cost-effective to develop and implement, but as with preventive controls, they may be complex. The development of preventive and detective controls requires a thorough knowledge of the process being controlled as well as of the potential negative impact of data errors in processing.

Corrective Controls

Corrective controls can be developed and implemented to fix an error once it has been detected. Corrective controls follow detective controls. In general, it does no good and wastes time to identify an error if the facility will not correct it. However, the very nature of corrective controls is that they occur retrospectively to the error. Thus, if an error report identified an invalid date such as July 45, the date would have to be corrected after the fact.

Nevertheless, some errors, such as administration of incorrect medications, are not effectively correctable once they occur. In such cases, analysis of the error is necessary in order to determine whether sufficient controls are in place to prevent the error in the future. For example, if a patient received an injection of an incorrect medication, the medication cannot subsequently be withdrawn. However, the events leading up to the administration of the drug can be thoroughly examined to determine why the error occurred. Did the physician order the wrong medication? Was the order transmitted incorrectly to the pharmacy? Did the health care provider check the patient's wristband prior to administering the medication? Once the source of the error is determined, the appropriate correction in the process can take place. Employee education and disciplinary action are two examples of typical corrective actions that may take place if procedures were in place but were not followed.

Earlier in the chapter we used an unsigned progress note as an example of incomplete data. Authentication of the note was missing. In a paper-based environment, the HIM professional would have to physically obtain the record and read all of the progress notes in it in order to identify the incomplete note. In a computer-based environment, preventive controls such as noises and verbal prompts can be built into the program to encourage the authentication of the note, at the time the note is originally recorded and also on subsequent access to the record. The computer can also be programmed to review the record and to identify incomplete notes. In both paper-based and computer-based environments, the corrective control consists of alerting the physician to the omission and providing the physician with the opportunity to complete the note.

HIT BIT

Computerization has had an impact on the HIM profession. The terminology of computerization can be confusing. The terms "electronic," "computerized," "computer-assisted," and "computer-based" are sometimes used interchangeably. For the purpose of clarity in this text, we use the following definitions:

- *Electronic:* The collection, transmission, or storage of data via electronic media, such as telephone wires, cables, and computer. A paper document that has been faxed can be considered electronic. An e-mail is electronic.

Hit Bit Continued

Hit Bit Continued
- *Computer-assisted:* The collection, transmission, or storage of data that is aided by the use of the computer, but is not completely performed on the computer. Some surgical procedures are computer-assisted. Some types of quantitative analysis are computer-assisted (see later in chapter).
- *Computerized:* The collection, transmission, or storage of data by a computer. For example, a word processing document is a computerized record.
- *Computer-based:* The collection and storage of data in a relational database.

The health care profession is shifting from using paper-based to computer-based health records. Terminology used to describe the health record varies, and the terms *electronic patient record, computerized patient record,* and *computer-based patient record* all are currently used. You should be alert to the variety of terminology and pay particular attention to how the terminology is used as you are reading and learning about health information management.

Correction of Errors

The correction of errors is an important consideration in patient record keeping because nothing that is recorded should be deleted. Corrections must be made in such a way that the error can be seen as easily as the corrected information. In a paper-based record, errors are corrected by drawing a line through the erroneous data and writing the correct data near it. It is important not to obscure the original entry. The correction must be authenticated and dated.

In a computer-based record, errors can be corrected in several ways, depending on the type of error and the data that are being changed. For example, suppose that a patient admitted to a facility was previously treated there. A record of the previous visit exists. The patient registration specialist looks at the previous record and discovers that the patient has moved. The address and telephone number are now incorrect. Therefore, the patient registration clerk may delete the old data and re-enter them with the new data. In doing so, the computer may be programmed to create a historical file of the patient's previous addresses. Alternatively, the previous address could be wiped out completely, replaced by the new address. Because the patient's previous address may not be of future interest to the facility, either method is acceptable. However, in both cases, an **audit trail** should be created to indicate that the correction was made. An audit trail is a list of all activities performed in a computer. In addition to the date and time, the audit trail contains a list of the activities, the computer in which the activity took place, the user who performed the activity, and a description of the activity itself. In the case of changes, such as the one previously described, the audit trail may also be programmed to contain the pre- and postchange data.

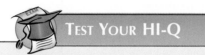

TEST YOUR HI-Q

The physician accidentally entered an order into the computer to request a cardiology consultation for the wrong patient. A staff nurse noticed the error. How should the correction be handled?

Postdischarge Processing

The understanding of data concepts and control issues is critical for the development and implementation of **postdischarge processing** procedures (Fig. 4–2). Postdischarge processing is what happens to the patient data after the patient is discharged. In a paper-based environment, postdischarge processing is a series of procedures aimed at **retention** of a completed record. In a computer-based environment, the goals are the same, but the procedures are different. Concepts to understand in the retention of records include storage, security, and access. Table 4–3 summarizes the components of record retention.

Postdischarge processing is traditionally performed by the health information department of a facility. In a small physician's office or long-term care facility, the entire process may be performed by one person. In a group practice or small inpatient facility, the process may be divided into functions and distributed among several individuals. In a large facility, many individuals may perform the separate functions of the process. Even though you may never work in a health care facility, it is useful to understand the process by which records are processed for retention, because the data concepts and control issues are relevant to many other health information environments.

In Chapter 2, we discussed the clinical flow of data in a physician's office. In Chapter 3, we reviewed the same process in an acute care facility. In those discussions, we focused on the collection of data: what is captured, who collects it, and how it is collected. Now we turn our attention to preparing the data for storage. The following descriptions pertain to inpatient facilities, and although the principles are similar for outpatient facilities, the application of the principles may vary.

TABLE 4–3. Components of Record Retention	
Component	**Description**
Storage	Compiling, indexing or cataloging, and maintaining a physical or electronic location for data (see Chapter 5)
Security	Safety and confidentiality of data (see Chapters 5 and 8)
Access	Ability to retrieve data; release of data only to appropriate individuals or other entities (see Chapters 7 and 8)

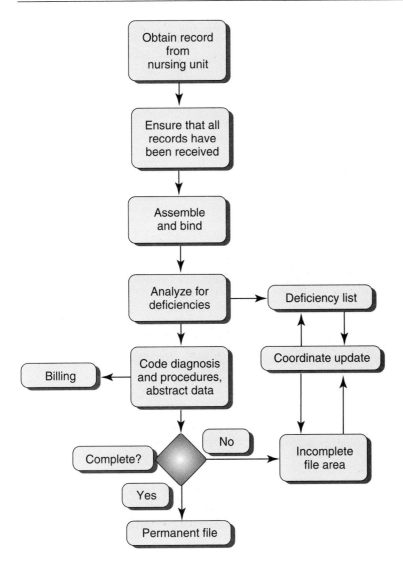

FIGURE 4–2.
Postdischarge processing in a health information management department.

Identification of Records to Process

Before the data can be prepared for storage, the HIM professional needs
to know which records require storage. This can be accomplished by reviewing
a list of the patients who have been discharged. This list is called the **discharge
register** or **discharge list.** The discharge register is compiled throughout
the day, as patients leave the facility. It may be compiled automatically by
the computer system or manually, usually by staff on the appropriate nursing

TABLE 4–4. Discharge Register						

Discharge Date: June 5, 2000

Admission Date	Patient Identification Number	Patient Name		Attending Physician	Discharge Disposition	Room Number
		Last	*First*			
6/2/00	234675	Johnson	Thomas	Bottoms	Transfer LTC	313A
6/4/00	234731	Kudovski	Maria	Patel	Home	303A
6/4/00	234565	Kudovski	Vladimir	Thomas	Home	Nursery
5/31/00	156785	Macey	Anna	Flint	Home	213B
6/3/00	234523	Mattingly	Richard	Johnson	Home	202A
6/5/00	274568	Ng	Charles	Kudro	Home	224A
5/15/00	234465	Rodriguez	Francisco	Benet	Deceased	ICU-4
6/1/00	198543	Rogers	Danielle	Patel	Home	226B
6/2/00	224678	Young	Rebecca	Muniz	Home	325B

unit. Sometimes, a combination of methods is used. However it is compiled, the discharge register contains a list of the patients who have been discharged on a specific calendar day (see Chapter 2). A day is from 12:01 AM to 12 midnight (00:00:01 to 24:59:59), so discharges may include a patient who died at 11 PM or one who left against medical advice (AMA) at 5 PM. Table 4–4 illustrates a discharge register.

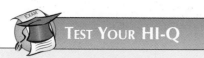

TEST YOUR HI-Q

Answer the following questions after examining the discharge register shown in Table 4–4:

- What is the length of stay for each of these patients?
- What is the average length of stay?
- Why do we want to know the room number if the patient has already been discharged?

Bear in mind that ambulatory care records are not tracked by a list of discharges but rather by a list of visits or encounters. Nevertheless, there should be some centrally prepared document that identifies patients whose records should be available for processing.

In a paper-based environment, patient records move from the nursing unit to the HIM department. The process by which the records move varies from facility to facility. Some of the considerations that determine what process is used include the distance from the nursing units to the HIM department, the staffing levels on the nursing unit, the staffing levels in the HIM department, and the availability of alternative personnel, such as volunteers. For example, nursing unit personnel can remove the records from their binders and leave them in a pile for pickup. The records can then be picked up by any authorized person and delivered to the HIM department. Alternatively, the nursing unit personnel can deliver the records. Some facilities use physical transportation systems such as pneumatic tube systems and elevators.

HIT BIT

Pneumatic tube systems are widely used today at banks for drive-in banking customers. The customer drives up to a stand that contains a container. The checks or other documents are placed in the container, which is then shipped at the press of a button, by forced air, to the teller inside the bank. Larger documents, such as health records, require larger containers. These systems are quick and generally efficient; however, the tendency of containers to get stuck in the tubes and the relatively short range of the system limit their appeal for this purpose. However, they are still used to transport records and for other uses, such as physical delivery of physicians' orders to the pharmacy.

Once the record arrives in the HIM department, processing can begin. The first step is to ensure that all records have been received. This can be accomplished by checking the records received against the discharge register. If a patient was discharged but a record was not received, the nursing unit should be contacted to obtain the record. If a record was received but the patient is not on the discharge register, the record may have been sent in error, because the patient may not have been discharged. Alternatively, the discharge register may be incorrect: The patient was discharged, but he or she was not added to the discharge register. The nursing unit should be contacted to verify the patient's status and correct whatever error was made. Although the physician orders the patient's discharge and prepares a final progress note to that effect, it is the nursing staff that is usually responsible for recording the actual discharge of the patient. This is a nursing responsibility because there is often a time lag of many hours between the order to discharge the patient and the physical movement of the patient out of the facility. This process is greatly facilitated by computers.

TEST YOUR HI-Q

What type of control is provided by the first processing step of receiving the records, as previously described?

Assembly

Assembly is the set of procedures by which a record is reorganized and bound for storage. The extent to which a record is reorganized varies among facilities and arises from the differences between the order of the record as filed on the nursing unit and the order of the record used in the storage process. For example, the nursing unit may organize the chart in chronologic order. If facility policy is storage of records in source-oriented order, the record would have to be reorganized for postdischarge processing. Sometimes, the difference is subtler.

For example, the nursing unit may use source orientation, placing the most recent page first in each section (reverse chronologic order). If facility policy states that each source section be organized in chronologic order, then each section of the record would have to be re-sorted.

Reorganization of a paper record is done manually and can take a long time, particularly in the case of large records that have to be substantially reorganized. An obvious solution to the problem is to store the record the same way as it is kept on the nursing unit. This is called **universal chart order.** Universal chart order is in theory a practical idea. However, because the uses of the record vary dramatically between the nursing unit and storage, universal chart order is not always implemented.

It may seem obvious that in a computer-based environment, assembly is not performed because there is nothing to assemble. However, even hospitals that have a high percentage of records in computer-based format still print out much of the record. The assembler must be aware of which parts are received from the nursing unit and which parts are printouts directly from the computer.

Once the record has been organized, it is bound. Binding consists of affixing the pages of the record within a permanent cover, usually a manila folder. The front of the folder usually contains the name of the facility. It may also contain warnings about the confidentiality of the record and other pertinent facility record policies. (Confidentiality is discussed in Chapter 8.) The front and tabs of the folder contain the patient's name and medical record number. Sometimes, the front of the folder also shows the discharge date.

You may be familiar with file folders that have a tab on the long open side of the folder. This enables the user to label the folder and identify the contents when the folder is placed in a drawer. Health records are generally stored in open shelves (or shelves that can open), so the tab is on the short side of the folder. This enables the user to identify the contents of the folder when it is standing on a shelf. See Chapter 5 for a complete discussion of paper file storage.

Quantitative Analysis

One important detective control in place in health care facilities is called **analysis.** Analysis is the process of reviewing a health record to ensure that the record is complete in every respect. We know from our discussion of data concepts that completeness refers to the entirety of data: Are all of the data elements accounted for? Therefore, this type of analysis is called **quantitative analysis.** The HIM professional who performs this function is frequently called a medical record analyst, medical record analysis specialist, health information specialist, health information analyst, or similar title. This person's responsibility is to review the patient's record and determine whether there are any missing reports or notes and to check if or any critical signatures are missing.

The extent of quantitative analysis performed in a facility depends on the type of facility and the rules of its licensure and accreditation. However, there are three guiding principles:

- The record must contain all of the elements required by the clinical services pertaining to that patient's treatment as well as the elements common to all patients.
- Each element of the record must be properly authenticated and the authors clearly identified.
- The record must contain all of the elements required by the licensure and accrediting bodies for the particular type of facility.

ELEMENTS OF THE RECORD

Different clinical services may have special forms that pertain to that service. Physical therapists may have special assessment and progress forms that differ from those used by nursing. Ambulatory surgery may use different operative records than inpatient surgery. The analyst must know which forms are used in each service and be able to identify any forms that are missing. The analyst must also be able to identify forms that are incomplete.

The absence of the author's authentication or of identification of authorship is easily recognized, as long as the analyst is aware of when and where a signature must appear. However, the analyst must also know who *should* have authenticated the document. This becomes critical if a document has been signed, but not by the correct individual. Perhaps a countersignature is required. A **countersignature** is authentication by an individual in addition to the author. For example, an unlicensed resident may write (author) a progress note, which the attending physician must then countersign to evidence supervision of the resident.

HIT BIT

The author of a verbal order may be a registered nurse, who then authenticates the entry by initialing or signing it. The physician then authenticates the order to evidence that it has been reviewed. Both parties can be identified by their unique signatures. Therefore, a signature can verify identity as well as represent an activity, such as review or approval.

Finally, the analyst ensures that the record is complete with respect to licensure and accreditation rules. Sometimes this requirement overlaps with the requirement for authentication. Again, the complete absence of the element is not as difficult to identify as the partial absence. For example, an H&P must be documented on every patient record. Failure to perform an H&P is a serious error. If the history or physical examination typed report is missing, it may not have been performed. More often, however, the H&P was performed, noted in the record, and dictated, but the dictation has not been matched with the chart. The same is true of operative reports and consultations. In addition, on some records, a hand-written H&P is acceptable. The analyst must know the rules and be able to identify noncompliance. Table 4–5 summarizes the major record elements for which quantitative analysis acts as a detective control.

	TABLE 4–5. Elements of a Record	
Element	**Analysis to Determine**	**Common Deficiencies**
Existence	Do the data exist?	Missing operative report
		Missing discharge summary
Completeness	Are the data entirely present or are there missing components?	Missing reason for consultation
Authentication	Is the author's or other appropriate signature/password present?	Unsigned H&P
		Unsigned discharge summary
		Unsigned order

As the analyst identifies missing elements, the pages are flagged and the missing elements are noted along with the responsible party. Flagging consists of affixing stickers to the pages of the record. The stickers come in multiple colors so that many different clinicians can be identified uniquely in a single record. Many facilities analyze only the physician portions of the record. Other facilities choose to analyze many sections or all of the clinical documentation.

In a completely computer-based record, most of the quantitative analysis can be performed by the computer. The analyst would then receive a computer exception or error report for follow-up. Analysts can then turn their attention to other data quality issues, such as extent of patient/family education documentation and consistency of diagnostic statements between caregivers and other departments (see Chapter 6).

RECORD COMPLETION

Once the missing elements, or **deficiencies,** are identified, the responsible parties are then required to complete the record. Time limits for completing the record vary from state to state. The Joint Commission on Accreditation of Healthcare Organizations (JCAHO) requires that acute care records be completed within 30 days of discharge; therefore, JCAHO-accredited facilities will have policies that fall within that time frame. If a state requires quicker completion, for example, 15 days, then the facility will have policies that fall within the shorter time frame.

There is some degree of controversy over the usefulness of requiring clinical staff to authenticate records after discharge, because the lack of authentication has no clinical significance for patient care. For example, if a physician forgot to sign a progress note but the patient has already been discharged, what possible impact could that signature have on the patient 30 days later? Any control function that would have been effected by the physician's signature has been lost. A small benefit may be obtained in the event that the entry is later questioned. These arguments, of course, are not relevant as long as licensure and accrediting agencies are still reviewing stored records for compliance with such standards. On the other hand, the argument has prompted some facilities to implement analysis procedures while the patient is still being treated. Called **concurrent analysis,** because it occurs concurrently with the patient's stay, such procedures better facilitate compliance with the intent of authentication rules and may speed postdischarge processing of the record.

It should be noted that a concurrent analysis can only look for deficiencies that will have occurred to that point. For example, if the chart is being reviewed 48 hours after admission, there should certainly be an H&P on the report, but no one would be looking for a discharge summary because the patient is still in the facility. If the analyst is reviewing the chart after the patient has gone home, this is called a *retrospective* or *postdischarge analysis.*

There is a great deal of benefit to be derived from obtaining other data elements after the patient's discharge. In some cases, there may have been a delay in obtaining a particular report. For example, the results of a radiology examination may have been communicated verbally to the physician; however, the typed report did not arrive at the nursing unit prior to discharge. Because the record is used primarily for communication, the lack of a report must certainly be resolved.

DEFICIENCY SYSTEM

Once the patient's record has been reviewed and it has been determined that there are missing elements, the corrective control procedure is initiated. The responsible party—that is, the individual who was responsible for preparing the report or for signing the note or report—is notified and is asked to complete the record. The most common deficiencies that exist in inpatient records are lack of a discharge summary, operative report, formal consultation report, and signatures. This process of completing missing elements in a record is called the **deficiency system.** In some facilities it is called the **incomplete system.** The deficiency system consists of procedures to record, report, and track deficiencies that have been identified. This system applies to retrospective analysis. Concurrent analysis is not generally recorded and tracked, because the clinician is expected to see the flag, whether manually or computer-generated, the next time he or she reviews the record.

Keeping track of "who did not do what" is a classic application for computerization and was one of the first HIM department functions to become computerized in many facilities. In order to track deficiencies, the name of the clinician and the type of the deficiency must be captured and recorded on the record, and it must be reported to the clinician. Manual systems of tracking may require multipart forms or rewriting deficiencies on separate forms. Performance of this task with a manual system engenders a healthy appreciation for computerization. Figure 4–3 illustrates a deficiency sheet, the form used to capture deficiencies.

When deficiencies are tracked manually, the analyst frequently records a separate slip for each physician, in duplicate, which can then be given to the clinician to inform him or her to complete the chart. When tracked in a computer, screens are generally organized by chart, with different lines or pages for each physician. In many cases, the deficiencies are first captured on a paper form and then transferred to the computerized tracking system. This is an example of a computer-assisted function, which we defined earlier. In either case, the analysis form is kept with the chart and enables clinicians to quickly reference their deficiencies and facilitates the distribution of the records to different clinicians. Incomplete charts are routinely maintained in a special area of the department in

<table>
<tr><td colspan="2">

Community Hospital
City, State

</td><td>

Frank Bright
ID #354792
Admission Date 05/02/00
Discharge Date 05/07/00

</td></tr>
</table>

DEFICIENCIES

PHYSICIAN:					
H&P					
Report					
Signature					
Discharge Summary					
Report					
Signature					
Face Sheet					
D/C Diagnosis & Procedures					
D/C Disposition					
Signature					
Orders					
Signature					
Operative Report					
Report					
Signature					

Partial list of deficiencies for which analysts review the record. Can you think of additional deficiencies?

FIGURE 4–3.
Deficiency sheet.

order to provide clinicians easy access to complete the charts. When a record seems complete, it is analyzed again to ensure that nothing was missed. If it has been completed, then it is passed to permanent storage. Incomplete records are returned to the incomplete chart area.

On a regular basis, typically weekly or biweekly, clinicians are reminded of their incomplete records. This report of incomplete records must be compiled at least monthly for accreditation purposes. JCAHO-accredited facilities must comply with maximum allowable incomplete record rules. Because acute care records must be completed within 30 days of discharge, all records incomplete after 30 days of discharge are considered **delinquent**. Acute care facilities are permitted maximum delinquent records equal to 50% of average monthly discharges. Therefore, a facility with an average of 2000 discharges per month would be allowed to have 1000 delinquent records. Specific deficiencies, such as missing H&Ps and operative reports, are very serious. Some facilities track these deficiencies as well to ensure 100% compliance with completing them on a timely basis (within 24 hours of admission for H&Ps and immediately after surgery for operative reports).

Each facility has its own policies and procedures for ensuring that records are completed, depending on the number of incomplete charts there are, the location of the HIM department, and the historical compliance of clinicians with record completion policies.

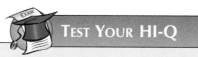

TEST YOUR HI-Q

Because physicians are often not actually employees of the facility at which they have privileges, what incentive do they have to complete their records?

Computerization lends itself to ensuring the completeness of charts simply because when data are entered into a computer, they can automatically be authenticated. However, this works best with orders, notes, nurses' recordings of vital signs, nursing assessments, and admission data. There still remains the issue of dictation of reports and progress notes, which are difficult at best to capture in the database format.

Coding

One of the topics that we are not discussing in detail in this book because you will be having an entire course in it is **coding.** Coding is the representation of diagnoses and procedures as alphanumeric values in order to capture them in a computer-based manner.

NOMENCLATURE AND CLASSIFICATION

There are two basic types of coding systems: nomenclature and classification. A **nomenclature** is a system of naming things. Scientific and technical professions typically have their own nomenclatures. In medicine, nomenclature is the naming of diseases and/or procedures. A number of different nomenclatures are in use in medicine. The most common nomenclature with which HIM professionals are generally familiar is Current Procedural Terminology (CPT). CPT is a nomenclature developed and maintained by the American Medical Association. It is used primarily in the representation of procedures that are performed on an outpatient basis, whether in a physician's office, clinic, ambulatory surgery facility, emergency department, or rehabilitation facility. Because it has been modified four times, CPT is often referred to as **CPT-4.**

CPT is part of a larger system of coding called the Health Care Financing Administration Common Procedure Coding System (HCPCS). HCPCS consists of

TABLE 4–6. Health Care Financing Administration Common Procedure Coding System	
	Description
Level I—CPT	Current Procedural Terminology manual is developed, maintained, and copyrighted by the American Medical Association. The CPT is the primary coding system used in the outpatient setting to code professional services provided to patients.
Level II—National codes	Approved and maintained jointly by the Alpha-Numeric Workgroup consisting of the Health Care Financing Administration, the Health Insurance Association of America, and the Blue Cross Blue Shield Association. Level II codes represent physician and nonphysician services that are not represented in the Level I codes.
Level III—Local codes	Developed by insurance companies for use at the local level. These codes represent physician and nonphysician services that are not represented in the Level I or Level II codes.

Adapted from Buck CJ: Step-by-Step Medical Coding, 3rd ed. Philadelphia, WB Saunders, 2000.

three levels. Level I is CPT, as we just mentioned. Level II is a group of codes, simply called HCPCS, that represent the procedures, services, and durable medical equipment that is not included in CPT. Level III is a group of codes that are devised by local insurance companies to represent services that are provided in their area but are not included in either of the other two levels. Level I and Level II codes are national codes represented in documents that can be obtained by anyone. Level III codes are specific to individual carriers and vary from carrier to carrier, as well as from state to state. Table 4–6 lists the levels of HCPCS.

In addition to nomenclatures, **classification** systems are very important in health care. The primary classification system used in health care delivery systems is the International Classification of Diseases (ICD). ICD is used worldwide and is in its Ninth Revision. In the United States, it has been modified (Clinical Modification, CM) to increase its level of detail. We usually refer to the system as **ICD-9-CM.** As we write this book, the health care industry and the federal government are considering the implementation of the Tenth Revision—**ICD-10**—which is already in use elsewhere in the world.

Two other classification systems should be mentioned also. One of them is the International Classification of Diseases–Oncology, or **ICD-O,** which is an oncology classification system used primarily by tumor registrars in reporting tumors as they are identified. The other one is the Diagnostic and Statistical Manual of Mental Disorders, **DSM-IV,** which is the classification system used in behavioral health. ICD-9-CM encompasses diagnoses and procedures, whereas ICD-O and DSM-IV involve only diagnoses. It is very likely that an HIM professional would use the ICD-O coding system if employed in tumor registry (see Chapter 9) and the DSM-IV if he or she works in the behavioral health profession. It is also important to know DSM-IV because behavioral health professionals often express their diagnoses in terms of the way DSM-IV is structured. Table 4–7 summarizes these coding systems.

TABLE 4–7. Coding Systems Used in the Health and Behavioral Professions	
ICD-9-CM	All diagnosis coding; inpatient procedure coding
CPT-4	Outpatient procedure coding
ICD-O	Oncology diagnosis codes
DSM-IV	Psychiatric diagnosis codes

Other coding systems are used for specialty settings, such as dental and veterinary settings. HIM professionals must be knowledgeable about the coding systems used in the setting in which they are employed.

INPATIENT CODING

There are three times during a patient's encounter with the facility that coding routinely occurs, all of which relate to the physician's development of the diagnosis: on admission, during the stay, and at discharge.

When a patient is being admitted, whether it is to an acute care, rehabilitation, or mental health facility, the patient states a reason for the admission. The physician also states the reason for admission when making the arrangements for admission. The physician's statement of the reason for admission is expressed as a diagnosis: the admitting diagnosis. At the time of admission a code is frequently assigned to the diagnosis so that computer-assisted tracking of the patient's stay can take place. If the admitting diagnosis is expressed only as words, the computer cannot match and track the patient's diagnosis with known lengths of stay and clinical treatment plans. The responsibility for coding an admitting diagnosis may rest with the patient registration department. However, if the patient registration department merely writes out the words, it is frequently left to the HIM department, after the patient is discharged, to assign a code to the admitting diagnosis.

Codes may also be assigned during the patient's stay in the facility. While the patient is in the facility there are a variety of reasons for HIM professionals to review the patient's record and assign codes to it. For example, computer matching and tracking of the patient's diagnosis is useful to help estimate the patient's length of hospital stay and thus can help control the delivery of health care. Coding that is done while the patient is still in the facility is called **concurrent coding.**

The most common point at which patient charts are coded by HIM professionals is after the patient's discharge. Coders then read the entire record and assign their codes. In acute care, rehabilitation, and mental health facilities, this postdischarge coding process generates the patient's bill. For more information about reimbursement, see Chapter 9. Because it is not the discharge of the patient that generates the bill to the payer but the coding, the function of assigning postdischarge codes has become critical. Even in a physician's office, the postvisit assignment of a code is critical to determining the reimbursement.

The importance of coding cannot be overemphasized. The capture of diagnosis and procedure codes enables facilities, payers, government agencies, researchers, and other users to analyze health data on a large scale. In the Uniform Ambulatory Care Data Set (UACDS) and the Uniform Hospital Discharge Data Set (UHDDS), the diagnoses and procedures are conveyed by code.

Retrieval

In Chapters 5 and 6 we discuss the storage and uses of health data. It is appropriate here to mention that in a paper environment, storage is a very critical function in the facility. The storage and retention of health records as well as the ability to retrieve those records efficiently is traditionally the responsibility of Health Information Technology (HIT) professionals.

Once the records are complete and they are filed, the necessity for retrieving them is based on a number of different issues. If no one ever needed to look at the record again after the patient went home, then we could probably discard it. But, as we've already mentioned, the health record itself is a critical communication tool and will be reviewed many times after the patient leaves the facility.

The function of retrieving the health record and providing it, or parts of it, to individuals that need it is commonly called *release of information* or *correspondence*. It is extremely important that HIT professionals understand who is allowed to receive a record, who is allowed to receive a copy of a record, and how to prepare a record for review. The function of releasing a record is discussed in Chapter 8 under confidentiality.

Abstracting

HIM professionals are uniquely suited to perform functions that require identification of the best source of data. Coding is one such function. **Abstracting** is another. Abstracting refers to a number of activities in which specific data are located in the record and transferred to another document. The necessity for abstracting arises for several different reasons, including data transfer, volume reduction, and analysis. First, if the data in a paper-based record are to be transmitted electronically, then the data must be transferred from the paper record to the electronic medium. The data are located in the record and copied into a computer via data entry. Sometimes, an interim step is performed in which the data are transcribed onto the form as they are located, then entered all at once into the computer. Diagnosis and procedure codes are often captured this way, as are surgical procedure dates and physician identification numbers.

Another reason for abstracting is to reduce the volume of data. There are often far more data in a health record than are needed for a particular user. For example, a patient keeping a file of his or her health records at home would not usually need an entire copy of the record. The patient may need only a copy of the discharge summary and/or the operative records. This data could be abstracted for the patient.

Finally, health data are frequently analyzed for research, performance improvement, and other uses. These activities are described in detail in Chapters 6 and 7; we want to emphasize here that HIM professionals are well suited by their training to be involved in these functions.

Tracking Records While Processing

While the patient is in the facility, the responsibility for maintaining his or her record rests with the clinical staff, particularly nursing. Traditionally, in a paper-based environment, once the patient is discharged, the HIM department assumes control. In a computer-based environment, there may be a number of departments that control aspects of the record. Because the record never actually "moves" from the computer, the physical location of the record is not in question. However, a paper-based record moves virtually every time an individual touches it. Therefore, keeping track of it requires control procedures.

Batch by Days

One way to keep track of records while processing is to batch the records together by day. In this manner, all records of discharges from April 15 would be gathered together and kept together while processing. These records would move as a group through assembly, analysis, and coding. After coding, they would be separated. Completed charts would move to the permanent file area; incomplete charts would move to the incomplete chart area. A *batch control form* lists the processing status of each record. This is particularly helpful if the record must be removed from the processing cycle for any reason.

Records may be removed from the processing cycle for a variety of reasons. The patient may have been readmitted, requiring review of the previous record. The record may need to be reviewed by any of a number of different departments—for example, quality review. When the record is removed from the processing cycle, a *batch control sheet* clearly highlights the status of the record and facilitates its return to the appropriate processing step.

Loose Sheets

In a paper-based record, some reports, test results, and other data have not been compiled with the record prior to the patient's discharge. While the patient is in the facility, it is the responsibility of the clinical staff, usually nursing, to compile these pages into the record. This is not an issue in a completely computer-based record. Because many reports and other data are delivered to the area that requested them, there may be some delay in rerouting the data to the HIM department. These noncompiled pages are frequently called **loose sheets.**

Loose sheets may arrive in the HIM department hours, days, or weeks after the patient has been discharged. By that time, the record has been processed and must be located. Handling the volume of loose sheets arriving on a daily basis may be a full-time job in a large facility. Sometimes, considerable creativity is required to ensure that the loose sheets are properly filed. Bear in mind that in an ambulatory care facility, most reports arrive loose and must be compiled. Regular, systematic sorting and distribution of loose sheets is necessary to ensure a complete record.

Efficiency

Health records must be processed on a timely basis that facilitates the many uses of the record, as discussed in Chapter 6. Common sense tells us that we must obtain the record in order to assemble it; we must assemble the record in order to analyze it; and we must analyze the record in order to facilitate coding. In some facilities, all personnel perform all of the steps. In other facilities, the chart is coded prior to analysis. Each facility processes the health record in the way that best suits its needs. For efficient processing, the record should be moved as little as possible, and each step should be performed in its entirety before the next step. Many facilities maintain a central staging area where records in process are kept between steps. This facilitates the location of records and the movement to the next processing step. Figure 4–2 illustrates the postdischarge processing flow.

Other Health Information Management Roles

HIM professionals are employed in a variety of roles and settings in the health care industry. In the remainder of this text, you are introduced to many activities and the professionals who perform them. As some of the traditional, paper-based activities are replaced by computer-based activities, exciting new opportunities arise for well-trained professionals with an eye to the future and a willingness to learn new skills. Opportunities in pharmaceuticals, insurance, and research are increasing, along with new roles in health care. We encourage you to explore the traditional as well as the new in planning your career in HIM.

Suggested Reading

Abdelhak M, Grostick S, Hanken MA, Jacobs E: Health Information: Management of a Strategic Resource, 2nd ed. Philadelphia, WB Saunders, 2001.

Andress AA: Manual of Medical Office Management. Philadelphia, WB Saunders, 1996.

Buck J: Step-by-Step Medical Coding, 3rd ed. Philadelphia, WB Saunders, 2000.

CHAPTER SUMMARY

Accuracy, validity, timeliness, and completeness are important data qualities. Prevention, detection, and correction of errors help to promote data of the best quality. HIM professionals are traditionally responsible for the postdischarge processing of health data. The focus of postdischarge processing of a health record is the retention of health data, that is, storage, security, and access.

After the patient's discharge, records must be obtained, assembled, analyzed, coded, and completed. Some data are abstracted for data transfer, volume reduction, and analysis. Once control over the health record has been obtained, the record must be tracked and controlled throughout the processing cycle. Ultimately, control passes to the permanent file area. HIM professionals are employed in these traditional functions and also in many other functions throughout the health care industry.

REVIEW QUESTIONS

1. List and explain the elements of data quality discussed in this chapter.

2. List, explain, and give examples of the three types of processing controls.

3. Explain the flow of postdischarge processing of health information.

4. List and explain the major functions of a health information management department.

5. Explain the principles and process flow of an incomplete record system.

6. Design a paper-based data collection device to capture medication administration. How would data collection differ in a computer-based device?

PROFESSIONAL PROFILE
Coder

My name is Shamees, and I am a coder in the health information management department at Community Medical Center. There are six coders in our department: four inpatient coders and two outpatient coders. In addition, there is a coding supervisor, who trains us and checks our work.

I started out as an assembler in the department. I assembled records for a year. I had to learn the postdischarge order of the record and how to file loose sheets. When an opening came up in the analysis section, I applied for it and was promoted. I enjoyed analysis, but I also began to understand the importance of the data contained in the records. I was really interested in the clinical data and decided to go to school to learn about coding, because coders work with the data.

Our local community college has a health information technology department and I enrolled in their Coding Certificate Program. I studied medical terminology, health record development and retention, anatomy and physiology, and disease pathology. I took several coding courses, learning ICD-9-CM and CPT. While I was a student, the coding supervisor allowed me to study completed records so that I could practice coding. When I finished the program, I was promoted to outpatient coder. I kept practicing inpatient coding with the completed records and I asked a *lot* of questions. Now, I code inpatient records most of the time and help out with the outpatient records.

After 2 years as an inpatient coder, I sat for and passed the Certified Coding Specialist (CCS) examination that is offered by the American Health Information Management Association. I am now a CCS! I really enjoy coding. It's challenging and interesting and there are a lot of opportunities for me as I learn more about clinical data and how to manage health information.

APPLICATION

Merging Expectations

You are the director of health information management at Community Hospital, a small hospital that has just merged with another hospital in your area. The facilities are roughly the same size. About half of the physicians at your facility also have privileges at the other facility. With some exceptions, both facilities have similar departments and services. Both facilities are partially computer-based and fortunately use the same computer vendor. Full computerization will not take place for at least 5 years. The administration of the two facilities would like to standardize the data collection with the intent of reducing the cost of forms and facilitating communication between the two facilities. As the senior director, you have been asked to coordinate this effort. What issues do you think should be addressed first? Who will you ask to assist in the project? What impact does this standardization project have on the health information management department?

Unit Two

STORAGE, USES, and REPORTING of HEALTH INFORMATION

5

Storage of
Health Information

Chapter Outline

The Paper Explosion

Master Patient Index
Manual Master Patient Index
Computerized Master Patient Index
Retention of Master Patient Index

Filing
Computer Files
Physical Files
Identification of Physical Files
   Alphabetic Filing
   Unit Numbering
   Serial Numbering
   Serial–Unit Numbering
   Family Unit Numbering
Filing Methods
   Alphabetic Filing
   Straight Numeric Filing
   Terminal-Digit Filing
   Middle-Digit Filing
Computer Indexing
Record Retention
   Retention Policy
   Facility Closure
Filing Furniture
   File Cabinets
   Open Shelves
   Compressible Shelves
   Revolving File System
File Rooms

Alternative Storage Methods
Microfilm
   Microfilm Equipment
   Document/Optical Imaging
On-site Storage
Off-site Storage
Selection of Storage Method

Chart Locator Systems
Manual Systems
Computerized Systems

Security of Health Information
Disaster Planning
Security from Fire
Security from Water Damage
Security from Theft or Tampering
Destruction of Health Information
   Restoring Information Lost Inadvertently

Suggested Reading

Web Site

Chapter Summary

Review Questions

Professional Profile

Application

By the end of this chapter, the student should be able to:

- Explain the use of the master patient index.

- Determine whether a patient has a previous health record at the facility.

- Compare and contrast numbering systems for identification of patient records.

- Compare and contrast filing systems for patient records.

- File health records appropriately according to the file system used by the facility.

- Maintain accuracy of filing methods.

- Identify the alternative storage system best suited for a particular health care facility when it is running out of file space for records.

- Determine the appropriate file space for a given set of circumstances.

- Given a specific type of health information, determine the retention schedule.

- Identify ways to ensure the physical security of health information.

- Explain a chart locator system.

Vocabulary

chart locator system	index	record retention schedule
computer-based patient record	master patient index	scanner
computerized patient record	microfiche	serial numbering
family unit numbering	microfilm	serial–unit numbering
file folder	middle-digit filing	straight numeric filing
	optical disk	terminal-digit filing
	outguide	unit numbering

Storage of health records is critical to the management of health information. Health information management (HIM) professionals systematically collect and organize each patient's health information to create a timely, accurate, and complete record. Health information is vital to the patient, health care provider, and community; therefore, it must be stored in a secure, accessible, organized environment. The patient's health record must be retained for the continuation of patient care and for reimbursement, accreditation, potential litigation, research, and education purposes. HIM departments demonstrate excellence by providing health information on request to authorized users. To provide health information, we must first be able to locate the information requested. To locate patient health information, we must ensure the systematic organization of all health record files.

The health data (collected on forms) for each patient are organized in the patient's health record. The record may be in a paper file or computer file. This chapter explores issues in health record storage including file identification, filing systems, filing furniture, and security of the file environment.

The Paper Explosion

Physicians, clinics, hospitals, and other health care facilities provide health care to hundreds or even thousands of patients each week. The number of health records that can accumulate is staggering.

HIT Bit

Imagine that a busy clinic sees 75 patients each day and is open just 5 days a week.

$$75 \text{ patients} \times 5 \text{ days} = 375 \text{ records per week}$$

$$375 \text{ records per week} \times 52 \text{ weeks} = 19{,}500 \text{ records annually}$$

If each record is only one sheet of paper, then 19,500 records could amount to approximately four cases of paper.

How many records would this facility have in storage after 2 years? The answer, of course, is 39,000 records (19,500 × 2). How would you locate a record for a patient who was seen in the clinic last year and is coming for a return visit, if you had to look through 39,000 records?

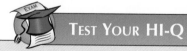

TEST YOUR HI-Q

How many records would this facility have in storage after 5 years?

In Chapter 3 we mentioned the necessity of recording patient data for communication. Previous patient data may communicate to a physician important information that is necessary for a patient's current treatment. What happens if the physician cannot locate the patient's health record from the last visit? What if the notes from the previous visit compared with the present information reflect that the patient has had significant weight loss? This information may be important in the care and treatment of the patient. For example, it could change the patient's dosage of a particular medication. A patient's health care can depend on the review of previous health records. Therefore, it is important to make sure that once a patient's health data are recorded, organized, and analyzed, the health record is stored in a way that allows the information to be retrieved when the patient returns to the facility for follow-up care. Organized storage of health records begins with appropriate identification of each patient's record. Let's begin with a discussion of health record identification.

HIT Bit

Other reasons that a health record may be retrieved include

- A physician specialist may review a patient's record before providing care
- Insurance companies request copies of reports prior to paying the claim (reimbursement)
- Facilities review their own records to assess quality of care
- Accrediting bodies review records to evaluate compliance with standards
- Litigation—lawyers present a health record during a lawsuit to represent their client
- Research—health records may be used to investigate disease trends

Master Patient Index

The **master patient index (MPI)** is the key to locating a health record in the HIM department. The MPI contains information on every patient admitted to the facility. The MPI is the primary tool for identifying each file for all patients who have been seen at a particular facility. HIM departments use the MPI as the source of information correlating the patient to his or her health record file. An MPI may be a manual system that is kept on index cards organized in a file cabinet in alphabetic order, or it may be a computerized system.

The information contained in the MPI is first collected during the patient registration process. During registration the patient provides demographic information to the facility (see Chapter 3). This information is used to individually identify each patient within that health care facility and initiates the patient's health record. In the process of creating the patient record, an identification number is assigned (the *medical record number [MR#]*) and correlated to the patient's health record.

To envision an MPI, think of the catalog index at your local library. To locate a book in your library, you must first access the catalog to determine whether the book is available in the library. If it is available, then you must know the catalog number specific to that book. The library catalog index correlates the book to its catalog number. This allows you to locate the book on the shelf in the library, because the books are filed by catalog number (Fig. 5–1).

To relate this example to health information, each health care facility has an MPI. The MPI is a list of all patients who have had encounters at the facility. When looking for the health record of a particular patient, you must first know that the patient was previously seen at the facility, and then know the patient's file identification number. You must use the MPI to obtain this information. The MPI correlates the patient to the facility's medical record number to identify the patient's health record. Figure 5–2 lists recommended and optional contents of

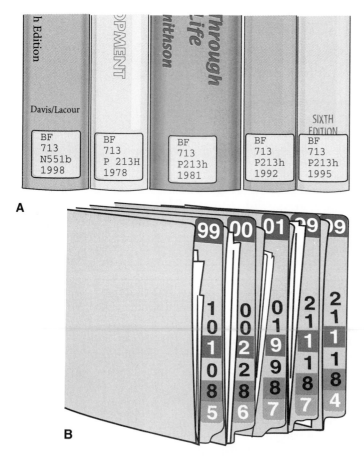

Figure 5–1.

Books with catalog numbers *(A)* and file folders with medical record numbers *(B)*.

CONTENTS OF A MASTER PATIENT INDEX

RECOMMENDED DATA ELEMENTS

- Patient's name
- Alias/previous name
- Address
- Date of birth*
- Social Security number
- Gender
- Race
- Ethnicity
- Medical record number, hospital identification number
- Patient's account number
- Admission date(s)*
- Discharge date(s)*
- Type of service for the encounter
- Patient disposition

OPTIONAL DATA ELEMENTS

- Marital status
- Physician
- Telephone number
- Mother's maiden name
- Place of birth
- Advance directive and surrogate decision making
- Organ donor status
- Emergency contact
- Allergies/reactions
- Problem list

* When capturing dates, it is important to record the year as four numbers, i.e., MMDDYYYY or YYYYMMDD.

FIGURE 5-2.

Contents of a master patient index. (From AHIMA Practice Brief No. 433.)

an MPI. Notice that the information contained in the MPI is a combination of the demographic, financial, and clinical data.

Each patient is entered only once in the MPI. All visits for a particular patient are listed in the MPI under the patient's name. It is extremely important to prevent duplication of patients within the MPI because it may cause confusion and delay when retrieving patient files.

Manual Master Patient Index

In a manual MPI system, each patient who is registered in the health care facility has an index card in the MPI located in the HIM department. As patients are registered in the facility, the HIM department is notified of the admission: The notification can be a copy of the face sheet, a computer printout of the admission, or the admit log. To locate a record for the patient, the HIM clerk researches the MPI to see whether the patient has been treated at the facility before.

HIT BIT

Do you know how a facility distinguishes a new patient from an old patient?

- *New:* New to the facility as a patient; not registered or treated at the facility on a prior occasion.
- *Old:* The patient is a returning patient; therefore, he or she has an MPI card and has been registered or treated previously in the facility. The new visit is added to the patient's existing MPI card.

An MPI card is created for each new patient registered. If the patient has been treated at the facility on a previous occasion, the patient's MPI card is retrieved from the card file. The MPI card is reviewed to make sure that the patient's information is correct, and the new admission information is added (admit date, type of service, account number for that visit, attending physician, discharge date). The MPI must be updated each time the patient has an admission to the health care facility. Figure 5–3 illustrates a manual MPI card.

HIT BIT

A manual MPI system does not allow you to capture all of the recommended data elements, because it is limited by the size of the index card. The manual system will not typically have all of the items listed in Figure 5–2.

The advantages of a manual MPI system are that it can be inexpensive, implemented quickly, and accessible regardless of energy supply to the facility, unless the MPI cards are stored in a revolving file system (see Filing Furniture). One disadvantage of the manual MPI system is that the amount of information for each patient in the MPI is limited by the size of the index card. The manual index is also inefficient if the index cards are labeled incorrectly or if they are misfiled, and it can be accessed only from the HIM department.

Last Name, First Name, Middle Initial		Date of Birth ___ / ___ / ___	Medical Record #
Address		Phone # (___) ___ - ___	Married ___	Death ___
City, State	Zip Code	Social Security # ___ - ___ - ___	
Gender ___			
Race ___	Financial Class ___		
Admit Date	Discharge Date	Service	Physician	Patient Account #

FIGURE 5–3.

MPI card in a manual system.

HIT BIT

It is important to note that when the MPI file cabinet is full, the HIM department may need to remove, or purge, MPI cards and store them in another location or format, discussed later in the chapter under MPI retention. How does a purge begin? The department must set criteria for which MPI cards to remove from the file cabinet. The decision may be made to remove all cards for patients who are deceased. It is important to inform all facility employees and to update the department's policy and procedure manual (discussed in Chapter 10) when an alternative storage site exists for MPI cards. Employees will need to know the criteria used for MPI card removal. This facilitates locating old charts and ensures that new numbers are not assigned to patients who are readmitted to the facility.

Computerized Master Patient Index

A computerized MPI is often more flexible than a manual system. It captures more patient information and can be accessed from areas outside the HIM department, such as the emergency room or patient registration. A computerized MPI system uses computer software to capture and store patient identification and admission information. The computerized MPI software is typically one feature of a larger computer system or is interfaced with other computer systems in the health care facility.

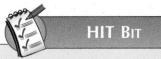

HIT Bit

A computer *interface* allows two different computer systems or software products to exchange information.

As stated previously, the facility begins collecting identification information on the patient at the time of registration. Information entered into a computerized MPI creates a demographic history for each patient. At registration, the admitting clerk searches the MPI history files to determine if the patient has been treated at the facility on a previous occasion. If the patient is new, a new history is created by entering the information (as prompted by the system) listed in Figure 5–2. If the patient has been treated at the facility on a previous occasion, the admitting clerk identifies the patient's history and reviews it to ensure that all of the information is correct. For example, if the patient's address has changed, this information must be updated in the patient's MPI history file. If his or her insurance company has changed, this information is also updated. The new admission information is also entered into the MPI, that is, admit date, type of service, account number for that visit, and attending physician. Figure 5–4 shows computerized MPI screens.

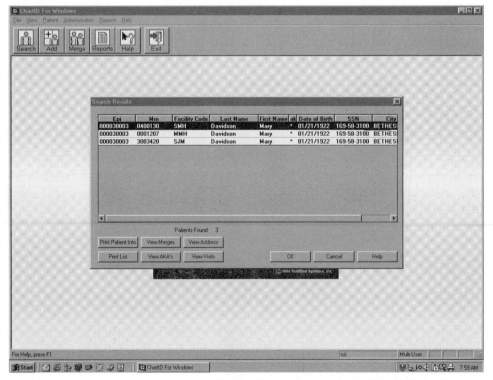

Figure 5–4.

MPI screens in a computerized system. (Courtesy of SoftMed Systems, Inc. Bethesda, Md.)

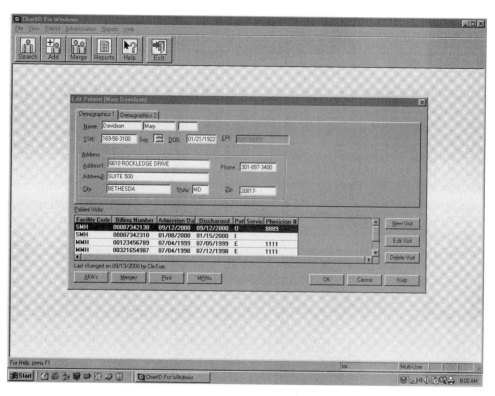

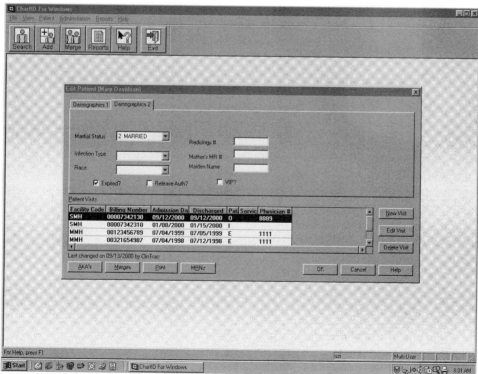

FIGURE 5–4.

Continued

There are advantages and disadvantages to a computerized MPI. The computerized MPI provides the opportunity to store more patient identification information for each admission, for example, patient financial class, marital status, social security number, and "also known as" (AKA) functions, which link the patient to another name resulting from divorce or marriage or to a pseudonym. More information is stored in a smaller space combined with greater search capabilities that can access possible matches for a name using phonetics, date of birth (DOB), Social Security number (SS#), or age. Computerization also allows the MPI to be linked to other departments within the facility, for example, the emergency department or the patient registration area. A computerized MPI system may be more expensive than a manual system, and uninterrupted access to the MPI requires a connection to an emergency power supply. However, after consideration most HIM departments find that the benefits of a computerized MPI far outweigh the disadvantages.

HIT BIT

Phonetic searching is the function in a computer system that queries the database for all names that sound like the name that has been entered. For example, all forms of the name Steven sound the same, even though they are spelled differently. With a phonetic feature the computer can search for all sound-alike spellings of the name, such as Stephen, Stefan, Stephan, and Steven.

Retention of Master Patient Index

The MPI must be retained permanently. This index is extremely important in the everyday operations of a health care facility and the HIM department. It must not be destroyed. In a numeric filing system, you must know the medical record number to retrieve the patient's health record. The MPI is the easiest way to access the patient's medical record number.

When a facility implements a computerized MPI, it must decide what to do with the manual system. Because the information in an MPI is never destroyed, the facility must consider how to convert the information from the manual file into the computerized system. When a computerized MPI is installed, the data on the manual MPI cards are entered into the computerized system. This creates computer access to all MPI information. HIM professionals should monitor the accuracy of the manual MPI conversion. If the information on even one patient or encounter is omitted or entered incorrectly, the MPI is not accurate. The omission or error may cause great difficulty when accessing patient records. Maintenance of the original MPI information secures the validity of the data in the computerized MPI and provides a reference if a discrepancy arises in a patient's file that originated prior to the conversion. The ability to reference the original MPI cards allows the correction of any discrepancies caused by an error or omission. In this type of conversion, the facility should consider storing the manual MPI in the original format or microfilming the original MPI cards for future reference. The minor inconvenience caused by storing the manual system can prevent serious problems with record discrepancies in the future.

HIT Bit

During a conversion, if the manual MPI information is not entered into the computerized system, then the manual card index must be checked each time a patient is admitted to be certain that the patient does not have a previous record.

TEST YOUR HI-Q

When you receive a request for an old patient health record, what is the first step to take in locating the record?

TEST YOUR HI-Q

What should you do if you are unable to access the computerized MPI? How can you locate a medical record number to find a patient's record?

Filing

Computer Files

In the computerized record environment, patient documentation may be computer-based, computerized, or a combination of both. In summary, the **computer-based patient record** is the patient's information in a compilation of data elements, health information, and various media forms, all connected for fast access to patient information. The **computerized patient record** is a digital form of the patient's paper record. In the computerized format the paper record is scanned into a computer system so that the data on the paper documents are digitally stored in the computer for future use. In both of these file formats the patient's health record is stored in the computer with the capability to retrieve the information by searching the patient's name, medical record number, encounter number, and various other methods, as discussed earlier in the computerized MPI scenario. When the paper record is scanned into the computer system, the images are *indexed* or *named* so that they can be retrieved at a later date. The creation of an accurate **index** facilitates future retrieval of the images. By correctly identifying (indexing/naming) the document for each patient, the computer system is able to locate the correct image when you perform a search. For example, when you scan a document into a computer using a standard flatbed scanner, you must name the file to identify the information stored. Because you name the file when you save it, the next time you access the file index, you are able to identify the contents without opening each file. Therefore, indexing in the computer environment facilitates future retrieval.

What happens if the image is indexed by the wrong patient's name? How do you find the missing images of a record in the computer? All computer systems have various search methods to aid in the retrieval of the images. Additional methods to locate missing files require searching the discharge list to identify other patient records that were indexed on the same day. When records are scanned into a computer system, they are typically scanned in groups or batches. A typical group or batch of records would be one day of discharges. Therefore, looking through the images of all the patients' records scanned the same day may retrieve the missing image. Once the missing image is identified, it is renamed and indexed appropriately.

Physical Files

In the paper record environment, health data captured during the patient's stay are organized on appropriate forms, for example, the face sheet, history and physical (H&P), nursing admission assessment, laboratory reports, or progress notes. In order to file these forms in the correct patient file folder, the patient's name and identifying medical record number must be labeled on each form. This can be accomplished several different ways: by using an addressograph, by affixing printed labels, or by hand-writing the data.

HIT BIT

Prior to computerized technology, health care forms were manually stamped with the patient's name, medical record number, account number, and room number by using an *addressograph*. The addressograph is a machine that uses a plastic card imprinted with the patient's identification information. The imprint on the card resembles the name imprinted on a credit card. The plastic card is put into the addressograph machine, the patient's forms are placed one at a time on top of the card, and an ink roller is passed over the paper and card to mark the patient's information on each piece of the record. The addressograph card contains enough information to identify the patient so that the forms can be placed in the correct patient record. Although this system is still used, technology has replaced it in many facilities with printed labels, computer-generated forms, and bar code technology.

All of the forms for each patient are assembled (see Chapter 4) in a file folder. The **file folder** is the container used to store the forms that document the patient's health information. A few housekeeping rules and recommendations apply to the file folder and its design and labeling.

The file folder must be durable to protect the forms containing the patient's health information. File folders are available in many different weights and sizes, varying from very thin (onionskin) to thick (card stock). The heavier the weight, the more durable the folder. The HIM department must be sure that file folders are strong enough to handle daily use. A file folder that is accessed repeatedly shows wear over time. The file folder must also expand wide enough to allow for the thickness of the patient's record. In an acute care environment for a patient stay of 5 days, the record may be 1 inch thick. Therefore, the folder should be heavier than the standard manila folder to withstand the weight of the forms and the frequency of use. Files that are thin (physician's office records) may be adequately stored in lighter-weight folders.

A fastener on the inside of the folder is used to secure the forms in the folder. The fastener usually has two prongs and may be positioned in several different places within the folder, for example, on the top right side or on the inside right (see Fig. 5–17). The fastener keeps the record assembled in the appropriate order and prevents pages from falling out of the folder.

Health record folders commonly have a tab that protrudes from the edge of the folder. The tab may be on the top or on the side of the file folder. The tab is used to label the folder for easy recognition within the file cabinet or on the shelf. Top tabs are used for folders filed in a file cabinet, that is, for alphabetic filing. Side tabs are used to label the patient's medical record number filed on shelves, and they may even include a bar code, the patient's name, date of service, volume numbers, year-band labels, etc. The medical record number labeled on the side tab of a folder may also be color coded. Normally colors are assigned to each alphabetic or numeric character. This easily identifies a section of files by the colors associated with the number or alphabetic character. Color coding aids in accurate filing because misfiled folders are easily recognized. Figure 5–5 shows the different labeling styles for file folders.

Health record file folders must be clearly labeled with appropriate patient identification information, such as the patient's name and medical record number, if applicable. Clear labeling of the patient's file folder is important for accurate filing and storage. Use ink or marker, not pencil. The patient's name should be printed on the outside of the folder; do NOT use script or fancy handwriting. If applicable, the medical record number should also be printed on the outside of the folder.

When a patient's record is too thick to fit into the file folder, or when the patient has multiple visits, several file folders may exist for that one patient. Labeling each of the patient's folders by the volume number identifies how many file folders exist for the patient.

HIM professionals also use colored file folders to differentiate one type of file from another. Color coding of a patient's file folder can identify the type of documents contained in the file folder; for example, outpatient records may be in a folder of a color different from that of inpatient files. The color of file folders may also indicate the record type, such as skilled nursing facility, acute care, same-day surgery, or rehabilitation, or it can be coordinated in some way with the medical record number.

File folders can also contain information about the facility to which the files belong, for example, "Property of Southern Hospital, CONFIDENTIAL. If found please return this record to Southern Hospital, 615 Medical Center Blvd., Orange, Texas 77777."

The following is a list of things to consider when choosing file folders for a health care facility:

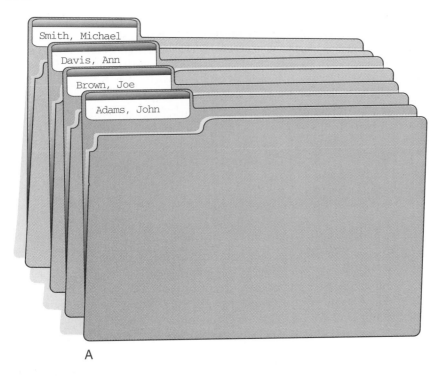

Smith, Michael

Davis, Ann

Brown, Joe

Adams, John

A

FIGURE 5–5.

File folder labeling showing top *(A)* and side *(B)* tabs.

- How often will the folder be accessed and handled by file clerks? For example, do the patients typical to the facility have repeated visits requiring retrieval of the old record for patient care?
- Are the records in the facility thick or thin? For thick files be sure to purchase a file folder that expands wide enough to contain and cover the documents in the record.
- Choose a fastener to secure the forms inside the folder. Be sure to have the fastener in the correct position for the documents within the folder. Make sure that the fastener does not require holes to be punched through the patient information.
- Consider identifying the facility to which the file belongs on the cover of the file. Other information that can be printed on the file folder includes the address of the facility, a confidentiality statement, and a place to highlight patient allergies.
- The folder should accommodate labeling for the file system used in the facility—for example, patient's name, discharge date, and medical record number.
- Be sure that the tab is in the correct place; end tabs are used in shelf filing and top tabs are used in cabinet filing. Also be sure the tab is large enough to accommodate the medical record number or the patient's name.

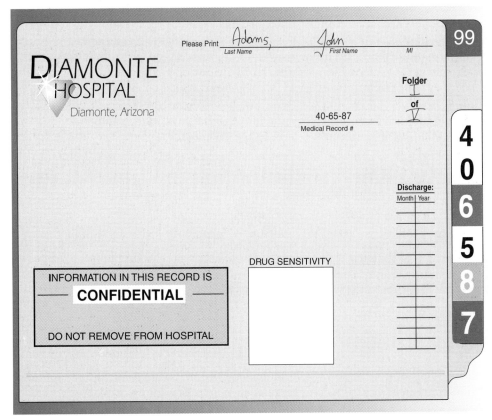

B

FIGURE 5-5.

Continued

HIT BIT

Some health care environments may retain patient health records in manila folders, binders, envelopes, pocket expandable files, and the like.

Identification of Physical Files

For easy identification and filing, the file folder containing the patient's health information is labeled with alphabetic or numeric characters. In a small health care facility or for physician's office records, the file folder may be identified alphabetically with the patient's name. In a large health care facility the medical record number is used to identify the patient's health record file. Medical record numbers vary in length: Some are only six digits, others are eight or nine digits, and some may even be longer. Currently, the number of digits or type of number used by a facility is not mandated. However, accreditation agencies such as the Joint Commission on Accreditation of Healthcare Organizations (JCAHO) require facilities to use a system that ensures timely access to patient information when requested for patient care or other authorized use. Additionally, the facility chooses the system (alphabetic or numeric) that best suits its purpose for identification and storage of patient files. We discuss five types of health record identification: *alphabetic filing, unit numbering, serial numbering, serial–unit numbering,* and *family unit numbering.* As we discuss these identification methods, keep in mind that (except for alphabetic filing) a numbering (identification) system is not the same as a filing method (discussed later in the chapter).

HIT Bit

Medical record numbers are assigned by the facility in which the patient is registered to receive health care. Patients do not have the same medical record number for their files when receiving care at another facility. However, if a patient receives care in a large multifacility health care system, owned and operated by the same organization, patients may be assigned a system-wide medical record number, one that is used in all the facilities.

ALPHABETIC FILING

A typical setting for filing of patient records in alphabetic order is a small physician's office, clinic, home health care facility, or nursing home. The patient's file folders are labeled using the patient's name with the last name followed by the first name. The name *John Adams* converted to file in the alphabetic system becomes *Adams, John.* File folders are arranged on the shelf in alphabetic order, beginning with the patient's last name (Fig. 5–6). In the alphabetic system in which records are filed in a cabinet, the folder is labeled with the patient's name, preferably on the top tab. For those records stored on a shelf, the patient's name is color coded on the side tab, often using the first three letters of the patient's last name. The records are still filed alphabetically, but the labeling is different.

Alphabetic filing works well in health care environments where the number of patient visits or records is relatively low. The file folders are easy to label, and pulling a patient's file can be accomplished if the patient's name is known. Alphabetic filing does not require an additional system, such as the MPI, to correlate patient names and numbers to identify the file folder.

Problems can arise when two patients have the same name. Common names like Michael Smith, José Cruz, or Ann Davis require careful attention to be certain the correct patient record is found. Think about the names Michael, Joe, and Ann. How many other ways may these names be identified? Mike, Michael, Jo, Joe, Joseph, José, Josef, Ann, Anne, Annie, and Annette are common versions of Michael, José, and Ann. When duplicate names occur in an alphabetic filing system, procedures must be specified to further organize the records by the patient's middle name, by titles (Jr., Sr., III), or by the patient's date of birth (DOB). Common rules for alphabetic filing are as follows:

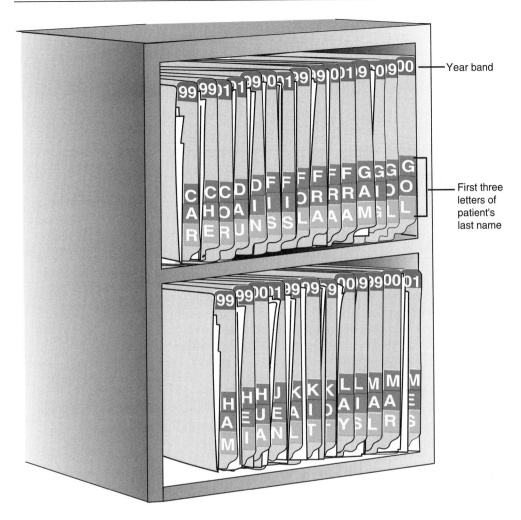

FIGURE 5–6.

File folders in alphabetic order.

1. Personal names are filed last name first; for example, the name John Adams is filed by *Adams* first, followed by *John:* Adams, John. The first name is followed by the middle initial (e.g., *E*) or name if necessary: Adams, John E.
2. All punctuation and possessives are ignored. Disregard commas, hyphens, apostrophes. In the last name, prefixes, foreign articles, and particles are combined with the name following it, omitting spaces (e.g., *De Witt* is filed as *dewitt*).
3. Abbreviations, nicknames, and shortened names are filed as written (e.g., Wm, Bud, Rob).
4. Suffixes are considered after the middle name or initial. Titles are considered after suffixes. Royal or religious titles follow the given name and surname; the title is indexed last.

TABLE 5–1. Advantages and Disadvantages of Alphabetic Filling	
Advantages	**Disadvantages**
Easy to learn.	Illegible handwriting may cause problems with filing.
Does not require additional cross-reference to locate a patient chart.	Space within the popular letters of the alphabet can fill quickly.
Works well in smaller facilities.	Can be inefficient for a large facility with a large patient population.
	Many alternative spellings of names.

5. When identical names occur, consider the date of birth for filing order and proceed chronologically.

Patients' files must be clearly labeled. It is important to print clearly when labeling the patient's file folder. This is not an occasion for fancy script or calligraphy. Illegible or fancy handwriting may cause a file folder to be misfiled. Table 5–1 lists the advantages and disadvantages of alphabetic filing.

Space is a common problem in the alphabetic filing system. The shelves or cabinets that hold the files of patients' names beginning with common letters become full very quickly, so be sure to allow adequate file space for these letters of the alphabet. Filing in a section that is full of records is difficult and requires shifting of the records for further filing. Alphabetic filing systems can become inefficient in a facility that serves a large population with a high volume of patient records.

Another consideration with this system is the spelling of patient names. Sometimes even the easiest names are misspelled. In an alphabetic file system, a folder labeled incorrectly because of misspelling will not be filed correctly on the shelf. When the HIM employee attempts to locate the patient's folder, efforts will involve searching for a misspelled, misfiled record. A review of your community's phone book provides examples of the many different ways a last name may be spelled. If you are unsure of the spelling of the patient's name, ask for identification (driver's license) to clarify the spelling.

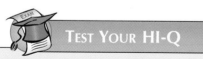

TEST YOUR HI-Q

File the following names in alphabetic order:

P. B. Josh
Hannah Curelle
Ginger Dugas
Lauren McIntyre
Beth Katerina Von Amberg
Sister Gabrielle Brown

Drew B. LaPeu
Cecelia Lower
Wm. Bill Matata
Amanda Modelle
Aubrey Bartolo, III
Brett Thomasse, Jr.

UNIT NUMBERING

In a **unit numbering** system, a patient receives the same medical record number for each admission to the facility. Therefore, the numeric identification of each individual patient is always the same. For example, if a person is born in a facility that uses unit numbering, at birth (admission) the patient is assigned a number (e.g., MR# 001234). Any subsequent admissions of this patient to the facility would use the same medical record number. In a unit numbering identification system, the patient's medical record number remains the same, in that facility, throughout the lifetime of the patient. Medical record numbers are not shared and are not reused after a patient dies.

Let's present a scenario: Molly Brabant was born at Diamonte Hospital on January 1, 2001. At birth, Molly is assigned MR# 001234. Her birth record is filed in a folder identified with the MR# 001234. At age 7, Molly returns to the same facility to have a tonsillectomy. Molly's new records are stored in the same folder identified as MR# 001234. Any subsequent admissions, for example, a hip replacement later in life, are filed under the same identification number (Fig. 5–7).

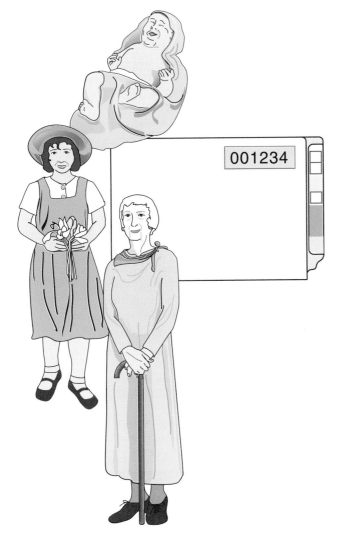

FIGURE 5–7.
Unit medical record number.

Serial Numbering

In a **serial numbering** system, each time a patient has an encounter at the facility a new medical record number is assigned. In this type of system, the patient's file folders containing the health record for each encounter are not filed in the same folder. Therefore, the records are not located together on the file shelf.

Using the previous scenario in a serial numbering system, at birth Molly is assigned MR# 001234. However, when she returns at age 7 for a tonsillectomy, a new number, MR# 112233, is assigned (Fig. 5–8). In this system, Molly's records are not stored in the same folder, and they are not located near each other on the file shelf. Molly now has two separate folders containing her health record, and she receives a third medical record number and a new folder when she visits the facility for a hip replacement in later years.

Serial–Unit Numbering

A **serial–unit numbering** system is a combination of the first two numbering systems discussed. In this system, the patient receives a new medical record number each time he or she comes into a facility. The difference is that each time the patient receives health care, the old records are brought forward and filed with the most recent visit, under a new medical record number. This system requires a cross-reference system from the old medical record number to the new number in order to locate records. To cross-reference, the MPI must be updated so that each encounter reflects the corresponding medical record number, and a file guide is placed in the old file location referring HIM employees to look for the current medical record number to locate the patient's health record.

In the serial–unit numbering system, Molly is assigned MR# 001234 at birth, and on return 7 years later for a tonsillectomy she is assigned a new number, MR# 112233. When Molly returns for the tonsillectomy, the birth record (MR# 001234) is retrieved from its place in the files and combined with the file folder numbered MR# 112233. A cross-reference can be set up by placing an outguide (see Fig. 5–18) in place of the old MR# 001234 to indicate that the record is now filed at MR# 112233 (Fig. 5–9). Molly's records are transferred and cross-referenced a third time when Molly has a hip replacement later in life.

Family Unit Numbering

In health care settings where it is common for an entire family to visit a physician or clinic, an entire family's records may be contained in one file folder. This family file is then identified by assigning one medical record number to the entire family (father/husband, mother/wife, and children). This system is called **family unit numbering.** The family unit number requires that within the family unit number, each family member receives his or her own modifier number, which is attached to the family number. The modifier is a number attached to the MR# using a hyphen. Each member of the family can be identified by a modifier associated with his or her position in the family: head of household,

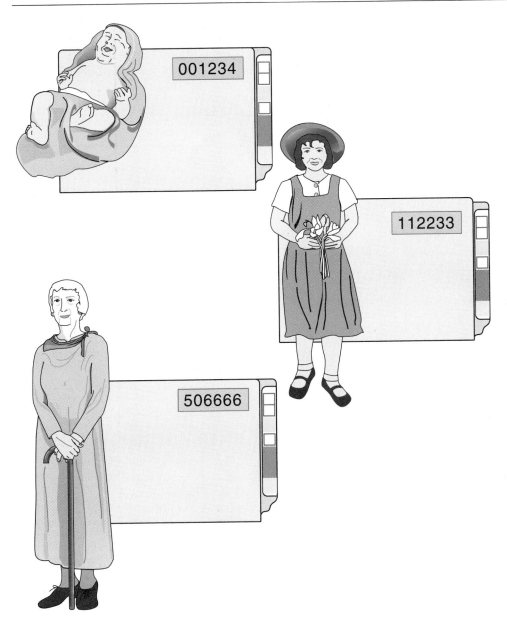

FIGURE 5–8.
Serial medical record number.

01; spouse, 02; first born, 03; second born, 04; etc. With this system all of the family members' records may be contained in one file folder. If you think about all members of a family having the same last name, and then being identified individually by their first names, you may see the similarity to family unit numbering.

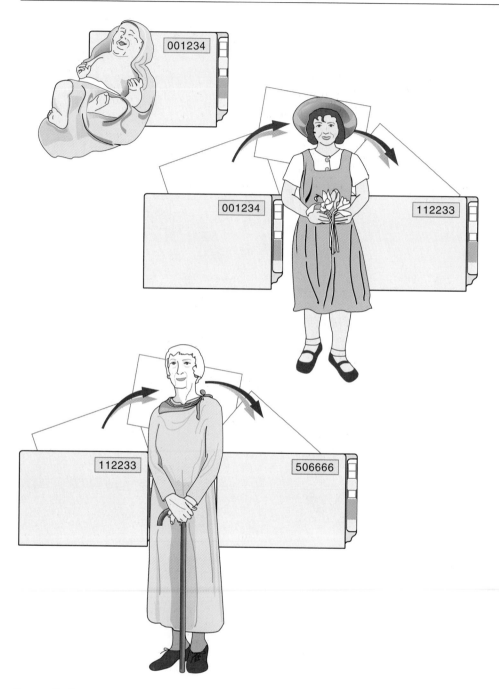

FIGURE 5–9.
Serial–unit medical record number.

TABLE 5–2. Family Unit Numbering			
Family member	**Family number**	**Modifier**	**Patient number**
John Smith	123456	01	123456-01
Mary Smith	123456	02	123456-02
Molly Smith	123456	03	123456-03
Tommy Smith	123456	04	123456-04

In our example, Molly's family unit number is MR# 123456. At birth Molly, being the first-born child, is assigned MR# 123456-03. Molly's mother has MR# 123456-02. The last two numbers after the hyphen indicate to which family member the record belongs. Table 5–2 provides an example of family unit numbering.

This system is beneficial in a small clinic or physician's office setting where clinical and financial records are combined for claims processing. There are potential problems with this numbering system. Families change, they undergo divorces, and grown children marry into other names. When members of the family divorce, die, marry, or remarry, the medical records for those patients must be renumbered. This process can be tedious and time-consuming. Even in a family unit numbering system, the facility is responsible for maintaining the confidentiality of each patient's health information. Safeguards must be taken to ensure that husbands and wives are allowed access to each other's information only with appropriate authorization (see Chapter 8). Likewise, procedures should exist to safeguard the confidentiality of a child's information after the legal age of majority.

Each facility should examine the positive as well as negative aspects of each numbering identification system in order to choose the system that allows efficient delivery of health care for the patient. The system should have a positive impact on both employee and facility productivity. Table 5–3 summarizes the advantages and disadvantages of each numbering system.

TABLE 5–3. Advantages and Disadvantages of Numbering Systems		
System	**Advantages**	**Disadvantages**
Unit	All patient records can be located under one number.	Filing of all encounters in one folder can cause problems with incomplete records.
Serial	Each admission is filed in a single folder.	Retrieving all the records for one patient involves going to multiple places in the files.
Serial–unit	Each admission has a unique number, but they are all filed with the most recent.	Time-consuming.
Family unit	Records are combined for clinical and financial processing of claims.	Confidentiality can be compromised; divorce, remarriage, etc. complicate this system.

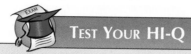

Using your knowledge of how numbers/identifiers are assigned to patient files in each of the following numbering systems, answer the questions below.

Numbering System	Next MR# Assigned
Unit	123456
Serial	234567
Serial–unit	345678
Family unit	456789

Scenario: Green Oak Hospital uses a serial numbering system to identify patient health records. Jane Creason is admitted to Green Oak facility for repair of a broken ankle. On a previous admission to Green Oak for a tonsillectomy, Jane was assigned MR# 012345.

1. What number will be assigned to Jane for the broken ankle admission?
2. If Green Oak uses a unit numbering system, what medical record number would be assigned for the broken ankle admission?

Filing Methods

Now that we know how medical records are numbered we can discuss how those numbers are used to file the records. Filing is the process of organizing the health record folders on a shelf, in a file cabinet, or in a computer system. There are three methods for organizing paper-based health records in a file area: *alphabetic, straight numeric,* and *terminal digit.* In a computer system patient health information is indexed, as discussed previously.

ALPHABETIC FILING

Alphabetic filing has already been discussed under identification of files.

STRAIGHT NUMERIC FILING

Straight numeric filing involves placing the folders on the shelf in numeric order, for example, MR# 001234, MR# 001235, MR# 001522, etc. This filing system is easy for HIM staff to understand. Straight numeric filing is best used in a system in which there is minimal activity in the records once they are filed in the permanent file area.

Straight numeric methods usually work well in long-term care facilities. In this filing method the activity is concentrated at the end of the file shelf. The filing shelves are filled as records are added. Increased filing in the older records (lower numbers) will cause growth in shelves that may already be full. This causes a need to shift records. Shifting records involves the systematic, physical relocation of files so that they are more evenly distributed on the shelves. In large file rooms, this is a time-consuming task.

TERMINAL-DIGIT FILING

Terminal-digit filing is a system in which the patient's medical record number is divided into sets of digits for filing purposes. Each of the sets of digits is used to file the health record numerically within sections of the files, beginning with the last set. Terminal-digit filing, and other variations of digit filing, is very common in health care facilities. The easiest example of terminal-digit filing uses a six-digit medical record number. The six-digit number is separated into three sets of two numbers before filing. For example for MR# 012345, the sets would look like this: 01-23-45. The sets of digits have names: The first two numbers are called the *tertiary digits,* the second two numbers are called the *secondary digits,* and the last two numbers are called the *primary digits* (Table 5–4). To file in terminal-digit order (TD order) you must locate the section of files that correspond with the sets, beginning with the primary digits, then within the primary section locate the secondary digits, and finally file the record in numeric order by the tertiary digits. Let's review an example, because filing in TD order is easy once you understand how to separate the digits in the medical record number, and then which digit set to use first.

In our example we begin by using the last two numbers of the medical record number, the primary digits.

Step 1. Separate the medical record number into the necessary sections. For this example we are using a six-digit number separated into three sections with two numbers each: MR# 012345 converts to 01-23-45. To file this health record (#01-23-45) you would begin with the primary digits 45, the last two digits of MR# 01-23-45. In the file area, you must locate the primary section 45. All files in primary section 45 will end with the number 45.

Step 2. In primary section 45, you then search for the middle digits, 23. Remain in section 45, where the bottom two numbers are all the same, and be sure not to venture into another primary section on the shelf. Find middle digits 22 to 24 because 23 is going to be filed between middle digits 22–45 and 24–45.

Step 3. Once you have located the appropriate middle-digit section, file the record numerically by the first two digits.

It is important to recognize that terminal-digit filing can be modified in sev-

TABLE 5–4. Terminal-Digit Sorting of Medical Record Number 01-23-45		
Medical record number	**Number in section**	**Filing**
0	Tertiary	Finally, file in numeric order by this number.
1		
2	Secondary	Then find number 23 in section 45.
3		
4	Primary	First find section 45 in the files.
5		

eral different ways. Some facilities use a larger nine-digit medical record number or the social security number. There are several different ways to separate a nine-digit medical record number for filing:

- One method is to have three sections with three numbers each; for example, MR# 111222333 converts to 111-222-333 for filing.
- Another method is to separate the number like a Social Security number, for example, MR# 012345678 converts to 012-34-5678.

In a six-digit filing scenario there are 100 primary sections of record, 00 through 99. In a nine-digit filing system there are 1000 primary sections, 000 through 999. Primary sections reaching 1000 require a tremendous file area!

MIDDLE-DIGIT FILING

Terminal-digit filing can be modified into another filing method, **middle-digit filing.** As in terminal-digit filing, the six-digit number is separated into three sets of two numbers before filing; MR# 012345 sets would look like this: 01-23-45. The sets of digits, however, have been renamed (Fig. 5–10); the first two numbers are the secondary digits, the second two numbers are the primary digits, and the last two numbers are the tertiary digits (Table 5–5).

The following shows middle-digit filing for MR# 012345.

Step 1. Separate the medical record number into three sections with two numbers each. MR# 012345 converts to 01-23-45. In middle-digit filing, begin with the middle set of digits and use that set as the primary digits; in our example, number 23. Locate the primary section 23 in the file area. All files in primary section 23 will have middle sets with the number 23.

Step 2. Remain in section 23. Be sure not to move into another primary section on the shelf. Find the second set of digits, 01.

Step 3. Remain in section 01-23, and then file the record numerically by the tertiary digits 45.

Figure 5–10 shows an example of terminal-digit filing and of middle-digit filing.

Each facility should examine the positive as well as negative aspects of each filing method. An organized filing system allows you to efficiently retrieve patient health records. Quick retrieval of health records can improve the quality of patient care. A good system should have a positive impact on both employee and facility productivity. Table 5–6 lists the advantages and disadvantages of each filing method.

TABLE 5–5. Middle-Digit Sorting of Medical Record Number 01-23-45		
Medical record number	**Number in section**	**Filing**
0 1	Secondary	Then find number 01 in section 23.
2 3	Primary	First find section 23 in the files.
4 5	Tertiary	Finally, file in numeric order by this number.

TABLE 5–6. Advantages and Disadvantages of Filing Methods		
Filing method	**Advantages**	**Disadvantages**
Alphabetic	Easy to learn; does not require additional cross-reference to identify a file number.	Illegible handwriting can cause problems; space requirements for popular letters also problematic.
Straight numeric	Easy to learn.	File activity is concentrated.
Terminal-digit	Equalizes filing activity throughout the filing sections.	Challenging for some file clerks to learn; misfiles are often difficult to locate.
Middle-digit	Equalizes filing activity throughout the filing sections.	Even more challenging for some file clerks to learn; misfiles are often difficult to locate.

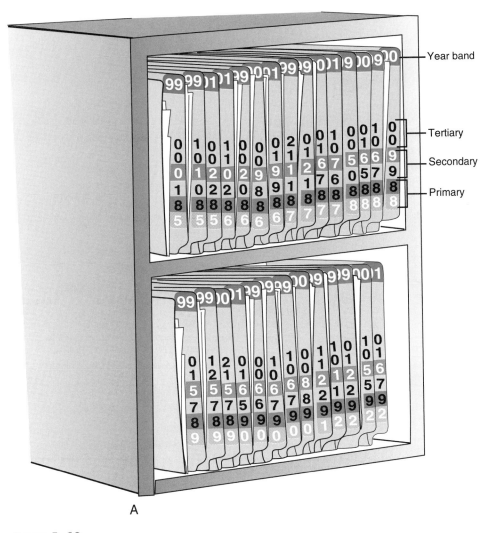

FIGURE 5–10.

Filing by terminal digit (A) and middle digit (B).

Illustration continued on following page

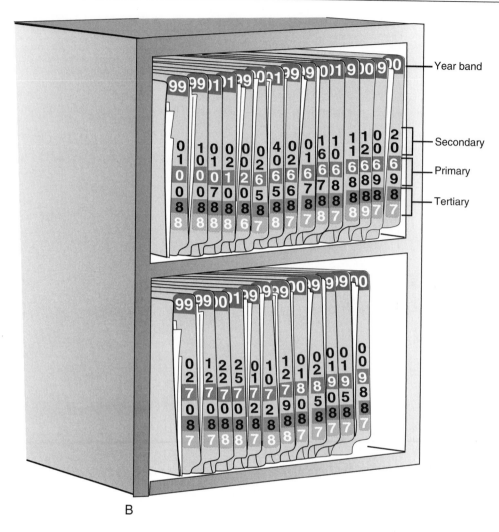

FIGURE 5–10.

Continued

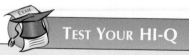

TEST YOUR HI-Q

1. In a terminal-digit filing system, MR# 658925 would be located in which primary section? (Remember to separate the medical record number into three sections with two digits each.)
2. In a middle-digit filing system, MR# 658925 would be located in which primary section? (Remember to separate the medical record number into three sections of two digits each.)
3. Design a filing method for a facility that uses a 9-digit medical record number.

Computer Indexing

Some health care facilities have patient health records in a computer system. These files may be in several different formats, for example, optical disk, digital imaging, or a database.

Optical disk and digital imaging of patient health records allow a facility to scan original pages of patient records into a machine that saves the image to an optical disk, platter, or magnetic tape. This type of system does not require the specific filing of patient records, but it requires indexing. Indexing, as previously discussed, is the naming of an image so that the computer can identify the file. HIM employees index the patient information so that the computer system recognizes the patient's record and attaches the location of the images for that patient.

An example of indexing is the creation of a file in a word processing software application. When you finish, you must save the work so you can find it on the system later. In order to differentiate it from other saved work, you must name your work. Indexing allows future retrieval of the images, without a lengthy search. Another example of indexing is a music compact disk (CD) that has the songs listed with a number next to each song; this is the order in which each song can be found on the disk. To locate a song on the CD, you look at the cover and find the corresponding number. After putting the CD in the player, you forward through the songs until the song is reached or simply press the number on the keypad for the song.

Indexing—attaching specific numbers to the images on the optical disk—allows an employee to go directly to the appropriate patient record. To retrieve information stored on an optical disk, the HIM employee enters the patient's name or identifying information into a computer that references the index to locate the appropriate point on the individual disk storing the patient's record. The patient's record may then be printed or sent to another station for viewing.

Indexing reinforces the importance of organized maintenance of patient health records. Patient files, images, and information must all be linked by the correct identifying information. Failure to accurately index a patient's information results in what we call a misfile in a paper-based system. When the patient's computerized records are retrieved, they will not be in the appropriate location. The employee then searches the computer files for the patient information, just as in a search for physical paper files. When the information is found, it has to be relocated (re-indexed) to the appropriate patient.

Record Retention

Having discussed the methods of record storage, it is important to know how long a health care facility must keep health records. The length of time a record is kept by a facility is the **record retention schedule.** Health records must be maintained by a facility to support patient care; meet legal and regulatory requirements; achieve accreditation; allow research, education, and reimbursement; and support facility administration. The duration of record retention differs for the various types of records kept (e.g., laboratory data, radiology reports and films, fetal monitor strips, birth certificates, MPIs) and for different facilities (e.g., physicians' offices, hospitals). Most states have a law that mandates how long a facility must maintain health information. In the absence of state law, the facility must follow the federal requirements stipulated by the Health Care Financing Administration, which is to save them for 5 years. A facility should also consider extending retention time to allow for cases in which malpractice, patient age, or research activity requires review of the record.

The retention time for patient health records (stipulated by law or regulation) may be a specific number of years, or it can be counted from the date of the patient's last encounter. For example, if the retention schedule in a state is 10 years and includes all previous records, when Jane Ryan has an appendectomy at age 20, a broken ankle with repair at age 25, and a motor vehicle accident (MVA) at age 29, the appendectomy record—a previous visit within 10-year limit—cannot be destroyed until 10 years have passed from the patient's last encounter. On admission for the ankle repair, the appendectomy record would be retained for another 10 years, and the same for the MVA. Jane's records are maintained until the retention time 10 years has lapsed from her last visit. However, if the retention schedule does not include previous visits, then the appendectomy can be destroyed when the retention period expires. Refer to Figure 5–11 for the retention schedule for health information suggested by the American Health Information Management Association (AHIMA).

RETENTION POLICY

HIM departments must have a policy explaining the storage of health records specific to that facility. The policy describes which health records are maintained in the department, how each type of record is organized (by number and/or filing system), the storage medium used (optical disk, microfilm, paper, computer), and the length of time each record is to be retained. The retention policy is very important to a facility that has many records that may be stored in different locations. The policy must state that a record is maintained on all patients registered to the facility; provide the retention schedule; indicate how the records are identified, organized, or filed; state their location; and document alternative locations or media, if necessary.

FACILITY CLOSURE

What happens when a facility, physician's office, or clinic closes its operation? Where do the records go? In the event of a facility's closing, the retention schedule remains in effect. The facility must investigate the applicable laws to determine the best method for retaining the records. If the facility or practice is purchased, the records are managed by the new owner. However, if the practice or facility closes, the records must be maintained for the duration of the retention schedule in an appropriate, secure, confidential location.

RETENTION SCHEDULE OF HEALTH CARE RECORDS

Type of Health Information	Retention Schedule	
Acute care facility records	Adults	10 years
	Minors	Age of majority + 10 years (or statute of limitations)
Birth, death, surgical procedure registers	Permanently	
X-ray films	5 years	
Fetal monitor strips	10 years after the patient reaches the age of majority	
Master patient index	Permanently	
Diseases index	10 years	
Emergency room register/log	Permanently	
Employee health records	30 years	

FIGURE 5–11.
Retention schedule for health care records. Medicare Condition of Participation (MCOP) requires retention of records, films, and scans for at least 5 years. Each provider should develop a retention schedule for records in that facility. (Modified from AHIMA Practice Brief. Retention of Health Information.)

The facility must notify its patients when it is closing. There are several excellent methods to inform patients of closure. One method is to run an advertisement in the local newspaper explaining the closure and what will happen to the patient records (Fig. 5–12). Another method is to notify patients through letters or notices mailed directly to the patients informing them of the closure. It is also important to post similar notices in and around the facility to notify patients of the closure. Because patient information is important in the continuity of

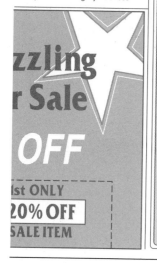

FIGURE 5–12.

Newspaper advertisement of facility closure.

care, it is important to maintain patient access to the records even after the facility is closed. This may be accomplished by transferring the records to another
local related facility or physician's office, as appropriate.

Filing Furniture

Now that we can identify and file health records, let's review the different furniture found in file areas of health care facilities. These include file cabinets, open
shelving, revolving systems, and movable shelves.

FILE CABINETS

A file cabinet (Fig. 5–13) can be a vertical or lateral drawer system for filing
records. This type of furniture is secure in many ways because it is easily locked,
keeps records out of plain sight, and is typically a good way to secure records

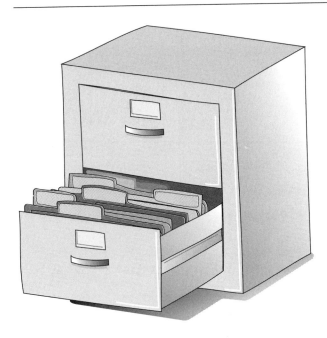

FIGURE 5–13.
File cabinet.

from fire or water damage. The disadvantages associated with this type of filing furniture are

- File cabinets are large (bulky) and require more space than shelving systems.
- They are not efficient if the department has a large number of records that need to be accessed frequently.
- Only one drawer of records in each file cabinet can be accessed at a time.

When file cabinets face each other in rows, always leave enough room for facing drawers to open. Approximately 5 feet between rows is necessary unless aisle space is not required.

OPEN SHELVES

This type of filing furniture is simply a shelf that is always open to the file area (Fig. 5–14). Open shelves allow the filing of many health records on shelves with open access to all records at all times. Open shelves require less space than filing cabinets; they may be 16 inches deep and require an aisle space of only 4 feet. Therefore, two shelves can face each other and allow good

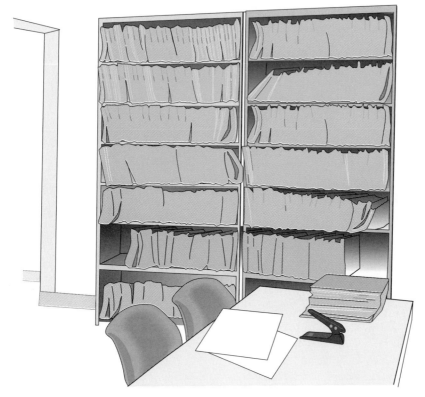

FIGURE 5–14.
Open shelves.

access with only a 4-foot aisle. The disadvantages are that the records are always visible to visitors in the file area and they are exposed to potential fire or water damage.

COMPRESSIBLE SHELVES

Compressible or movable shelves allow storage of files on shelves that can be compressed so that more shelves will fit in a smaller file space (Fig. 5–15). This type of shelving can move back and forth or side to side. This file furniture works well in a file room where space is limited and there are numerous patient files. The problem encountered with this filing furniture is that it provides access only to those sections of the files that are open. If a file area is very busy, compressible units may hinder filing productivity. This furniture also allows some visibility of records to visitors in the file area and potential exposure of the records to fire or water damage.

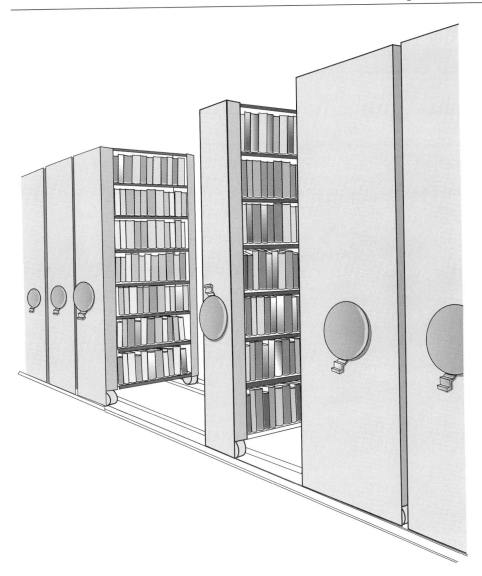

FIGURE 5–15.
Compressible shelves.

REVOLVING FILE SYSTEM

A revolving file system looks like a Ferris wheel (Fig. 5–16). This system can revolve laterally or horizontally. On a revolving file shelf a record cannot be retrieved until the relevant file shelf rolls around to the opening. The system may use a computer to correlate the medical record numbers to a file. When a record is needed, the file identification (MR#) is entered into the system. The revolving system presents the shelf on which that record is located so that the record may

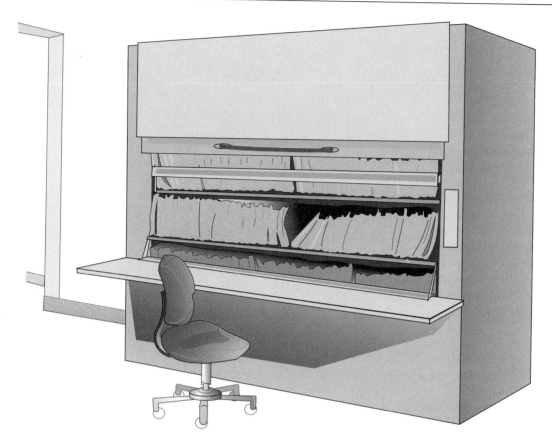

FIGURE 5–16.
Revolving file system.

be pulled from the shelf. This system provides a secure environment for storing records; however, access is limited to only one shelf at a time. In a horizontal revolving system, if the power supply is out, only one shelf can be accessed.

There are many types of file furniture capable of storing health records. Table 5–7 compares the advantages and disadvantages of each type of filing furniture and the most appropriate setting for each.

File Rooms

Although there are many types of file furniture for storage of health information, it is important to consider the Occupational Safety and Health Administration (OSHA) space requirements for filing areas. The OSHA requirements specify the appropriate space to provide a safe environment for employees working in the file area. OSHA mandates an aisle at least 3 feet wide between filing units or shelves, and the exit aisle must be at least 5 feet wide. Other requirements specify the amount of space required between the top shelf and the ceiling of the file room.

TABLE 5–7. Advantages and Disadvantages of Filing Equipment		
Filing equipment	**Advantages**	**Disadvantages**
File cabinets	Protects information from exposure to the environment. Conceals information from public view. Typically provides ability to lock/secure information.	Can access only one drawer of information at a time. Requires additional space to open for access to information.
Open shelves	Allows easy access to records.	Open to environment. Requires space for aisle access to each shelf.
Compressible shelves	Increases file space in small area.	Limits access to information.
Revolving file system	Accommodates file personnel, reducing time spent looking for file on shelf.	Limits access to files.

When one is designing a file area, the first item of business is to measure the file space. Before you can consider cost for filing furniture and other supplies you have to ensure that the area has adequate space that complies with OSHA guidelines to store the files. Do you have a room by itself for files or will you be using part of the space in the department? If you are relocating a file room, you can measure your existing file area to determine whether the files will fit into the new space. If you plan to order new file furniture, be sure that the new furniture will accommodate all of your files and includes room for growth. When ordering shelves or file cabinets, be sure to figure the filing space within each shelf unit (see Figs. 5–14 and 5–15). Count the number of shelves per unit. This will be important later when you are trying to calculate the correct number of shelves to purchase. If each shelving unit has 8 shelves at a width of 36 inches, you will have 288 inches (8 shelves × 36 inches = 288 inches or 24 feet) of file space on each shelving unit.

Calculation of file space is equally important if you plan to enlarge or reorganize an existing file area. It may be inaccurate to assume that each record will occupy 1 inch. It is best to measure a sample of files to determine (approximately) how many files will fit on a shelf. Rather than counting an entire shelf, count the files in several 1-foot sections. For each sample section, note how many records you counted. Then average the total number.

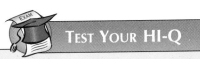

TEST YOUR HI-Q

Marcus counted the number of records in ten 1-foot sections in the file area prior to reorganizing the files. His findings were as follows:

Section #1—12 records, #2—8 records, #3—16 records, #4—6 records, #5—10 records, #6—24 records, #7—15 records, #8—14 records, #9—7 records, #10—11 records.

Using this information, calculate the average number of records in a 1-foot section of files.

Once you know the average number of records that occupy 1 foot of file space, you can calculate the file space needed for the entire room. We can use the answer to Test Your HI-Q example: Marcus calculated an average of 12.3 records per 1 foot of file space. The next information necessary is how many years of records are stored in this location? Let's assume that at Marcus' facility the file area contains 3 years of files. Knowing the facility's average number of discharges (12,000) allows an approximate calculation of 36,000 files in the file area. Knowing that 1 foot equals 12.3 records, dividing 36,000 by 12.3 equals 2926.8 or 2927 feet of file space to accommodate 3 years of records at Marcus' facility.

Before ordering furniture, you must determine how many shelves are necessary to store 2927 feet of files. Measure your current file space to determine whether you can use the current furniture. Using the 8-shelf unit that allows 36 inches of file space on each shelf, we know that one shelf unit (8 shelves) can hold 288 inches or 24 feet of records. For 2927 feet of files you will need 122 shelving units to accommodate these files (2927 divided by 24 feet for one 8-shelf unit equals 121.95 or 122 shelving units). This calculation is adequate for current files, but it does not allow room for expansion in the future. The facility should plan for an increase in the number of patient files. Planning for an increase by overestimating the necessary space may avoid overcrowding of records in the future. To determine an appropriate amount of growing space, recall how much the files have grown over the past several years. That may help you project for the future. Sometimes a facility has a strategic plan for growth, and the financial planners in the facility can provide you with information on expected growth of discharges for the coming years.

If you are planning file space in a new facility, you will have to work with estimations. An easy method for estimating is to contact the HIM professional at facilities in your area providing a similar type of health care. The HIM professional should be able to provide information regarding the facility's chart size, which you can use in your calculations. If another facility does not exist in your area, create a mock chart. A mock chart is a made-up record that includes an example of each document that could exist in the patient's health record. Keep in mind whether you will require one or more pages for a specific document, such as progress notes, operative reports, and the like. Remember that length of stay has an impact on the size of a record. After you create a mock chart, measure it. How thick is the record? Multiply this measurement by the number of patient records estimated and allow enough space in the file area for a specific time period. If you have a space shortage, you will need to evaluate alternative storage methods, discussed next.

TEST YOUR HI-Q

Calculate the filing space necessary for a new ambulatory surgery facility. The facility will average 45 surgeries each day, Monday through Friday (closed on holidays). Remember to create a mock chart to figure out the thickness of each file (e.g., 12 records per inch). Then be sure to allow for enough space for additional years of files. Your answer should consider how long the facility will store the records.

Alternative Storage Methods

It is common for an HIM department to store health records in an alternative site or format, either because of limited space or because the records are inactive. Activity of patient records refers to the facility's need to retrieve the record. A record is considered active as long as it is needed within the facility or for patient care. In the paper environment, a patient's health record may be termed inactive after it is complete and a specified number of years have passed since it was last needed.

The most common reason an HIM department needs alternative storage is a shortage of filing space in the department. In the paper record environment, health records can quickly fill all of the filing space available in an HIM department. Health care facilities maintain increasing amounts of patient health information. Remember, the patient health record must be retained for several reasons: state and federal laws, the continuation of patient care, reimbursement, accreditation, potential litigation, research, and education.

A likely solution to provide a significant amount of room for new files is to store the patient records in a new location or in a format that takes up less space. When space is limited within a facility, sometimes even active records are relocated. Microfilm, optical imaging, and on-site and off-site storage are discussed as alternative storage choices available to health care facilities.

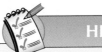

HIT BIT

Active records are regularly accessed for patient care. *Inactive records* are those that are rarely accessed for patient care or other activity.

Microfilm

Microfilm, simply described, is the reproduction of the original paper record into miniature pictures stored on plastic film, either on reels or on sheets. To microfilm patient records each page must be carefully prepared. The pages in each record must be free of staples, tears, and adhesives. Failure to prepare the documents before scanning the images to microfilm can cause the document to become jammed in the machine or torn, or it may obscure the image. The prepared pages are scanned, both back and front as necessary, into the microfilm machine, much like a copy machine. The image of each page is stored on film, and the film is developed to produce the final microfilm product (Fig. 5–17).

At first glance, microfilm looks like a negative from pictures taken with a camera. Further study reveals that the image looks like a small picture of the original document that was scanned through the machine. After processing, the images are assembled on roll film or sliced into a sheet of film and put into a jacket. The film that is sliced and put into jackets is also known as **microfiche.** Careful attention is required to ensure that each page in the patient record is scanned. Loss of one page of a record could eliminate valuable patient information and ultimately affect the completeness of the patient's record. Likewise,

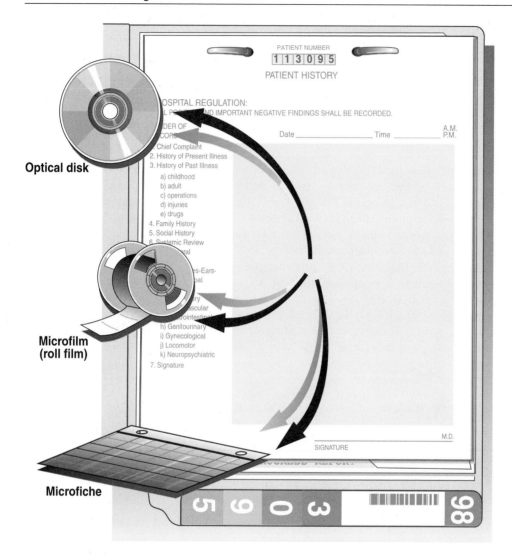

FIGURE 5-17.

Microfilm and microfiche.

once the image is processed onto microfilm, the image cannot be updated or altered. A facility should microfilm only complete patient records. Like other formats, microfilmed records are carefully labeled with the patient's identifying name or number. Each roll or sheet of film is labeled so that HIM employees are able to determine which patient records are stored on that roll or sheet. In the file cabinet, microfilm records are filed in the same way as files were stored in their original format, using either alphabetic, straight numeric, or terminal-digit filing systems.

MICROFILM EQUIPMENT

When using microfilm storage of records, some equipment is necessary to maintain access to the files. A printer is needed to reproduce a paper copy of the patient's record for release to another facility or authorized individual. The microfilm or microfiche health record must be maintained in appropriate storage equipment. Microfilm should be stored in a file cabinet or drawer capable of being locked, or it is kept enclosed in a locked room. The cabinets should also protect the records from the environment and from temperature and water damage.

Important things to remember:

- Microfilming can be performed at an on-site or off-site location.
- If an off-site contract company is chosen, the off-site company is responsible for maintaining the confidentiality of the information while it is being processed.
- The contracted company must also allow the necessary access to the information in a timely manner should it be required.
- The quality of the microfilm must be checked prior to destroying any of the original records.

DOCUMENT/OPTICAL IMAGING

Optical imaging is the reproduction of the original paper record into miniature pictures stored on **optical disk.** As with microfilm, each page (front and back) of the original health record must be prepared for scanning. By scanning the original pages of the patient health record into a computer system the record may be saved on a disk similar to a computer CD. The actual scanning process is similar to sending a piece of paper through a copy machine. In this format the machine, called a **scanner,** does not produce the image onto another piece of paper or plastic; instead the image is digitally stored in a computer system, on magnetic tape, or on optical disk.

Interestingly, this form of storage does not typically require a separate MPI system to locate the patient's health record. Patient identification by name or number is still a very important factor in the indexing of the patient information. The medical record number is still used to name or identify the records; however, an optical imaging system is capable of searching for the patient's health information via patient name, discharge date, or any other identifying data known to the system. Likewise, if one page of the record was not scanned with the original record, it can be added later and remain identifiable by the system as a part of the patient's original record within the system. With this system it is possible to scan records prior to completion. Loose work, transcription, and sometimes signatures can be added at a later date.

This format requires the use of a reader and printer to reproduce a paper copy of the patient's health record. However, some systems are capable of electronically sending the image to another authorized location for reproducing a paper copy.

On-site Storage

Space may limit the number of records that can be stored in the HIM department. Therefore, some facilities maintain their records in storage space in a separate room or building owned by their facility. This concept is called *on-site storage.* Storing medical records on-site allows a facility to maintain security, confidentiality, and timely access to its health care records. The HIM department simply relocates specified records to the new location, ensuring that the records are in a secure environment and organized as they were in the HIM department. The new location of the files should be updated in the MPI and in the department policy and procedure manual.

On-site storage of health records is usually the least expensive method for alternative storage. It is also the alternative that allows the HIM custodian to maintain direct control over the files. Costs associated with this type of storage include additional filing furniture, improvements to the environment, employee time, and filing supplies. If a facility chooses on-site storage, it is very important that a plan of action be developed so that the transferring of the records happens in a secure, timely, and organized manner.

HIT BIT

In a health care facility centralized and decentralized file areas reflect the number of separate locations within or outside the facility that store health records.

A *centralized file area* describes a file room where ALL health records for the facility are in one location.

A *decentralized file area* describes one or more locations outside the HIM department or outside the facility that are used to store the health records of a facility.

Off-site Storage

In addition to the choices previously mentioned, off-site storage is an alternative in which the original health records are stored at a separate location outside the facility that may be owned and operated by some party other than the facility. The off-site company that maintains the original records operates much like the file room in the health care facility. Patient health records can be requested when needed for patient care, release of information, record review, billing, or any other appropriate reason and brought to the facility. The records no longer take up space at the facility. The records are no longer under the direct control of the facility's HIM custodian but are relocated to another secure environment. Within this new environment, the facility HIM custodian must ensure that appropriate measures are taken to secure and organize the patient records.

There are many things that must be considered before choosing to store records off-site. The off-site storage facility signs a contract with the health care facility to maintain its health care records. All of the facility's concerns should be addressed in the contract. The contract must be reviewed thoroughly and clarified if anything is unclear. The following is a list of issues to consider before choosing an off-site facility:

- Be sure that the site has appropriate security for the storage of health information.
- Personally go to the site and examine the security system.
- What are the operating hours?
- How will you request a record in an emergency, for patient care, or other review?
- How often will the requested records be delivered to your facility?
- How will records be transported from the off-site facility to yours and back again? In secure vehicles, taxi, fax only, courier?
- Is there a charge for immediate delivery of a record in case of emergency?
- How will the company charge your facility—by linear foot of storage space or by record storage type?
- How will the company store your records: in boxes or open shelving?
- What are the training procedures for their employees?
- What are the safety and confidentiality procedures?

Selection of Storage Method

Before choosing an alternative storage method, analyze the amount of records that you plan to store and the length of time you plan to store the records. This analysis should focus on the initial cost of storing the records and include maintenance of the records in the storage site. For example, if you choose microfilm or optical imaging you will have to consider the cost of converting the records, storing the records in the new format, and purchasing reader-printer machines (including maintenance contracts) to produce paper images of the records. On-site storage is ideal if your facility has adequate space. With off-site storage, the length of time you will have to pay the off-site storage company to maintain the records is a factor. The annual cost to store 1 year's worth of health records in an off-site storage company over the length of the retention period may eventually be more than the original price of microfilming or optical imaging. This concept is called the pay-back period.

Chart Locator Systems

Health information is useful only if it is available for review. A **chart locator system** keeps track of the location of all records in the health care facility. Many people in the health care facility have authorized need and access to patient records. As a result, records are not always on the shelf in the permanent file location. Records may be signed out to a health care unit when a patient is readmitted. Records may be requested for research or for patient follow-up care. The quality management (QM) department may need to review records to ensure that the care provided to the patient was appropriate. Copies of records may be requested for litigation, which requires removing the health record file from the file system in order to copy it for authorized users. Because all of this use is necessary to the function of the facility, it is important that the HIM department be able to locate and retrieve patient records.

HIT BIT

Chart locator systems apply primarily to the paper health record. In a computerized or computer-based environment, records are tracked using an *audit trail*. The computer system keeps a log (known as the audit trail) of all transactions by recording the employee performing the task, what information is sent and to which location, the recipient, the date, the time, and other pertinent facts. This audit trail is an important tool in the computer environment for tracking the use of patient health records and information.

A chart locator system allows the HIM department to keep track of the facility's patient health records. Records that are removed from the department or from the normal processing flow in the department are "signed out" to the location to which they are being sent. Once the records are returned, they must be "signed in" to the department. This allows anyone in the HIM department to easily determine when a record is available for review and when it is out of the department. A chart locator system also allows faster retrieval of a record from another location in an urgent time of need—for example, for a patient care emergency. It has been said that the HIM department is only as good as the information that it can provide. If an HIM department can easily access and retrieve information, that department is functioning productively.

Manual Systems

Manual systems for chart location of the paper record use an **outguide** and a log or box to identify that a patient's health record file folder has been removed and sent to a new location. An outguide is a physical file card or jacket identifying that the record is out of its expected location (Fig. 5–18). The log or box is used as a quick alphabetic reference of all records that are signed out of the HIM department. When a patient's health record is needed in another location, the HIM file clerk completes an outguide slip as shown in Figure 5–18 to put in place of the file when it is removed. The outguide informs anyone who comes to that location to look for the patient's file that it has been moved to a new loca-

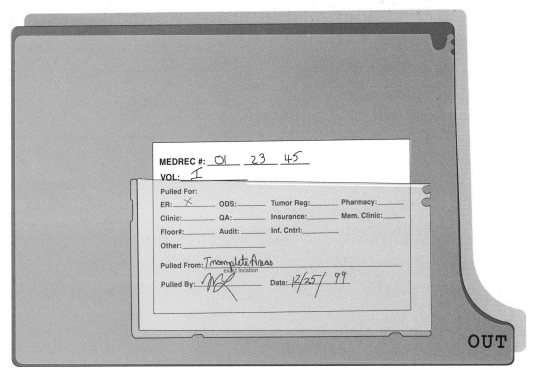

FIGURE 5–18.

Outguide identifies a record removed from its usual location.

tion. Outguides prevent HIM employees from spending unnecessary time searching for a file.

How does the manual system operate? When the HIM department receives a request for a health record, the clerk retrieves the patient's medical record number by looking up the patient's name in the MPI. The clerk locates the health record in the department. This may be the clerk's thought process: Is the record old enough to be in the permanent files? Is it just a week old and probably in the incomplete record area? or Is it a recent discharge and possibly in the coding area? Once the record is located and pulled, the clerk will sign the record out to the new location, meaning that the clerk notes where that record is going. In a manual chart locator system small duplicate outguide forms are completed with the following information: medical record number, discharge date(s) for that record, and the location to which the record is being sent, with the date the record was sent. The date the record was sent is important so that the date of expected return is known. The duplicate copy of the outguide is filed alphabetically in a box for all patient files that were signed out of the department. The department may also require that the person requesting the records sign for them on pickup.

Computerized Systems

Computerized chart locator systems can eliminate the need for physical out-guides and cards, although some HIM departments simultaneously use the manual chart locator system and the computer system. In a computerized chart locator system, the new location to which the record is being signed out is entered into the computer system. Therefore, if a chart is pulled from the permanent file location and sent to a clinic, in the computerized chart locator system that record is signed out to the clinic. The chart locator system must accurately reflect the current location of each patient record.

HIT BIT

As a rule of thumb, in a large HIM department, all records should be listed in the chart locator system as the record progresses through each function in the HIM department. When a record moves from one location it must be "signed out" of that location and "signed in" to the new location. This method allows personnel to determine the location of a patient file without spending time searching through the various sections of the HIM department.

Sign-in is done to check records back into the department, which involves updating the computerized chart locator system to note that the record has been returned. On a daily basis, records returned to the department must be signed in and placed back into their appropriate location. It is also very important to perform a regular audit (weekly) of the health records that are checked out to each location. For example, if 10 records are signed out to the clinic and upon inspection of the clinic you do not locate all 10 records, it is necessary to search for the missing records. Did they come back to the HIM department but not get checked in? Were the records transferred to a unit within your facility because that patient was admitted? Always know the location of your records, to ensure and maintain the security of patient health records.

A beneficial feature of some computerized chart locator systems is an automated prompt for the return of patient files. For example, patient files should leave the HIM department only when they are needed for continuity of patient care. The system prompt notifies the HIM staff of any files that were due back in the department but not yet signed in on the chart locator system. This prompt cues the clerk to locate the record.

The following scenario illustrates the computerized chart locator system. Mary Davidson has been a patient at the Diamonte facility several times over the past 5 years. In the course of her treatment, physicians have noted that Ms. Davidson is allergic to penicillin. On one particular evening in October, Mary is brought to the emergency room (ER) unconscious. Review of her personal belongings gave health care workers her name and DOB. The ER makes a routine call to the HIM department for her old records. The HIM department clerk enters "Mary Davidson" into the MPI system and quickly several patients with that name appear on the screen. Because the clerk has the DOB, she can easily check the MPI to find the correct patient file. With the medical record number for Mary Davidson, the clerk goes to the file room to look for the old record. She goes to the appropriate shelf in the terminal-digit order but the record is not there. The clerk then returns to the computer to enter Ms. Davidson's medical record number in the chart locator system (Fig. 5–19).

On doing so, the clerk learns that this record is signed out to the QM department for review. Knowing the routine of the facility, the clerk can go directly to the section of records set aside for the QM staff and retrieve Mary Davidson's record. The clerk then makes an entry into the chart locator system telling the system that the record is being sent to the ER and on return to the HIM department should be returned to the QM staff record section. Appropriate notes should also be made to tell the QM section that this record has been removed.

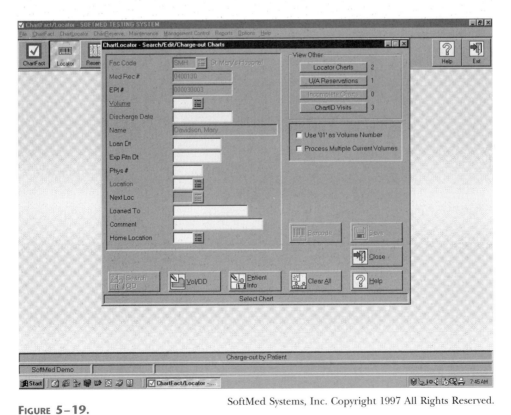

FIGURE 5–19.

Chart locator screens. (Courtesy of SoftMed Systems, Inc. Bethesda, Md.)

Illustration continued on following page

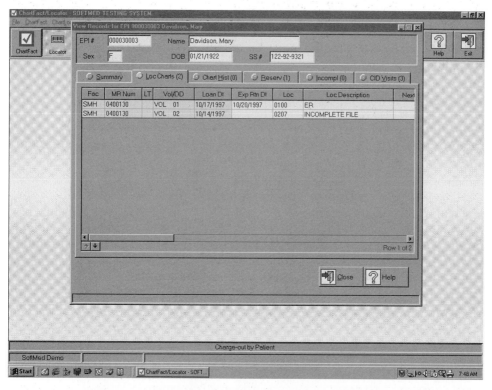

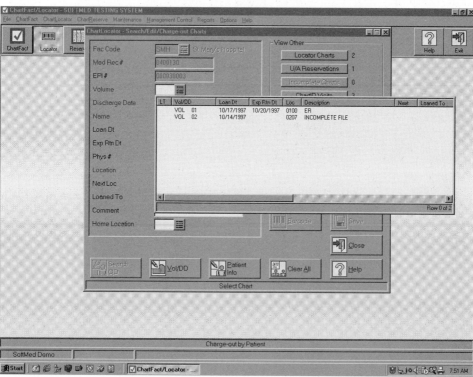

FIGURE 5–19.

Continued

HIT Bit

In a computer-based patient record environment, HIM file clerks are able to send a copy, a viewable image, of the patient's record while maintaining the original in the computer system. Once a patient's record is in the system, it can be shared by many users simultaneously. HIM professionals should be aware of the security concerns in the computer environment. Patients' health records must be secure from potential for loss, computer tampering, deletion, and unauthorized access.

Security of Health Information

Storage of health information involves its security. HIM professionals are considered custodians of patients' health information. They are responsible for ensuring that the information is complete, timely, accurate, and secure. HIM practitioners also ensure the physical security of health information. We discuss issues of security in the storage of health records, such as damage of records by fire, water, theft, tampering, and destruction. Every HIM department has policies to safeguard records from these hazards. It is the specific responsibility of HIM practitioners and all delegated employees to safeguard this information. Careful forethought and preparation for security of health records can prevent every HIM practitioner's worst nightmare.

HIT Bit

Read these two HIM nightmare scenarios, and you can see the importance of taking precautions with patient records.

Case 1. Your facility is caught unprepared during an unexpected torrential rainstorm, on a Sunday afternoon. On entering your department Monday morning you notice puddles of water on the floor in the file room. Further inspection reveals that the file room had been flooded with 16 inches of water.

Case 2. An HIM department receives a request for a patient record from the emergency room. After thorough search of the files, department, and facility, the HIM practitioner is unable to locate the requested patient record. Furthermore, failure to provide this patient record in a timely manner results in the patient's being treated with a medication to which the patient is allergic. The patient dies as a result of this treatment. When it is finally located, the patient's previous record documented the patient's allergy.

Disaster Planning

Unfortunately there are few solutions for a nightmare, once it occurs. However, careful forethought and policies can be established by facilities to protect health information. This is called disaster planning. *Disaster planning* is a method for dealing with catastrophes and other emergencies that occur in the health care environment. A disaster can be a large number of patients' requiring medical attention as a result of an explosion or a plane crash. Disasters include explosion and bomb threats, power failures, earthquakes, hurricanes, tornadoes, flooding, fires, patient abduction, and theft. All JCAHO-accredited facilities are required to maintain a disaster plan. Facilities must also educate HIM employees on the security procedures and make sure that they are prepared to follow procedure if a disaster occurs.

Security of health records is mandated by regulatory and accreditation agencies. HIM practitioners must protect all health information, including records; diagnosis, procedure, and physician indices; the MPI; computerized health information databases; x-ray films; and admission, discharge, and transfer logs.

Security from Fire

Providing protection from fire for the health information environment can prevent irreversible damage to the facility's health records. Some of the systems and barriers that can assist in the protection from fire are chemical systems, sprinkler systems, fire walls, fire compartments, and fire extinguishers.

Chemical systems deplete the oxygen from the air in an area where a fire exists. File rooms and computer facilities may be equipped with this type of system. The chemical system is designed to sense fire and release a chemical that removes oxygen from the air in the room. Removing the oxygen smothers the fire to prevent further damage to files or facility. (All personnel need to leave the area immediately when the alarm sounds.)

Building structures such as fire walls or fire compartments are designed to contain a fire within a facility. Fire walls prevent a fire from moving side to side on a particular floor of the building. Recall your last visit to a health care facility. When walking down the hallway you may have passed through double doors in which the doors were held open by magnets on each wall. When the fire alarm is triggered in a health care facility with fire walls, those double doors close to seal the fire and prevent it from spreading to other areas of the facility. A fire compartment is a structure in a building in which all sides of a room or area are protected by fire barriers. This means that the walls, ceiling, and floor are all fire resistant. If a fire begins in a fire compartment, the compartment contains the fire; likewise, if the fire is outside the compartment, the contents within the compartment are protected from the fire. A fire compartment is the ideal solution to protect the permanent file area or your central computer system if a fire occurs in another part of the facility.

Sprinkler systems release water to extinguish fire when activated by heat or smoke. When a sprinkler system is used to safeguard files, it is important to have at least 18 inches of clearance between the top of the file space and the ceiling. Failure to keep these areas clear blocks the water sprinklers from extinguishing the fire at a lower level. In the event of a fire, sprinkler systems may extinguish the fire and cause minimal water damage to your records.

All health care facilities are equipped with fire extinguishers. HIM employees must be familiar with the location of the nearest fire extinguisher. Employees must be able to operate the fire extinguishers in case of emergency. It is possible that a fire may begin in a very small trash can or near an electrical outlet. With a fire extinguisher, the fire can easily be controlled without activating a sprinkler system or chemical system.

Security from Water Damage

Water damage to health records, whether paper-based or computerized, can occur because of flooding, storms, or fire control. A plan must be established to protect health information from water damage. For example, is your facility in an area where flooding is common? Some options for this scenario may be to relocate the file area to a higher floor of the facility, elevate the file room a few feet, or, if the need arises, be capable of activating an emergency plan to move records on low shelves to a higher location in the facility. Health records maintained in file cabinets or on shelves that are closed or covered also need to be considered for protection from flooding. Although damage to file cabinets from a sprinkler system is usually minimal, sprinkler systems cause damage to open shelving. In case of flooding, the bottom drawers in file cabinets are likely to flood. Evaluate the health record environment and potential for flood or water damage. Remember to protect computer terminals and to have a plan in case of emergency.

On a positive note, processes exist to assist in the restoration of paper health records that are damaged by water. If paper records are soaked with water or other fluid, be sure to act immediately to restore and protect the information. Once the paper records dry, the opportunity to salvage them may be lost. Remember that wet paper may be salvaged, but records destroyed by fire are gone forever.

Security from Theft or Tampering

The issues to consider when protecting health records from theft or tampering are the location of files, access to files, and security. Health information, paper and computerized, must be protected from theft or tampering by parties both within and outside the facility. Within a facility, only authorized, appropriate personnel should have access to patient health information. Paper documents are secured by allowing release of the original record from the HIM department only if it is needed for the patient's treatment. The HIM department maintains appropriate measures to track the location of patient records (discussed earlier in the section on the chart locator system). Other review of a patient's record must occur within the HIM department and is allowed only if the person reviewing the record is authorized to do so.

How do you maintain the security of the paper record when it leaves the HIM department? HIM professionals cannot follow every patient record checked out to every location in a facility. Therefore, it is important to have policies and procedures that secure the information to the best of your ability. This can be done by notifying others of the policy and procedure for security of information, by performing regular in-service training for facility employees to inform them of the rules regarding health information, and by restricting the reasons for which a record is allowed to leave the department. In-service training and policies are discussed under training and development (see Chapter 11).

Additional security measures include

- After office hours, the HIM department is closed and all access doors locked, and only those people authorized to enter the department are allowed entrance. Anyone with a key to your area must be aware of all HIM policies and procedures regarding appropriate use of health information.
- Areas may also be protected by a key code entry system. Access codes are assigned only to appropriate employees or physicians. After hours, an authorized physician can access his or her incomplete health records with this code.
- A swipe badge security feature allows entry into the HIM department only with the appropriate access card assigned to authorized physicians or employees.
- Computer passwords assigned to authorized users allow the facility to limit and monitor the persons who access health information.
- Biometric technology, such as fingerprinting and retinal scanning, is also a means for limiting access to health records. With this technology, the system scans a person's fingerprint or retina to evaluate his or her authority to enter an area or access a system.
- Cameras are another security feature found in health care facilities. In areas where there is increased need for security, cameras monitored by the facility security personnel guard unauthorized entry.

For computerized health information, a facility must secure records when transferring files from one system to another within or outside of the facility. When upgrading or changing computer software or systems, patient health information is transferred from one system to another. Copying of records from one system to another is acceptable; however, the HIM department must supervise this type of data transfer. Additionally, the department must validate that patient information is not deleted in the transfer. Failure to maintain complete patient information can affect future patient care. Likewise, an incomplete medical record may not be admissible in court as evidence in the event of litigation. Maintain an index of the old system to verify accuracy of the new.

Computerized health information must be protected from sabotage such as computer viruses. Equipment should be secure and precautions should be taken to prevent others from accessing the system. It is also important to ensure that the facility can update current systems and still retrieve information from obsolete systems. Otherwise, much time and energy are spent converting information from one system to another.

Destruction of Health Information

There are circumstances when it is appropriate to destroy health information. For example, records may be destroyed at the completion of the retention period or when paper-based records are successfully transferred to another medium like microfilm, diskette, or optical imaging. However, HIM employees must prevent negligent destruction. In a paper record environment, a common method of destroying health information is the shredding or incineration of the paper document. The destruction should be done in the presence of a credentialed custodian of the HIM department or its delegate. Do not leave health information to be destroyed without the proper supervision. In the computerized environment, destruction of health information may include entering a virus into the computer software system, destroying the equipment or software used to access the health information, or removing the information from the system.

To avoid premature destruction of health information in the paper environment, several things must be accomplished. Employees should be aware of the appropriate content of the health record, so that pertinent and valuable patient information is not inadvertently thrown out. Likewise, the employees should be aware of the record retention schedule for all health information in the HIM department. If the the facility has chosen to store records in an alternative format, the finished product—microfilm, diskette, or optical images— must be reviewed to ensure that all of the information is intact before the original paper record is destroyed. Once a paper record is destroyed, it cannot be recovered.

For computerized health information, a backup file of all health information in all systems must be completed daily. The backup copy allows information restoration to the time the backup was created. For instance, if you are typing a 10-page report, it is wise to save the report each time you step away from the computer or at certain intervals in the report. By saving the information that has been typed on the disk, the information will be retrievable when you return to the system. A procedure called backup is performed daily in health care facilities. The backup file copies the information from the computer systems in the facility. If the system crashes, at least the facility will have all of the information necessary to restore the system to the previous day's business.

Computerized health information should be maintained in an environment that supports the use of computers. The HIM department must maintain the computerized equipment so that it is free from harm by temperature, water, and other environmental effects. These considerations also apply to microfilm and optical disk storage. Microfilm and optical disks can be damaged by intense heat. Computers are affected by temperatures as well. Water can damage a computer and cause loss of function and information. Falling objects can damage computer equipment and disks, and drinks (liquid) spilled into keyboards or hard drives can impair or destroy a system.

RESTORING INFORMATION LOST INADVERTENTLY

What can be done when health records are lost or destroyed inadvertently? It is important to have a plan of action. In a computerized record system, daily back-ups of the information in the system should allow full recovery of all patient information (prior to backup). In the event of inadvertent destruction of paper records, the only information that can be reproduced is the duplicate paper documents maintained by allied health departments within the facility. For example, the laboratory and radiology departments usually maintain a duplicate copy of reports, the transcription department or service may be able to recover transcription of any dictated reports, and in some instances the billing office may maintain a file including patient information. As a last-resort effort, a facility may also find information in the attending physician's office. Often the attending physician needs copies of patient information for follow-up care or to bill for services. Obtaining a copy of information sent to the physician can assist the effort to recover this information.

Suggested Reading

Abdelhak M, Grostick, S, Hanken MA, Jacobs E: Health Information: Management of a Strategic Resource, 2nd ed. Philadelphia, WB Saunders, 2001.

Brandt MD, Rhodes H: Protecting patient information after facility closure (updated). AHIMA Practice Brief. Journal of AHIMA 70(3), 1999.

Claeys T: Medical Filing, 2nd ed. Albany, NY, Delmar, 1997.

Huffman EK: Health Information Management, 10th ed. Berwyn, Ill, Physician's Record Company, 1994.

Web Site

Definition of a computer-based patient record institute. May 24, 1999. **www.cpri.org/what.html.**

CHAPTER SUMMARY

HIM departments that maintain their health records in a neat and orderly manner provide a valuable service to the facility. Health records are valuable as long as they are available for access. Maintenance of an organized storage area facilitates timely retrieval of records for all authorized users. Records can be identified alphabetically or numerically. When numeric identification is chosen, the master patient index is the key tool to correlate the patient to his or her medical record number. Medical record (identification) numbers can be assigned as unit, serial, serial–unit, or family numbering systems. Filing methods use either the patient's name or the medical record number to organize the health record in the filing system. These filing methods are alphabetic, straight numeric, and terminal-digit order. The chart locator system allows the HIM department to keep track of the location of health records. HIM practitioners must consider the physical security issues of storing health records safely to prevent damage of records by fire, water, theft, tampering, destruction, and loss of confidentiality.

It is critical to secure all health information within a facility. HIM professionals pay special attention to the storage details so that all authorized users in the facility have efficient and effective access to health information. Storage of health records is a function that many take for granted in the health care facility. By now you should recognize the importance of this function and its impact on the entire health care facility.

REVIEW QUESTIONS

1. Compare and contrast the different record identification systems.
2. Compare and contrast the various filing systems.
3. Explain the use of a master patient index.
4. Describe a chart locator system.

PROFESSIONAL PROFILE
Document Imaging Manager

My name is Melissa, and I am the Document Imaging Manager at Foster Community Hospital, a 150-bed acute care facility. I am responsible for the document imaging of all emergency room (ER) and outpatient records. Prior to this position, I was the supervisor of the clerical and release-of-information functions in this department. As the Document Imaging Manager, I oversee the preparation, scanning, indexing, and quality of the document imaging.

On a daily basis, ER and outpatient records are prepared for scanning. Pages are smoothed, staples removed, and edges cleaned. Records are batched and scanned, and the images must be reviewed and indexed. The HIM staff verify each scanned image on the computer system to identify the document for each patient record. This process tells the system the identity of an image; for example, the image is identified as an H&P for the patient as opposed to the face sheet or consent form.

To maintain this system, I must keep a current list to identify every document in the health record. The document list (something like the chart order in a paper environment) allows the record to be indexed appropriately for document identification within each patient record.

My facility no longer uses the paper record. All personnel use the images in the computer system to reference the records, including coding, release of information, and patient care areas.

APPLICATION

File System Conversion

Diamonte Hospital is preparing to convert its current filing system. The old system uses a six-digit medical record number for file identification, and the records are stored in straight numeric order on the file shelf. The new system will maintain the six-digit medical record number, but it will use terminal-digit filing because of high volume of filing activity. The facility will also get rid of the compressible shelves and use open shelving.

Develop a plan for converting the straight numeric file system to terminal-digit filing. Remember that the medical record numbers will remain the same. The change will occur in the organization of the files on the shelves.

Determine how many shelf units and how much space will be needed to store the current records in an open-shelf system. Remember to allow for aisle space, as necessary.

The current records of Diamonte occupy 3000 linear feet.

Open-shelf units contain eight shelves, and each unit is 38 inches wide (allowing for 36 inches of file space per shelf).

6

Uses of Health Information

Chapter Outline

Health Information and Its Uses
Improvement of Patient Care
Support and Collection of Reimbursement
Licensure, Accreditation, and
  Certification
Administration
Prevalence and Incidence of Mortality
  and Morbidity
National Policy and Legislation
Development of Community Awareness
  of Health Care Issues
Litigation
Education
Research
Managed Care
Marketing

The Quality of Health Care

Quality Management Theories
Deming
Juran
Crosby

History and Evolution of Quality in Health Care
Medical Education
Standardization and Accreditation
  Accreditation Agencies
Federal Government

Monitoring the Quality of Health Information
Quality Assurance
Performance Improvement
  Benchmarking

Health Information in Quality Activities
Quantitative Analysis
Qualitative Analysis
  Record Review
  Computer Applications of Qualitative
    Analysis
Clinical Pathways (Patient Care Plans)
Utilization Management
Case Management
Risk Management

Organization and Presentation of Data
Meetings
Quality Improvement Tools
  Data-Gathering Tools
  Data Organization and Presentation
    Tools

Health Care Facility Committees
Medical Staff Committees
HIM Committee
Infection Control Committee
Safety Committee

References

Suggested Reading

Web Sites

Chapter Summary

Review Questions

Professional Profile

Application

By the end of this chapter, the student should be able to:

- Identify various uses of health information.

- Review health records for documentation in compliance with accreditation agency standards.

- Review records to obtain information specific to a request for committee review.

- Participate in a quality improvement project using health information to improve patient care.

- Identify appropriate requests for health information to be used within and outside the health care facility.

- Identify the uses of health information related to the quality of patient care.

- Provide examples of the types of record reviews conducted by health information technologists to assist in the quality of care for patients and documentation in the health record.

- Identify the steps in the quality assurance process.

- Understand the intent of various health care regulations and standards.

Vocabulary

American College of Surgeons (ACS)

benchmarking

brainstorming

case management

certification

clinical pathway

clinical pertinence

concurrent review

decision matrix

graph

incidence

interdepartmental

intradepartmental

litigation

marketing

morbidity

mortality

performance improvement (PI)

placebo

potentially compensable event (PCE)

prevalence

qualitative analysis

quality assurance (QA)

reimbursement

research

retrospective review

risk management

survey

table

utilization management (UM)

By now we know the data elements constituting health information and how the information is organized and stored in paper- and computer-based systems. Now that we have collected the health information, what can we do with it? In this chapter we discuss how health information is used for reimbursement, litigation, accreditation, marketing, research, education, and quality management.

Health Information and Its Uses

Health information is extremely valuable; health care facilities use health information to

- Improve patient care
- Support and collect reimbursement
- Support and prove compliance for licensing, accreditation, and certification
- Support the administration of the facility
- Provide evidence in litigation
- Educate future health care professionals

Agencies outside of the health care facility use health information to

- Study the prevalence and incidence of mortality and morbidity
- Support litigation
- Develop community awareness of health care issues
- Influence national policy on health care issues through legislation
- Educate patients and health care professionals
- Develop health care products

The above-mentioned uses are the most obvious, but they may not include every possible use of health information.

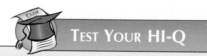

TEST YOUR HI-Q

Can you think of another use for health information besides those listed above?

Improvement of Patient Care

Health information is used to improve the quality of care provided to patients. Have you ever been treated by a physician or in a health care facility and thought that a few things could have been improved? For instance, did you wait too long to see the physician? Was communication inadequate between the health care professionals? Maybe you were given the impression that no one knew exactly what was going on with your care. Health care facilities review patients' records to determine whether patients received quality care.

Historically, health information management (HIM) professionals have reviewed the documentation of patient health care after the patient is discharged. Review of the patient's record after discharge is called **retrospective review;** it analyzes how, when, and where the patient received care. Retrospective reviews provide statistical information to support decisions that will improve care for future patients. Although retrospective reviews can be effective in improving future care, they cannot change or improve the outcome for patients who have already been discharged. The alternative to retrospective review is **concurrent review.** Concurrent reviews of patient health information provide timely information that is used to support decisions made while the patient is still in the hospital. Concurrent information provides an opportunity that *can* change or improve the patient's outcome. This process is discussed later in this chapter under Health Information in Quality Activities.

Support and Collection of Reimbursement

Reimbursement is the amount of money that the health care facility receives from the party responsible for paying the bill. Health care, although personal in service, has evolved into a large and sometimes very impersonal industry. All health care facilities have a vested interest in their financial operations. As with any other business, a health care facility provides a service or product and then charges a fee for that service or product. The facility may obtain reimbursement from several different parties—the patient, an insurance company, a managed care organization, or the state or federal government.

HIT BIT

Several different people may be involved in reimbursement for health care. You can pay for health care services yourself or through insurance. Paying yourself involves two people, or parties, making the transaction. However, if you choose to pay with insurance, a third party is introduced. The insurance company becomes a third party payer. In health care, a payer is the person or party responsible for the bill.

The patient's health record, with documentation of all of the patient's care, enables the facility to charge for services and supplies. The health record contains documentation of the type of product or service, the date and time at which the service was provided, and the employee who provided the service to the patient.

HIM coding personnel review the patient's health record to identify the correct diagnoses and procedure(s) and then assign the appropriate codes, found in the International Classification of Diseases, Ninth Revision—Clinical Modification (ICD-9-CM) and the Current Procedural Terminology (CPT). These codes are documented on the UB-92 or the HCFA-1500 form (see Chapter 9); they tell the payer why the patient received health care (the diagnosis) and if any procedures were performed that affect reimbursement. Accurate coding requires a thorough analysis of the complete health record. Inaccurate coding causes the facility to submit false claims for reimbursement. Submission of false claims is a crime punishable by law; therefore, HIM coders are educated in the review of records and the appropriate assignment of codes for reimbursement.

HIT BIT

Fraud is the term most often used to describe a false claim. The facility should have a compliance officer to ensure that the coding of health information and the billing comply with federal, state, and coding guideline requirements.

Licensure, Accreditation, and Certification

Health care facilities must have a license to operate. *Licensure* of health care facilities is performed by the state in which the facility is located. Among the many requirements necessary to receive a license, the facility must maintain documentation (a health record) on all patients.

As discussed in Chapter 1, health care facilities that provide care to Medicare and Medicaid patients receive reimbursement from the federal government. The Health Care Financing Administration (HCFA) oversees the federal responsibilities of the Medicare and Medicaid program. For a facility to receive reimbursement from the federal government, it must be certified under Medicare's Conditions of Participation (COP). The COP are the HCFA rules and regulations (standards) that govern the Medicare program. **Certification** under the COP, performed by the states, attests that the health care facility has met the HCFA standards.

Accreditation is another means by which some health care facilities may be approved to serve state and federally funded patients. Accreditation, like certification, recognizes that a facility has met a predetermined set of standards. However, accreditation is voluntary. Facilities are not mandated to attain accreditation, but they may be motivated by third party payer requirements for reimbursement and the perception that accreditation indicates a certain quality of care necessary to compete in the marketplace. Accreditation is performed by organizations like the Joint Commission on Accreditation of Healthcare Organizations (JCAHO), the Commission on Accreditation of Rehabilitation Facilities (CARF), and the American Osteopathic Association (AOA). In some health care settings a successful survey by JCAHO and some other accreditation agencies results in *deemed status* assignment by HCFA that accepts JCAHO accreditation in lieu of the Medicare COP certification.

What does any of this have to do with health information? Licensure, certification, and accreditation require that a facility prove compliance with regulations or standards. Much of the proof necessary to validate certification and accreditation standards is found in a review of the facility's patient records. The certification or accreditation survey of the facility records reveals the quality of care delivered to patients within a facility. The survey record review is coordinated to determine if the facility is providing care within the established guidelines. For example, JCAHO requires that an operative report be completed immediately after surgery. In cases in which the physician chooses to dictate the operative report, an operative note should be made part of the patient's chart and should include information pertinent to the operation that a health care professional might need to know in the absence of the detailed operative report. To check the compliance with this standard, a sample of surgery records would be pulled for review. The surveyor, HIM personnel, or others would review the record to determine the date and time of surgery. The date and time of the surgery are used for comparison with the date the operative report was dictated and the date it was transcribed, both of which are indicated on the operative report (Fig. 6–1).

OPERATIVE REPORT

Patient's name: Mary Davidson

Hospital no.: 400130

Date of surgery: 01/07/2000

Admitting Physician: Mark Ellis, MD

Surgeon: Fred Cotter, MD

Preoperative diagnosis: Nodular lymphoma
Postoperative diagnosis: Nodular lymphoma
Operative procedure: Regional lymph node excision

PROCEDURE AND GROSS FINDINGS: Under general anesthesia, after usual sterile preparation and draping, the patient was...

The patient tolerated the procedure well. Approximate blood loss 200 mL.

Fred Cotter, MD

DD: 01/07/2000
DT: 01/07/2000

FIGURE 6–1.
Operative report with date dictated (DD) and date transcribed (DT).

The date dictated is indicated by a DD: mm/dd/yy, and the date transcribed is shown by DT: mm/dd/yy at the end of the report. This information identifies when the report was dictated, when it was transcribed, and who the transcriptionist was. During record review, this information is very helpful in determining whether the facility has met the predetermined standards.

Administration

Administration is the common term used to describe the management of the health care facility. To manage health care, the services that are provided must be evaluated. Managers want to be certain that they are providing health care services in an efficient and effective manner. The administrators responsible for a facility are concerned with the personnel, financial, and clinical operations of the health care facility. Health information is used in administrative aspects to support reimbursement, make decisions regarding services, and analyze the quality of patient care.

The administrators of the facility rely on the review of health information to make decisions regarding the management of the facility. For example, review of health information may indicate that improper coding, which affects reimbursement, caused a significant decrease in revenue; or that patients who receive physical therapy soon after heart surgery recover in a shorter period of time. Health information is also used to make decisions regarding the health care services offered, to formulate policies, and to design an organizational structure.

Administrators also use health information to negotiate and evaluate contracts with managed care companies or other vendors, such as surgical supply companies and laundry companies. For surgical supply companies and laundry companies the facility uses statistics from its database (discussed in Chapter 7) to negotiate terms of a contract. The statistics help the facility determine how much to purchase from the surgical supply or laundry company.

Prevalence and Incidence of Mortality and Morbidity

Health care facilities are required to report statistics on communicable and infectious diseases to agencies of the federal government, discussed in Chapter 7. The agencies use this information to aid in the prevention and treatment of these diseases. In this use of health information, you need to understand some new statistical terms. **Prevalence** is the extent to which something occurs (Random House Webster's College Dictionary, 1991), that is, the number of existing cases. **Incidence** is the rate of occurrence (Webster's Tenth New Collegiate Dictionary, 1993), that is, the number of new cases (Abdelhak et al., 2001, p 317). Prevalence and incidence are very similar terms, but they differ in that incidence captures only new cases of a disease, and prevalence captures all existing cases of the disease. By studying the number of cases and how fast a disease is spreading in a given population, the government can target areas for prevention and treatment.

The other statistics that are reported as a result of the review of health information are mortality and morbidity. **Mortality** refers to death. **Morbidity** refers to disease or sickness. As a society we are very concerned with death and disease. As a population we are living longer, but some diseases remain fatal for many people. Federal agencies monitor, study, and determine the impact of diseases on the American public.

Within our national government the Department of Health and Human Services (DHHS) is responsible for overseeing many agencies that have an impact on health care. We reviewed the DHHS in Chapter 1, so you are familiar with the role of the Health Care Financing Administration. The mission of the Centers for Disease Control and Prevention (CDC) is "to promote health and quality of life by preventing and controlling disease, injury, and disability" (CDC, 2000). The agencies of the CDC use health information to study diseases and support their mission. There are 11 centers, institutes, and offices in the CDC that are responsible for a wide variety of health issues including minority health, human immunodeficiency virus, sexually transmitted diseases, tuberculosis prevention, occupational safety and health, chronic disease prevention and health promotion, infectious diseases and genetics (Fig. 6–2).

National Policy and Legislation

Federal and state governments use health information when making decisions related to health care. Sometimes their decisions have an impact only on Medicare and Medicaid beneficiaries; at other times their decisions influence the legislation that governs other areas of health care. For example, the Health Insurance Portability and Accountability Act (HIPAA) of 1996 affects health plans, health care clearinghouses, and providers. This legislation affects many aspects of health care including the portability of health insurance and standardization of electronic transfer of health information. Another type of legislation has an impact on health maintenance organizations (HMOs), which administer health insurance. In some states a patient has the right to sue an HMO; in other states it is illegal. On yet another issue, many insurance carriers reduced the length of stay (LOS) for obstetric deliveries: 48-hour LOS for a cesarean section, and a 24-hour LOS for a vaginal delivery. State legislation has an impact on the insurance carriers' decision requiring assessment and prevention of premature discharge for these maternity cases.

CDC CENTERS, INSTITUTES, AND OFFICES

Office of the Director

Epidemiology Program Office

National Center for Chronic Disease Prevention and Health Promotion

National Center for Environmental Health

National Center for Health Statistics

National Center for HIV, STD, and TB Prevention

National Center for Infectious Disease

National Center for Injury Prevention and Control

National Immunization Program

National Institute for Occupational Safety and Health

Public Health Practice Program Office

FIGURE 6-2.

The 11 CDC centers.

Health information is used to determine the type of coverage that Medicare or Medicaid patients receive. In other words, the government looks at the history of care provided to its beneficiaries and determines the cost and quality of that care to make decisions and enact legislation. These decisions and the legislation affect future coverage, reimbursement, and availability of services for Medicare and Medicaid beneficiaries.

Health care policy is another method that the federal government uses to influence health care. The Surgeon General is an advisor, spokesperson, and leader concerning many health issues that affect the U.S. public. For example, a familiar influence of the Surgeon General is the warning on tobacco and alcohol products manufactured in the United States (Fig. 6-3).

How did the Surgeon General's office decide that this warning was necessary? The incidence and prevalence of certain diseases, combined with research requiring review of health information, indicate that tobacco and alcohol products can cause harm to society. The warning statement is one way the government has tried to affect how and when people use these products. The Surgeon General also works to educate the public and advise the President about disease prevention and health promotion in the United States.

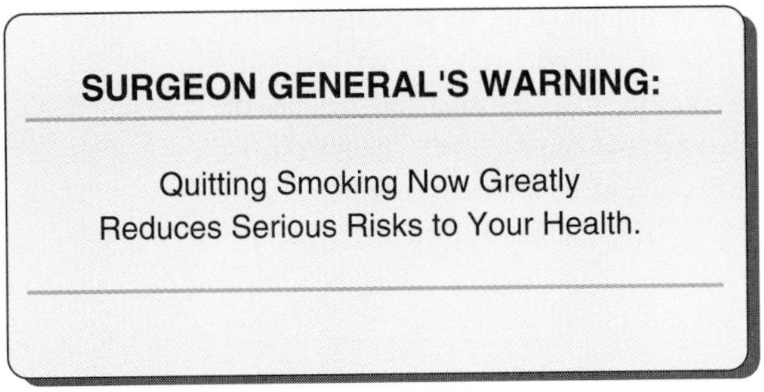

SURGEON GENERAL'S WARNING:

Quitting Smoking Now Greatly
Reduces Serious Risks to Your Health.

FIGURE 6-3.
Surgeon General's warning on tobacco and alcohol products.

Development of Community Awareness of Health Care Issues

Many diseases in our society have caused people to organize into groups to promote awareness, raise money for research, and increase prevention. Have you seen a person wearing a pink or red ribbon on a lapel to promote awareness of a particular disease? Breast cancer and acquired immunodeficiency syndrome (AIDS) awareness groups are very common. These groups use a widely known symbol to promote public education about their particular disease. Since the involvement of these groups in health care, more people are educated about the prevention, detection, and treatment of these diseases. These groups use health information, research, and statistics to inform the public. Health information in this case may relate to different populations' exposure to the disease. Health information about the prevention, cause, and treatment of a particular disease can improve the recognition of the disease in a population. Typically, a disease diagnosed at an early stage is easier to treat, and the patient's prognosis is better.

Litigation

Litigation is the term used to indicate that a matter must be settled in court. During litigation, health records or health information is used to support a plaintiff's or a defendant's case. Health records can support or validate a claim of physician malpractice. However, the opposite can be proved if there is complete and accurate documentation showing that the physician was not at fault. The health record, when admissible as evidence in court, provides evidence of the events that are alleged in a lawsuit. Chapter 8 includes more information about the use of health information in litigation.

Standards of care, expert testimony, and research are other sources of health information that may be used as evidence in a trial. Standards of care provide information regarding the typical method of providing services to a patient with a particular diagnosis. Expert testimony in health care provides the jury with information or an explanation that they may not typically understand by the words used in the health care profession. Research information provides information that the judge or jury can use to make decisions as well. Health information, whether specific to a patient or a disease, is very helpful in litigation that involves a person's health or injury.

Education

Health information is used in the education of health care professionals and patients. For example, physicians, nurses, physical therapists, and pharmacists need health information for instruction and examples as they learn how to perform their duties. The documentation of past occurrences provides an excellent opportunity to show others how to handle patient care in the future. Medical institutions use case studies of patients to teach new students about a disease process. Some health care professionals are required to maintain continuing education in their field. These professionals perform case studies on new and intriguing cases or present new technology for the education of their peers.

Likewise, health information is presented to patients and the community to inform them of the prevention, causes, incidence, and treatment for many diseases. This use of health information involves research, statistics, and information on new technology for treatment or prevention of disease.

Research

Research is the systematic investigation into a matter to obtain or increase knowledge. Health-related research requires a tremendous amount of investigation of health information. In the health care profession, documentation from previous patient care combined with the scientific process allows physicians and other researchers to improve, invent, or change patient care and technology. The intention, of course, is to affect health care by giving patients the technology, medication, or opportunity to live longer, healthier, happier lives.

Researchers review the health information from past or present patient health care. They retrieve data specific to their topic and analyze it to look for trends or suggested ways to enhance a treatment, disease, or diagnosis. They can analyze a patient's response to medication or treatment, prognosis, and the stages of a disease process; that is, how the disease develops. Health information is documented during the course of the research. Although the health information may not be reported in the traditional form of a health record, it must be organized and stored in a manner that facilitates its retrieval and reference at a later date.

HIT BIT

Pharmaceutical companies perform a great deal of research on medications before receiving approval to market them to the consumer. This research involves clinical trials in which patients with a known diagnosis or predisposition are given the medication or a **placebo** or routine treatment. While receiving the medication, the patients are monitored to determine the impact of the medication on their condition. In later clinical trials the new medication is administered to a wider group for more extensive study. Results of this monitoring are reported in the patients' health records.

Managed Care

Managed care is the coordination of health care benefits by the insurance company to control access and emphasize preventive care (see Chapter 9). Managed care organizations use health information internally and in their relationship with health care providers. A managed care organization chooses to use a health care provider's services based on an analysis of the provider's performance. The managed care organization requires the health care facility to provide information about its services, performance, patient length of stay, outcomes, and the like. The managed care organization uses this information to determine whether to choose the facility as a provider for the organization's beneficiaries.

This data gathering is part of the contract negotiation and evaluation. Before entering into a managed care contract, a lot of health information is exchanged between the managed care organization and the health care provider. While the facility is providing this information to a managed care organization, it also begins evaluating its own data to determine its ability to provide health care to this group of beneficiaries. With this information the facility can determine whether the contract is viable.

Managed care organizations can also be accredited by the National Committee for Quality Assurance (NCQA). The NCQA requires that managed care organizations comply with clinical and administrative performance standards, including a requirement for health records. Therefore, the use of health information within a managed care organization has an impact not only on the benefits of the group members, but also on the accreditation of the organization.

HIT BIT

The National Committee for Quality Assurance was founded in 1979.

Marketing

Marketing is promoting products or services in the hope that the consumer chooses those products or services over the products or services of a competitor. Health information can be used for marketing. Health care facilities are in business to make a profit. Regardless of their status, for-profit or nonprofit, they must make enough profit to sustain their business. Facilities routinely involve themselves in situations that allow them to compare their business to the competition. They analyze market share and compare usage and cost of particular services, and information about patient length of stay. In other words, they analyze statistical information obtained from health care information databases (see Chapter 7) to determine if there is a need for new treatment or technology in the community. Perhaps the study reveals that the facility has a significant share of the maternity market. There are methods that the facility can use to promote

TABLE 6–1. Uses of Health Information	
Use	**Example/Explanation**
Improvement in patient care	The health care facility uses the documentation in the health record to determine patient care.
Support and collection of reimbursement	Documentation of health care is used to support and collect reimbursement for services rendered to patients.
Licensing, accreditation, and certification	Health information must be maintained as a requirement of licensure. Likewise, it supports compliance with certification requirements and accreditation standards.
Administration	Uses health information to make decisions regarding the delivery of health care services.
Prevalence and incidence of morbidity and mortality	Statistics are reported to aid in the prevention and treatment of certain diseases.
National policy and legislation	Research and statistics are referenced to establish policy and legislation related to health care (i.e., Medicare and Medicaid).
Development of community awareness of health care issues	Research and literature are used to educate the public regarding health care issues (e.g., cancer awareness programs).
Litigation	Health information is used to support or prove a fact in a lawsuit.
Education	Health information is used to educate patients, clinicians, allied health professionals, and the public.
Research	Health information is used to support and document health care research.
Managed care	Managed care organizations evaluate health information (statistics) to determine whether to include a facility in their plan. Also, managed care organizations use health information to analyze services provided to their beneficiaries.
Marketing	Analysis of health information provides statistical information that the marketing department can use to promote the facility within a community.

other services to that group of patients. They also analyze trends that show a need for a specific type of health care, such as dialysis care, midwifery, sports medicine, or laser surgery.

The marketing department also uses successful survey by an accreditation agency as a method of promoting the facility in the community. Because the accreditation recognizes compliance with set standards, an accredited facility is perceived as better than one that is not accredited.

Table 6–1 reviews all of the uses of health information mentioned in the previous sections. We now turn our attention to the discussion of quality in health information.

The Quality of Health Care

For health information to be used effectively, it must reflect quality data. In Chapter 4 we discussed data quality characteristics (see Table 4–1). Now we discuss the meaning of quality. Common sense tells us that quality is a good thing. However, in health care, quality is determined by the person or agency that is evaluating the product or service. Some people define quality as "something that is excellent," while others may judge quality by the outcome of the service.

Customers are typically the people who judge quality. In health care we have many customers—patients, physicians, insurance companies, attorneys, accreditation agencies, and employees. Each of these customers analyzes quality from a different perspective. Therefore, a discussion of quality management in health care can lead in many different directions. Patients react to their perception of the quality of the services and care they receive. Physicians perceive the facility through the eyes of their patients, their office staff, and their professional and personal interactions with employees in the facility. Insurance companies perceive the quality of a facility through the cost and outcome of the services provided to their beneficiaries. Employees may perceive the facility through the competence of the staff and administration. Accreditation agencies perceive quality based on the facility's compliance with set standards. These examples are only a few of the methods by which a facility's quality is viewed, but you can see that a facility is judged from many different perspectives. The facility itself measures quality based on its priorities. The next section provides a simple explanation of quality theories and the use of health information in quality activities.

HIT Bit

Quality is perceived through the eyes of the patient based on the patient's priorities. For some patients, a prolonged life far outweighs the pain caused by a medical procedure. For example, a patient who suffers from persistent heart attacks requires bypass surgery to correct his heart dynamics and improve his chances for a longer life. The patient experiences tremendous pain from the

HIT Bit continued

HIT Bit continued

surgery; however, if after the operation he no longer has heart attacks, his condition is improved. The patient is probably pleased with the outcome, regardless of the intense pain experienced during the procedure. Therefore, quality was not determined by the amount of pain experienced by the patient.

For another patient, the health care experience may end with a healthy new baby. However, during the course of the patient's stay the nurses and employees of the facility were rude, uncooperative, and of little help to the new mother. For this patient, although the experience ended well, the quality is perceived as poor because of the patient's interaction with the staff.

Note that each circumstance is different, but in each case the quality of the service is determined by the customer.

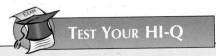

TEST YOUR HI-Q

What is quality? Take a moment to define quality and then discuss your thoughts with another person. Is that person's perception of quality the same as yours?

Quality Management Theories

Typically, in the health care industry, quality is not consistent unless it is managed. Therefore, health care facilities have a quality management department, typically staffed by HIM and nursing professionals. It is the primary responsibility of this department to ensure quality for all customers throughout the facility. This department performs a significant number of record reviews, participates on medical staff and facility committees, and coordinates performance improvement.

A commonsense approach to quality would say that to produce quality a facility must

1. Have a procedure or process in place that ensures quality. (Do things correctly.)
2. Periodically review the procedure or process and the product. (Check to make sure the facility is doing things correctly.)
3. Always document the review of the procedures, processes, and product. (When you check the procedure or process, write down your findings.)
4. Make any corrections to the procedure or process that are required to guarantee quality. (If you find an error, fix it!)

Common sense prompts the development of methods to prevent, detect, or correct flaws in a product or service to improve the quality. These methods are referred to as preventive controls, detective controls, or corrective controls, respectively (see Chapter 4). To control something, you must be able to affect or change it in some way.

To understand quality management we must mention those who are credited with the founding theories: Deming, Juran, and Crosby. Their theories have very similar and yet sometimes contradictory rules for managing quality. Each one has influenced the way that the health care industry monitors quality. Therefore it would be correct to say that they have influenced the necessity to use health information to monitor quality and, in doing so, have promoted the improvement of the quality of health information.

Deming

Of the three pioneers, Edward Deming was the first and is perhaps the most widely known. Deming gained his notoriety when the Japanese used his philosophy to rebuild their industry after World War II. As consumers increasingly chose products "Made in Japan," the American industry realized the value of adopting a quality management philosophy.

Deming's philosophy is process oriented, that is, it is necessary to evaluate *how* a task is performed or a product is produced. (This is different from the evaluation of the end product only once at the end of production.) A product that does not meet company standards must be identified before it is completed. If the problem is noted after the production is completed, the company may not be able to correct it. However, if a company inspects the process as the product is being developed, problems are more likely to be addressed and corrected before it is too late. Deming coined 14 principles to implement a successful quality management program and 7 deadly diseases that would harm a quality management program. Deming's quality principles (consolidated by Rudman [1997, p 10]) are

- Change plus innovation equals stability and organizational survival.
- Organizations have a responsibility to provide employees with appropriate education and resources.
- Organizations must foster employee empowerment and pride in work.
- Organizations should emphasize process and eliminate benchmark standards and performance evaluation.
- Quality is emphasized constantly.

Juran

Another pivotal quality philosophy is Joseph M. Juran's "quality trilogy." Juran says that every quality management program should have a strong yet balanced infrastructure of quality planning, control, and improvement. He also states that a successful program is one that is acceptable to the entire organization. The program should be as important to the employees as it is to the administrators.

Finally, Juran is credited with stipulating the value of documentation and data in the quality management program.

Crosby

Philip Crosby is best known for the term *zero defects*. The Crosby quality management philosophy requires education of the *entire* organization. Education of the entire organization requires that everyone—staff employees, supervisors, managers, and administrators—be knowledgeable about the program and capable of participating.

For a health care facility to effectively improve the quality of its care and services, it needs to adopt some method or philosophy similar to the three mentioned here. The idea of checking the quality of health care provided in the United States is not new. Quality, however, has evolved into a major focus for the health care industry.

History and Evolution of Quality in Health Care

In the 18th century, hospitals had a high incidence of deadly epidemics and relatively high death rates.

HIT Bit

The *death rate* is the number of patient deaths (over a period of time) divided by the total number of patients discharged, including deaths (over the same period of time) expressed as a percentage. Therefore, 6 deaths out of 1200 discharges is a death rate of 0.5%.

The poor received health care in hospitals, whereas the wealthy were visited in their homes. The concept of quality in health care can be traced to the 19th century. In the late 19th century hospitals finally became known as places that people could go to get well. During this time two important associations were founded, the American Medical Association (AMA) and the American Hospital Association (AHA). These two associations worked diligently to promote quality health care through standardized medical education and hospital functions. Figure 6–4 provides a time line of the evolution of quality in health care.

HIT Bit

The AMA was founded in 1847.
The AHA began as the Association of Hospital Superintendents in 1899. In 1906, the name was changed to the American Hospital Association (AHA, 2000).

18th Century	19th Century			20th Century					21st Century
Deadly epidemics Hospitals unpopular	AMA est. 1847	AOA est. 1897	AHA est. 1899	Flexner Report 1910	Club of Record Clerks 1912	ACS est. 1913	JCAHO est. 1950s	Medicare est. 1965	

FIGURE 6–4.
Time line of the evolution of quality in health care.

Medical Education

Before the existence of formal medical education, early physicians were trained through an apprenticeship. By the early 20th century many medical institutions existed to educate physicians. As the health care profession increased in size and number of physicians, quality of patient care was compromised. Although having more physicians seemed like a good solution to an ailing population, the facts suggested that more needed to be done to improve the quality of health care. Even after the establishment of the AMA in 1847, the medical education provided by many institutions remained questionable. Medical institutions needed a mechanism to standardize or guide the training of physicians.

Abner Flexner studied the quality of medical education in the United States. The Flexner Report of 1910 documented critical issues and discrepancies in medical education. The findings in the Flexner Report prompted the closing of many institutions, revising of the curriculum in those that remained, and implementation by the AMA of a mechanism for accreditation of medical education institutions.

HIT BIT

The proof is in the documentation. The old saying "If it isn't documented, it didn't happen" had an effect on the history of health care. The lack of documentation of health care prohibited the effective study of quality to improve health care.

TEST YOUR HI-Q

Which association was the first to recognize a need for quality in health care and was organized for the purpose of promoting quality health care?

Standardization and Accreditation

Not long after the Flexner Report, in 1913 the **American College of Surgeons (ACS)** was founded as an association of surgeons "to improve the quality of care for the surgical patient by setting high standards for surgical education and practice" (ACS, 1999). The ACS assumed responsibility for reviewing the quality of health care provided to patients in hospitals. Its efforts to analyze quality involved review of information from patient medical records. This effort revealed insufficient documentation of patient care. The contents of the patient health record needed to be standardized so that future reviews could provide useful information.

The ACS developed the *Hospital Standardization Program.* This program established standards, or rules, by which the ACS would review hospitals to recognize quality of care. The first survey following the establishment of the Hospital Standardization Program revealed that only 13% of the hospitals surveyed (with 100 beds or more) met the standards. The ACS then determined that for a facility to be considered a hospital it must meet a set of minimum standards. These minimum standards included the requirements for health records to be maintained in a timely, accurate fashion and specified the minimum content or required documentation for a health record (Fig. 6–5).

HIT Bit

As we move toward the computer-based patient record, standardization of information will become a prevalent issue. Standardized information allows for similar information to be shared as well as compared.

Test Your HI-Q

What was the name of the first program (set of standards) designed to measure quality in a health care setting?

By the 1950s the ACS was overwhelmed by the numerous hospitals that required surveying. The establishment of the Joint Commission on the Accreditation of Hospitals (JCAH) was a collaborative effort supported by the AMA, AHA, and ACS to relieve the ACS of the duty and responsibility of surveying hospitals. Over time, JCAH accreditation became popular in alternative health care settings, and in 1987 the organization was renamed the Joint Commission on Accreditation of Healthcare Organizations (JCAHO).

The JCAHO continued to use the Hospital Standardization Program. Current accreditation under JCAHO requires compliance with standards found in the JCAHO accreditation manuals for the various health care settings (Table 6–2).

MEDICAL RECORD SPECIFICATIONS — MINIMUM STANDARDS

A complete case record should be developed, including the following:

- Patient identification data
- Complaint
- Personal and family history
- History of current illness
- Physical examination
- Special examinations (consultations, radiography, clinical laboratory)
- Provisional or working diagnosis
- Medical and surgical treatments
- Progress notes
- Gross and microscopic findings
- Final diagnosis
- Condition on discharge
- Follow-up
- Autopsy findings in the event of death

FIGURE 6–5.
Minimum standards for medical record specifications.

TABLE 6–2. List of JCAHO Accreditation Manuals	
Setting	**Manual**
Health care networks	Comprehensive Accreditation Manual for Health Care Networks
Behavioral health	Comprehensive Accreditation Manual for Behavioral Health Centers
Home health	Comprehensive Accreditation Manual for Home Care
Hospitals	Comprehensive Accreditation Manual for Hospitals
Long-term care	Comprehensive Accreditation Manual for Long-term Care
Pathology and clinical laboratories	Comprehensive Accreditation Manual for Pathology and Clinical Laboratory Services
Ambulatory	Comprehensive Accreditation Manual for Ambulatory Care
Long-term care pharmacies	Comprehensive Accreditation Manual for Long-term Care Pharmacies
PPO	Accreditation Manual for Preferred Provider Organizations

Adapted from http://www.jcaho.org. List of publications, http://store.trihost.com/jcaho/dept.asp.

ACCREDITATION AGENCIES

Accreditation is a common indicator of quality and compliance with predetermined standards in today's health care industry. JCAHO is no longer the primary accreditation agency. Other examples of accreditation bodies are the Commission on Accreditation of Rehabilitation Facilities (CARF), which accredits rehabilitation facilities, and the American Osteopathic Association (AOA), which accredits osteopathic facilities. Table 1–6 provides a list of major accreditation agencies.

HIT BIT

The History of the American Health Information Management Association (AHIMA) can be traced back to the "Club of Record Clerks," organized in 1912 by a small group of women known as medical record librarians. The group officially initiated the Association of Record Librarians of North America (ARLNA), which included members from both the United States and Canada. The first president of this organization was Grace Whiting Myers. Eventually the members from Canada and the United States separated, and the U.S. organization became known as the American Association of Medical Record Librarians (AAMRL). In 1970 the association changed its name to the American Medical Record Association (AMRA). AMRA conferred the following credentials: Accredited Record Technician (ART) and Registered Record Administrator (RRA). Over the next 20 years the roles and responsibilities of the ART and the RRA reflected more diverse areas. By 1991, the association voted to change the name of the AMRA to the American Health Information Management Association (AHIMA). Since that time the credentials have also changed from ART to Registered Health Information Technician (RHIT) and from RRA to Registered Health Information Administrator (RHIA). The change from medical records to health information was motivated by the changing health care environment and the responsibilities of the association's members. HIM professionals hold positions in various roles, health care settings, and associated areas, such as hospitals, alternative health care settings, consulting, accreditation agencies, managed care companies, case management roles, quality management, insurance agencies, and attorneys offices.

AHIMA is a membership organization with offices in Chicago and Washington, D.C.

Federal Government

In 1965, the federal government established the Medicare and Medicaid programs. Medicare is federally funded health insurance for the elderly and some disabled people. Medicaid is federally and state-funded health insurance for the poor.

When the federal government began paying for health care, the quality and cost of care of the beneficiaries became a concern. Thus, the federal government began performing reviews of the actual care received by Medicare patients.

This was done through a review of the patient's health record. Reviewers traveled to health care facilities and looked at the health record documentation to be certain that Medicare patients were receiving appropriate quality care. If the documentation did not reflect appropriate quality, the facility was cited, asked to explain, and possibly required to return the reimbursement that was received.

In the 21st century, the health care industry is still heavily regulated and surveyed for compliance with standards and quality. Health records and health information remain a vital part of this process.

Monitoring the Quality of Health Information

In the history and evolution of quality in health care we reviewed the associations and organizations that were founded to promote quality. Some of them accredit or certify facilities. Health records are among the primary documents used by health care facilities to evaluate compliance with the standards set by the accreditation or certification agencies. In brief, health information is analyzed for quality as a part of patient care, and during this analysis the facility recognizes opportunities to improve its performance.

The HIM department is responsible for monitoring the quality of health information. Each function in the HIM department exists to enable quality; however, the functions must be monitored to ensure quality. The department, led by a credentialed HIM professional, coordinates several functions to ensure that the health information is timely, complete, accurate, and valid. Essential HIM functions are collection (assembly/abstracting), analysis, coding, storage, and retrieval. The director of HIM must manage the department functions in a manner that promotes quality information. The director and other personnel accomplish this by reviewing the functions of the HIM department.

HIT BIT

Timely Health Information

Timeliness of health information relates to documentation of an event close to the time it occurred. Health information should be documented as events occur, treatment is performed, or results are noticed. Delaying documentation could cause information to be omitted. Reports must be dictated and typed in a timely manner.

The following are examples of timeliness:

- In the physician's office, the patient documents the history before seeing the physician, and the physical examination is completed during the office visit.
- In an acute care facility, the history and physical (H&P) must be on the record within 24 hours of the patient's admission to the facility,

HIT Bit continued

HIT Bit continued

and progress notes must be documented daily. Physician's orders must be dated and timed. A discharge summary should be recorded when the patient is discharged and no later than 30 days after discharge.

Complete Health Information

Completeness of health information requires that the health care record contain all pertinent documents with all of the appropriate documentation, that is, face sheet, H&P, consent forms, progress notes, anesthesia record, operative report, recovery room record, discharge notes, nursing documentation, and so on (see Chapter 4 for the contents of a complete health record). A complete health record can be used in many more ways than an incomplete one. Review of health records to ensure that each record is complete is called *quantitative analysis.*

Accurate Health Information

Accuracy of health information requires that the documentation reflect the event as it really happened. This includes pertinent details and all relevant facts. Review of health records for pertinent documentation examines the content of each document. All of the pages in the health record must be for the same patient and also for the same visit.

Valid Health Information

Validity of health information requires that the data or information documented be of an acceptable or allowable predetermined value or within a specified parameter. This particularly pertains to the documentation of clinical services provided to the patient. For example, there are predetermined accepted values for blood pressure and temperature.

Quality Assurance

Several aspects of monitoring quality involve ensuring that the employees in the HIM department are performing their functions appropriately and that the functions work correctly to promote the employees' productivity. Assembly, analysis, coding, abstracting, completion of records, filing, release of information, and transcription all must happen within specified time frames in order to enhance the timeliness, completion, accuracy, and validity of the record. The monitoring of these functions is called quality assessment or **quality assurance (QA).** QA monitoring ensures that HIM functions are working effectively within the department's standards. Quality assurance is a retrospective analysis, performed at the end of a patient's visit.

The 1984 JCAHO standards outlined specific instructions requiring each department in the health care facility to develop a monitoring and evaluation program. By requiring the participation of all staff and departments in the facility, JCAHO planned to move health care facilities from retrospective quality assurance to quality improvement. Table 6–3 demonstrates the JCAHO 10-step plan, introduced in 1984, as used by an HIM department. The 10 steps required that

JCAHO 10 Steps	Health Information Department Example
TABLE 6–3. Transcription Example Using the JCAHO 10-Step Process	
1. Assign responsibility.	Someone must be designated to perform the audits of the identified aspects of care—transcription supervisor.
2. Delineate scope of care and service.	The transcription department converts dictated clinical information into reports for the health record.
3. Identify important aspects of care and service.	History and Physical (H&P) and operative reports must be typed with 98% accuracy within 12 hours of dictation, in order for the reports to be returned to the paper record within 24 hours of dictation.
4. Identify indicators.	H&P transcribed within 12 hours of dictation, 98% accurate. Operative report transcribed within 12 hours of dictation, 98% accurate.
5. Establish thresholds for evaluations.	Error rate 2%
6. Collect and organize data.	• Supervisor reviews random sample of H&P and operative reports for 98% accuracy. • Supervisor monitors the transcription system daily to determine compliance with the turnaround time of 12 hours. • Reports are generated from the transcription system monthly to determine compliance with the 12-hour turnaround.
7. Initiate evaluation.	The data described in step 6 are collected and reported to the HIM director monthly. All concerns and problems should be discussed in a timely fashion.
8. Take action to improve care or service.	Review of the data from step 6 determines whether the transcription department is meeting the quality standard. Failure to meet the standard requires action to improve compliance, i.e., increase of transcription staffing, appropriate assignment of transcriptionists to priority work.
9. Assess the effectiveness of actions and maintain the gain.	Continuous collection of the data in step 6, even after action is taken, will determine whether actions are effective.
10. Communicate results to affected individuals and groups.	Results of the audits should be reported to the employees in the transcription area during the monthly department meeting.

Modified from Abdelhak M, Grostick S, Hanken MA, Jacobs E: Health Information: Management of a Strategic Resource, 2nd ed. Philadelphia, WB Saunders, 2001, p 386.

the facility recognize and assign responsibility, identify important aspects of care and service, determine indicators of quality for these services, set thresholds that would require action when exceeded, develop an organized method for collecting the data according to the indicators, make an assessment of any actions taken to improve service, and communicate the results of the reviews and process to those affected.

According to the 1984 standards, HIM department managers set the standards for HIM functions. The HIM department had a written plan to monitor the effectiveness of its functions. HIM professionals determined for their facility (taking into consideration all of the regulations governing health records) the appropriate level of quality and productivity for each function. For example, the HIM professional determined that assembly and analysis should occur within 24 hours of the patient's discharge, and the records should be assembled correctly

TABLE 6–4. Quality Monitors for HIM Functions		
HIM Function	**Standard (Example)**	**How the Function Is Audited**
Assembly	Health records are assembled within 24 hours of discharge with 100% accuracy	Supervisor reviews a sample of records monthly to check accuracy
Analysis	Health records are analyzed (quantitative) within 24 hours of discharge with 100% accuracy	Supervisor reviews a sample of records monthly to check accuracy
Coding	All records are coded within 48 hours of discharge with 98% accuracy	Supervisor reviews a sample of records monthly to check accuracy
Abstracting	Health information is correctly abstracted on all patient records within 72 hours of discharge	Supervisor reviews a sample of records monthly to check accuracy
Filing	Health records are filed in the correct filing order 100% of the time	Supervisor reviews a section of the file area monthly to check accuracy
Release of information	Requests for information are processed according to law and hospital policy within 48 hours of the request, 100% of the time	Supervisor reviews a sample of requests monthly to check accuracy

100% of the time (Table 6–4). This standard required that the assembly of patient records be checked to make sure the function was happening according to the standard. If the review found that the records were not being assembled correctly 100% of the time, or that they were not being assembled within the 24-hour time frame, then action was taken to correct the problem. The same process was applied to the other standards set for HIM functions; reviews were performed, compliance was noted, and any problems were actively addressed to prevent recurrence. QA reviews of coding ensured that the coding staff was accurately coding all records in a timely fashion. In a QA review of the release of information function the HIM supervisor reviewed several requests to ensure that the release occurred in a timely fashion and that the facility's procedure for release of information was followed.

Today, the evaluation and monitoring of HIM functions is still an important process. JCAHO continues to require that facilities monitor the quality of their functions. The focus, however, is on quality improvement. The quality improvement process requires that the HIM department monitor its functions, thereby collecting data to identify things that need to be improved.

Performance Improvement

Performance improvement (PI), also known as *quality improvement (QI)* or *continuous quality improvement (CQI),* refers to the process by which a facility reviews its services or products to ensure quality. It is no longer acceptable to simply meet a standard; the facility should always seek to improve its performance. Performance improvement is a hospitalwide function that occurs intradepartmentally and interdepartmentally. Performance improvement is multidisciplinary because it involves the entire staff of the facility. The employees participate in teams to reach a solution to improve a process. All employees are encouraged to improve their work, surroundings, efforts, processes, and products. The philosophy of performance improvement implies that by improving the process, the outcome—patient care—will ultimately be improved.

HIT Bit

The prefix *inter-* means "between," for example, *inter*state highways, which run from state to state. **Interdepartmental** means between departments. The prefix *intra-* means "within," for example, *intra*venous injections, which are delivered within (into) the blood vessels. **Intradepartmental** means within a department.

The performance improvement process begins with a formal policy or statement of how the facility will conduct and document improvement efforts. The organization-wide performance improvement process is directed by a committee, the Medical Executive Committee (discussed later in this chapter) or by a committee established strictly for this purpose. All departments are required to improve processes both internally and in their relationships with other departments. Most facilities choose a model designed by a quality improvement philosopher. The model not only helps the facility document the performance improvement process to support accreditation and certification standards but also provides a measure for the facility to monitor its efforts internally. Multidisciplinary teams use the chosen model to do performance improvement.

There are several quality improvement models that provide a structure for a health care facility to follow. Ultimately, one model is chosen and the entire organization uses that model to facilitate and document performance improvement. A popular method for monitoring and improving performance is the *Plan, Do, Check and Act method*, also called the *PDCA method*, which was developed by Walter Shewhart.

HIT Bit

The JCAHO 10-step method can be used as a health care facility's quality improvement plan, but many facilities choose to go with a method that is simple or at least requires fewer steps. Methods other than PDCA are the seven-step method, recommended by Joiner Associates, Inc., and the six-step method of Re and Krousel-Wood (Abdelhak et al., 2001, p 393).

The PDCA method is easy to understand and use and therefore is one of the most widely used models (Fig. 6–6). The Plan phase consists of data collection and analysis to propose a solution for the identified problem. The Do, or implementation, phase tests the proposed solution. The Check phase monitors the effectiveness of the solution over a period of time. The Act phase formalizes the changes that have proved effective in the Do and Check stages (Abdelhak et al., 2001, p 393).

PDCA METHOD

P	Plan	**In this stage you:** ✓ Coordinate a team ✓ Investigate the problem: gather data ✓ Discuss potential solutions ✓ Decide on a plan of action
D	Do	**Here's where you test the plan of action:** ✓ Educate employees on the new process ✓ Pilot the new process
C	Check	✓ Monitor the new process during the pilot ✓ Did the plan of action work the way the team intended? ✓ Make necessary adjustments and continue the pilot
A	Act	**Once you are certain that the process is an improvement:** ✓ Change the policy ✓ Educate and train all affected employees ✓ Implement the new process

FIGURE 6–6.
PDCA method.

The key point to remember is that a process is being improved. The area of concentration is the process and not the employee performing the job. To improve a process all persons who are involved in the process must be part of the team. For example, an interdepartmental performance improvement team has employees representing each department involved in a process that affects them. An intradepartmental performance improvement team works to improve a process within a department; for example, an HIM department could organize a team to improve the effectiveness of the chart locator system (discussed in Chapter 5).

Let's discuss another example: A facility is required by state law to inform its patients about advance directives. At this facility, patients must sign a form stating that they received information about advance directives when admitted to the facility. This form is called an *acknowledgment form.* To improve the collection of the acknowledgment form for advance directives, all persons involved in the advance directive should be a part of the team.

HIT Bit

The Patient Self-Determination Act of 1990 promotes public awareness of patients' rights, health care options, and advance directives. The *advance directive* is a living will or durable medical power of attorney that allows a patient to inform health care professionals of his or her wishes if patient becomes incapable.

Because a customer's perspective must be considered to truly evaluate the quality of a process or product, a patient should be on the team for performance improvement of the advance directive's acknowledgment statement. Review Figure 6–7 for our scenario of an advance directive performance improvement team, as we discuss the additional members of the team.

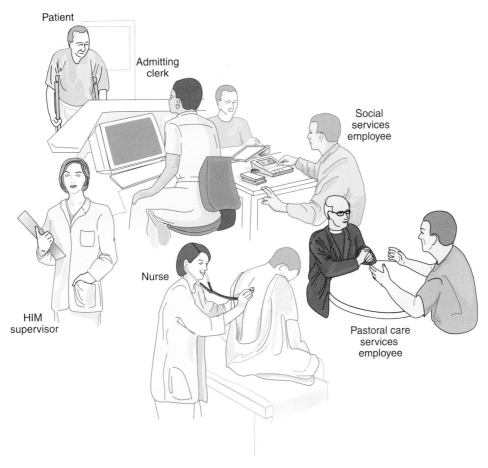

FIGURE 6–7.

Advance directive team members.

In our scenario, a patient is introduced to the advance directive at admission to the health care facility. State laws regarding advance directives vary dramatically. In our example the state assigns the responsibility of advance directives, patients' rights, and health care options to the hospital (this may or may not be the case in your state). The law does not require the patient to have an advance directive or to make any decisions immediately; it simply states that the patient must be made aware of his or her rights. To prove compliance with this state law, the facility has the patient sign an advance directive acknowledgment form. This acknowledgment form, signed by the patient and the admitting clerk, proves that the patient was given the advance directive information. A social services employee is called in to assess whether the patient has any questions regarding the advance directive. Therefore, the social service representative must be knowledgeable of both the content of the advance directive and the patient's concerns and other related issues. An advance directive is often an end-of-life determination. Pastoral care services assist the patient and family members with spiritual and emotional concerns. Their representation on the team may provide additional insight to other concerns affecting the patient or family during consideration of the advance directive statements. The nurse, being very involved in the patient care process and communicating often with the patient, is also an important member of the performance improvement team. From the HIM department, a quantitative analyst employee should be represented because of his or her knowledge of the record review process. To be effective, all people who are a part of this process must be included in the performance improvement team, and so a patient is also a key member of the team.

BENCHMARKING

Benchmarking is a quality improvement technique used by one facility to compare its process with that of another facility with noted superior performance. By reviewing a process that has proven effective in another facility, the HIM department may find methods or processes that would equally improve its own facility. Some processes are better served by throwing out the old model, the way things have always been done, and starting with a clean slate. Sometimes the benchmarking technique provides the facility with new and better methods for accomplishing the same thing.

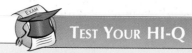

TEST YOUR HI-Q

What type of quality monitoring does JCAHO require health care facilities to perform?

Health Information in Quality Activities

Review of health records provides useful information to committees, physicians, administrators, and outside organizations. Quality analysis of health records involves two processes—quantitative analysis and qualitative analysis. Our focus in this chapter is on qualitative analysis. Typically, these two reviews are performed separately, but they can occur simultaneously.

Quantitative Analysis

To evaluate the quality of patient care, the health record must be complete, which means that all of the information must be included in the record. Analysis of the record to ensure that the documentation is complete is called quantitative analysis (see Chapter 4). An example of quantitative analysis is the review of an inpatient record for a history and physical (H&P) and discharge summary. Likewise the operative reports, laboratory reports, radiology reports, and notes must be present and authenticated by the health care professional who authored the notes, reports, or information. Quantitative analysis includes review of the record for the authentication or signatures. This analysis is performed on every health record.

Qualitative Analysis

Qualitative analysis is the review of the health record for accuracy and timeliness of contents. The information must be correct and appropriate as it pertains to the patient's care. In qualitative analysis, the patient's diagnoses, procedures, and treatment are analyzed. Qualitative analysis checks the validity of health information and the timeliness of data entries. A detailed review of the actual documentation in the record is performed to assess whether the clinically pertinent information has been recorded. Figure 6–8 provides an example of a generic (qualitative analysis) record review form that looks for basic information about the timeliness, completeness, accuracy, and validity of the health record.

The reviewer will use this generic form to determine whether the health record has the minimum requirements set by the JCAHO. Notice that the form captures information about the timeliness of the H&P: whether it was completed within 24 hours of admission. It also captures information about the content of the document: whether it contains the chief complaint, history of present illness, family history, mental status, and so on. This information is required by the JCAHO. When it surveys a health care facility, the JCAHO reviews the health records to see if this information is a part of the H&P. The record must be monitored before the survey to make sure the information is present.

Ideally, a qualitative review should be performed on every health record. However, it takes a significant amount of time to perform qualitative analysis on paper records, so a determination is made about which records to review. Accreditation agencies set the guidelines for this type of record review. Typically, qualitative analysis should be performed at least quarterly, or every 3 months. The records chosen for review should represent a sample, usually 30 records or 5% of the monthly average (whichever is greater). Record review may be based on the categories of medical staff in the facility or on specific diagnoses or procedures performed. To prevent a biased result, records must be reviewed for each physician on staff.

GENERIC RECORD REVIEW FORM

MR#_____ Attending physician: _____

Admit date: _____ Discharge date: _____

DRG: _____ Procedure:_____ Reviewer: _____ Review date: _____

CRITERIA		Y	N	N/A
Advance directive acknowledgement form signed by patient				
Patients with advance directives have copy on the health record				
H & P documented within 24 hours of admission (and prior to surgery)				
H&P contains:	Chief complaint			
	Medical history			
	Family history			
	Psychological status			
	Social status			
	Review of systems			
	Physical examination			
	Plan			
Initial nursing assessment documented within 24 hours of admission				
Discharge planning addressed				
All entries dated and authenticated				
Goals and treatment plans documented				
Progress notes documented daily				
Surgery/procedure performed				
Informed consent documented in the health record				
Preanesthesia assessment documented				
Immediately prior to procedure patient is reassesed for anesthesia				
Postoperative monitoring of the patient				
Postoperative monitoring includes:	Physiologic status			
	Mental status			
	IV fluids			
	Meds			
	Unusual events			
Operative report is documented immediately following the procedure				
Operative report includes:	Procedure			
	Findings			
	Specimen(s) removed			
	Postop Dx			
Surgical progress note documented immediately following procedure				
Discharge summary signed and documented within 30 days of discharge				
Discharge summary includes documentation of:	Diet			
	Meds			
	Follow-up			
	Activity			
	Diagnosis			

FIGURE 6-8.

Generic record review form.

RECORD REVIEW

The quantitative and qualitative review functions performed by HIM professionals to ensure quality of documentation in patient health records are also known as *record review* or *closed chart review*. The record review is required by JCAHO standards to be performed quarterly by a multidisciplinary team of health care professionals who are involved in patient care. HIM professionals read the JCAHO guidelines, understand them, and then coordinate the review of the patient records at their facility. The HIM professional typically has the responsibility for ensuring that the documentation in these records is in compliance with the standards set by the JCAHO.

This in-depth review of the health record according to standards enables a facility to determine if the appropriate care was delivered to its patients. This information is also invaluable when making decisions about future care, current practices, and legal cases involving health care.

Clinical Pertinence. The qualitative review that analyzes the patient's care specific to a diagnosis or procedure is known as **clinical pertinence.** Clinical pertinence is the review of patient health information to determine whether the care provided was appropriate, based on the patient's diagnosis. To determine which aspects of each diagnosis or procedure to review, HIM professionals work with physicians within the facility or use a published source to develop indicator screens.

The same rule for the record sample used in qualitative analysis applies to record review: Usually 30 records or 5% of the monthly average (whichever is greater). Be aware that both inpatient and outpatient diagnoses and procedures are reviewed. The generic review and the clinical pertinence review can be performed simultaneously, so that the reviewer does not duplicate his or her efforts.

An example of clinical pertinence is the review of a health record in which the patient comes to the emergency room (ER) with a productive cough and shortness of breath. The ER physician suspects pneumonia. A sputum culture is requested to identify the organism and to confirm the diagnosis of pneumonia. The review of the health record for documentation of the physician's order and test is an example of qualitative analysis. A thorough review of all pneumonia cases in a facility over a given period of time helps a facility determine whether patients are receiving pertinent care and how to improve the quality of care, if necessary. Figure 6–9 provides an example of the clinical pertinence form for the congestive heart failure (CHF) patient. Note that the indicators on the form are specific to the type of care and treatment that a CHF patient would receive.

Value of Record Review. Qualitative review of health information serves several purposes. The most important reason to perform this review is to evaluate the quality of patient care. Let's use the pneumonia scenario again. On review of a sample of patients with a pneumonia diagnosis, it is found that a sputum culture was ordered in 50% of the cases. Additionally, the culture was obtained immediately after suspicion of the diagnosis of pneumonia. The general treatment for pneumonia patients is to start them on some type of antibiotic. However, if the sputum culture returns a gram-negative specimen, normal antibiotics will not resolve the patient's pneumonia. The patient must be put on a more

CLINICAL PERTINENCE FORM—CONGESTIVE HEART FAILURE

MR#_____ Attending physician: _____

Admit date: _____ Discharge date: _____

Criteria		Y	N
Assessment			
H & P present within 24 hours of admission			
History contains documentation of:	Shortness of breath		
	Orthopnea		
Physical examination contains documentation of:	Lungs—rales		
	Heart—tachycardia		
	Liver—hepatomegaly		
	Extremities—edema		
Diagnostic workup			
Diagnostic workup includes:	Chest x-ray		
	ECG		
	Electrolyte profile		
	CBC		
	UA		
Orders			
Orders included:	Activities		
	Vital signs q 4 hours		
	Diet		
	Oxygen		
	Intake and output		
	Daily weights		
Complications documented			
Discharge status			
Discharge status includes:	Breathing improved		
	Clear x-ray		
	Potassium (K+) within normal range		
	Weight decrease		
Discharge plan			
Discharge plan includes:	Diet		
	Medications		
	Activities		
	Follow-up plans		

FIGURE 6–9.

Clinical pertinence form for congestive heart failure patient.

specific medicine. Early detection of the organism facilitates prompt medication and, ideally, a shorter period of recovery. The facility uses this information to educate the physicians and the clinical staff. The information shows the difference in patient outcome for those who received appropriate care versus those who did not. The information can also show the effect of the treatment on cost of health care or reimbursement.

These analyses—qualitative analysis, record review, and clinical pertinence—are also essential to the accreditation of the health care facility. Accreditation bodies expect facilities to analyze their compliance with predetermined standards. The quarterly review of health information to determine this compliance can prevent a facility from failing an accreditation survey. Noncompliance with standards detected early can be corrected before a survey.

During a JCAHO survey, the record review is performed by a surveyor on *open* patient charts. The results of this review are included in the accreditation decision. Therefore, it is important that facilities implement concurrent/open record reviews to ensure compliance with the standards.

Record Review Team. It is important to formalize your record review practices into a policy stating who will perform the record reviews. Multidisciplinary or interdisciplinary teams are organized for this function. Health care professionals who document information in the patient health record meet at least quarterly to review records against the standards. Record review teams include physicians, nurses, physical therapists, occupational therapists, radiologists, laboratory workers, dietitians, case managers, pharmacists, and others. Members of the record review team are challenged to determine if a record is in compliance with JCAHO standards. Record review requires review team members to become familiar with where and by whom health information is documented. In the multidisciplinary-team record review, health care professionals who document information in the health record are made aware of the importance of the documentation. For example, a nurse reviewing records to measure compliance with patient education standards may realize that the documentation in the records does not support that patient education is actually being accomplished.

The results of the record reviews must be communicated to the medical staff committee or a quality care review committee that understands the importance of health information and the effect it has on quality of patient care as well as on facility accreditation.

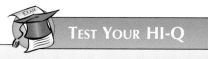

TEST YOUR HI-Q

Specify the number of records that would be reviewed at the following facilities using the rule of 5% or 30 discharges (whichever is greater).

Hospital A has 1200 discharges each month.
Hospital B has 400 discharges each month.
Hospital C has 150 discharges each month.

COMPUTER APPLICATIONS OF QUALITATIVE ANALYSIS

The computerized patient record also requires quantitative and qualitative analysis. The computerized patient record is only as good as the information that is entered. It is important that analysis of the health information remain a key function. However, it is expected that quantitative and qualitative analyses will primarily occur concurrently in the computerized patient record. Concurrent analysis provides information in a timely manner that can have an impact on patient care.

One anticipated aspect of the computer-based patient record is the decision support feature. We expect that computers will be able to be programed to recognize the data as information. This feature will allow the computer to determine or prompt the next course of action. In some cases, the computer will analyze each course of action. For example, in the pneumonia scenario, when pneumonia is entered as a suspected diagnosis, the computer searches for a physician's order to obtain a sputum culture. In addition, the computer recognizes the laboratory results of the sputum culture and is able to suggest the next course of action to the attending physician.

HIT BIT

The programing of decision support information will involve the HIM professional. Criteria must be established, decision support information entered, and scenarios analyzed to ensure that these functions work as expected in the health care environment.

TEST YOUR HI-Q

Health records contain demographic, socioeconomic, financial, and clinical data. If one of the JCAHO standards requires that the health record contain personal identification information for each patient, where could this information be found in the health record?

Clinical Pathways (Patient Care Plans)

A **clinical pathway** is the typical care provided to a patient with a specific diagnosis. After studying or reviewing a significant number of health records for patients with a particular diagnosis, a guide can be designed for most patients with that diagnosis. By doing so, a facility can streamline the patient's stay in the hospital and ideally eliminate any unnecessary time spent in the facility or in a particular level of care. The goal is to provide quality patient care in an efficient and effective manner. It is important to note that this does not mean that all patients will be treated the same. If the patient's condition warrants a change from the clinical pathway, appropriate treatment is rendered and, ideally, the patient's condition improves.

Utilization Management

Utilization management (UM), also known as *utilization review (UR),* is the function or department that ensures appropriate, efficient, and effective health care for patients. It also monitors patient outcomes and compares physician activities. "Appropriate" may also refer to what is covered by the patient's insurance plan. A health insurance plan may require a specific test in order to approve a specific treatment or procedure. The expectation is that the test will provide definitive information regarding the necessity of the treatment or procedure. For example, before approving arthroscopy of the knee, an insurance company may require magnetic resonance imaging (MRI). Historically, the physician made the sole determination of what procedures and treatments a patient would or would not receive. Today, this may be heavily influenced by the third party paying the bill.

Payers study historical patient treatment by analyzing patient health records to identify "best practices" or a specific plan of treatment that is most likely the best standard. This is not to say that physicians do not order tests that payers do not approve. Nor does it imply that payers overrule physician orders. However, there is significant controversy over the influence of payers in medical decision making.

Case Management

Case management is the coordination of the patient's care within the facility. Case management is performed by health care professionals within the facility as well as by the payers who send their employees into the facility to oversee or coordinate care. The health care professional coordinating the care is called a case manager. Case management in practice is multidisciplinary. The coordinator interacts with all of the health care professionals involved in the patient's care. With such a team, the expectation is that the communication among the disciplines (e.g., physical therapy, occupational therapy, nursing, physicians) will facilitate appropriate, effective, and efficient health care for the patient.

Typically, the case manager is the employee assigned to review the patient's care, interact with the health care team, and ensure that the services provided are covered by the patient's insurance. The case manager is assigned to the patient when the patient is admitted to the facility. Review of the patient's health information to determine the plan of care happens concurrently. Case management also includes multidisciplinary meetings of health care professionals to coordinate the patient's plan of care and to continually update each discipline on the patient's progress.

The team members in this multidisciplinary effort may include, but are not limited to, physicians, nurses, physical therapists, occupational therapists, respiratory therapists, speech therapists, HIM coders, and the patients (in some settings). Each person on the team attends the case management meeting to discuss the development or progress of the patient's care. Each team meeting is documented and becomes a part of the patient's health record. When necessary the plan of care is also updated.

Risk Management

Risk management is the coordination of efforts within a facility to prevent and control **potentially compensable events (PCEs)**. A PCE is any event that could cause the facility a financial loss or could lead to litigation. The health record serves as evidence of patient-related events that occur within the facility. The patient health record includes documentation of the facts of an incident as they are related to the care of the patient. For example, if a patient falls out of the bed during his or her stay in the health care facility, the documentation in the patient's record would indicate the time and date of the occurrence. It would also document the position of the patient's bed, use of side rails, and other pertinent information, such as the patient's diagnosis, medications administered, and instructions given to the patient before the incident.

This type of documentation in the health record is different from the *occurrence* or *incident report* that is completed when there is an inadvertent occurrence (Fig. 6–10). An incident report is a discovery tool used by the facility to obtain information about the incident. The incident report is *not* a part of the patient's health record, nor is it mentioned in any documentation. Incident reports should be completed immediately by the employee(s) most closely associated with the incident. The incident report is used to perform a mini-investigation into the facts surrounding the incident. Facts discovered immediately following the incident can significantly affect the facility's ability to defend, comprehend, or determine the cause of the incident and/or the liability of the parties in an incident. Examples of inadvertent occurrences are listed in Figure 6–11.

Occasionally, events are not recognized as incidents during the patient's stay. Review of documentation by the HIM staff may identify a PCE. As a result, health information is used in risk management to gather facts surrounding an occurrence, support the claim should it require litigation, or provide information to prevent a future occurrence.

HIT BIT

The HIM department maintains a sequestered file for all cases that are identified as PCEs or that are currently involved in litigation against the facility. This file is kept in a locked cabinet that contains the health records. Access to the file is generally limited to the department director. Records released from the file must not leave the department and can be reviewed only under direct supervision.

Incident Report

Do Not File in Medical Records

Name: _____ Employee ☐ Patient ☐ Visitor ☐

Facility name: _____

Attending physician: _____

MR # _____ SS # _____

D.O.B. ___/___/___ Sex: M[ ] F[ ]

Admission date: ___/___/___

Primary diagnosis: _____

Site (if applicable) _____

City _____

Facility ID# _____

State _____

Phone # _____

SECTION I: General Information

General Identification (circle one)

001 Inpatient
002 Outpatient
003 Nonpatient
004 Equipment only

Location (circle one):

005 Bathroom/toilet
006 Beauty shop
007 Cafeteria/dining room
008 Corridor/hall
009 During transport
010 Emergency department
011 Exterior grounds
012 ICU/SCU/CCU
013 Labor/delivery/birthing
014 Nursery
015 Outpatient clinic
016 Patient room
017 Radiology
018 Recovery room
019 Recreation area
020 Rehab
021 Shower room
022 Surgical suite
023 Treatment/exam room

Treatment Rendered (circle one):

024 Emergency room
025 First aid
026 None
026 Transfer to other facility
027 X-ray

SECTION II: Nature of Incident (Circle all that apply):

001 Adverse outcome after surgery or anesthetic
002 Anaphylactic shock
003 Anoxic event
004 Apgar score of 5 or less
005 Aspiration
006 Assault or altercation/combative event
007 Blood or IV variance
008 Blood/body fluid exposure
009 Code/arrest
010 Damage/loss of organ
011 Death
012 Dental-related complication
013 Dissatisfaction/noncompliance*
014 Equipment operation*
015 Fall with injury*
016 Fall without injury*
017 Handling of and/or exposure to hazardous waste
018 Informed consent issue
019 Injury to other
020 Injury to self
021 Loss of limb
022 Loss of vision
023 Medication variance*
024 Needle puncture/sharp injury
025 Paralysis
026 Patient-to-patient altercation
027 Perinatal complication*
028 Poisoning
029 Suspected nonstaff-to-patient abuse
030 Suspected staff-to-patient abuse
031 Thermal burn
032 Treatment/procedure issue
033 Ulcer: nosocomial stage III/IV

* Complete appropriate area in Section III

SECTION III: Type of Incident

If death, circle all that apply:

001 After medical equipment failure
002 After power equipment failure or damage
003 During surgery or postanesthesia
004 Within 24 hours of admission to facility
005 Within 1 week of fall in facility
006 Within 24 hours of medication error

Blood/IV Variance Issues (circle all that apply):

007 Additive
008 Administration consent
009 Contraindications/allergies
010 Equipment malfunction
011 Infusion rate
012 Labeling issue
013 Reaction
014 Solution/blood type
015 Transcription
016 Patient identification
017 Allergic/adverse reaction
018 Infiltration
019 Phlebitis

Dissatisfaction/Noncompliance (circle all that apply):

020 AMA
021 Elopement
022 Irate or angry (either family or patient)
023 Left without service
024 Noncompliant patient
025 Refused prescribed treatment

Falls (circle all that apply):*

001 Assisted fall
002 Found on floor
003 From bed
004 From chair
005 From commode/toilet
006 From exam table
007 From stretcher
008 From wheelchair
009 Patient states—unwitnessed
010 Unassisted fall
011 While ambulating
012 Witnessed fall

* For any marks in this field, Section V must be completed

Medication Variance Issues (circle all that apply):

013 Contraindication/allergies
014 Delay in dispensing
015 Incorrect dose
016 Expired drug
017 Medication identification
018 Narcotic log variance
019 Not ordered
020 Ordered, not given
021 Patient identification
022 Reaction
023 Route
024 Rx incorrectly dispensed
025 Time of dose
026 Transcription

FIGURE 6–10.

Incident report.

EXAMPLES OF INADVERTENT OCCURRENCES

- An employee falls in the hallway on a slippery floor, injuring his knee.
- A visitor entering the elevator is struck by the door as it closes.
- A missing patient is found on the roof of the health care facility.
- A patient falls out of bed; assessment of the patient found on the floor in the room reveals a broken arm.
- A nurse injures her back during transport of a large, uncooperative patient.

FIGURE 6–11.

Examples of inadvertent occurrences.

TEST YOUR HI-Q

What would you need to do if an employee reports that he or she fell while on a nursing unit, injuring his or her left knee?

Organization and Presentation of Data

To effectively communicate the information you have learned in the quality improvement activities and record reviews previously discussed, you need to know how to organize and present the data in a brief but effective format. The most common place that this information is presented is in a meeting.

Meetings

Meetings are an important method for bringing people together to improve performance. Meetings can be used to gather information or to impart information. At a meeting you can inform everyone of the purpose of your presentation: Everyone gets the same message at the same time. During a meeting, you can gather information about the process from the people who are involved, educate other members of the team, and keep the team focused on the goal of improving the process.

HIT BIT

The events of a meeting should be recorded and documented in the *minutes* of the meeting. The minutes help the team track its progress and stay focused on the goal. The minutes should also include meeting attendance, noting each member who is present and absent. Minutes also keep the team aware of any unresolved issues. We discuss meeting agendas and minutes in Chapter 11.

An important role in the performance improvement team meeting is that of the *facilitator*. The facilitator is the person who keeps the team focused on the goal, for example, to improve the collection of patient advance directives. During improvement efforts it is common for a team to get sidetracked by equally pressing issues that need to be corrected. A facilitator makes sure that the team does not deviate too far off course. Such deviation could impair the team's ability to accomplish its goal.

Quality Improvement Tools

Many tools facilitate the use of data in the quality improvement process. There are tools to gather information and to organize or present the information in a useful manner. Data-gathering tools assist the team in exploring or at least acknowledging issues surrounding the process of concern. Organization and presentation tools make a statement about the information that is gathered. We discuss two data-gathering tools, brainstorming and surveys; and several organization and presentation tools: bar graphs, line graphs, pie charts, decision matrices, and flowcharts.

DATA-GATHERING TOOLS

Brainstorming is a method by which a group of people get together to discuss ideas, solutions, or related issues on a topic or situation. It is a data-gathering tool used to identify all aspects, events, or issues surrounding a topic. This process encourages the involvement of everyone in the group. All ideas are accepted, no matter how insignificant they may appear. To perform brainstorming you need only to have a topic and a place to write down the ideas mentioned by the group. To begin the process, the team's facilitator explains that this tool is used to gather all ideas related to the issue—regardless of how unusual they may seem.

For example, a quality improvement team is organized to reduce the length of time that a patient waits to receive treatment in the emergency room. At the team's first meeting the members brainstorm all of the possible things that

TABLE 6–5. Survey Questions	
Open Question	**Limited Answer Question**
How would you describe your visit to our emergency room?	Choose one of the following to describe the emergency room during your recent visit: a. Very clean b. Adequately clean c. Unclean d. Very dirty
How long did you wait in the emergency room before being seen by a physician?	How long did you wait in the emergency room before being seen by a physician? a. Less than 1 hour b. 1–2 hours c. 2–3 hours d. Longer than 3 hours

could have an impact on the patient's wait in the emergency room. The team members are encouraged to mention anything that could affect the patient's wait time. Note that the members' ideas do not need to prove an impact. This is simply a data-gathering tool. Later you will learn the use of an organization tool to narrow your improvement effort.

A **survey** is set of questions designed to gather information about a specific topic or issue. A survey can be used routinely to gather information from a group, or it can be designed as part of a specific quality improvement team. For example, many facilities survey patients following a visit to the facility. They want to find out how the patient perceived the service. This type of survey can be used to measure patient satisfaction. When significant dissatisfaction is noticed, the facility may organize a performance improvement team to address the issue. In the emergency room example previously mentioned, the performance improvement team could develop a survey to ask patients why they perceive it took so long to receive treatment. The questions on a survey can be open, which means the response area is blank. With open questions patients are free to answer the question in their own words. However, this method of questioning may not provide enough information to determine how much improvement is necessary. Table 6–5 provides an example of the same survey question asked in two different ways.

DATA ORGANIZATION AND PRESENTATION TOOLS

Data organization and presentation tools are used to communicate information quickly to another person or group. Because quality improvement is a team effort, you will routinely need to organize information and display it so that the group can interpret or understand something. Such tools include graphs, tables, and charts. A **graph** is an illustration of data. A **table** has data organized in rows and columns. These visual tools can be very persuasive. You can emphasize positive information just as easily as negative information. Here is an example: The number of cigarette-smoking freshmen on our college campus has declined 40% between 1996 and 2000. However, overall smoking prevalence on our

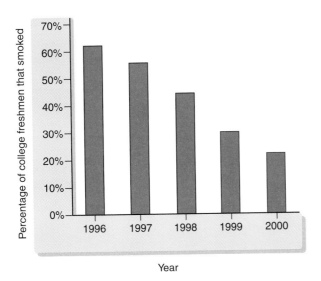

FIGURE 6–12.
Bar graph of college freshmen who smoked cigarettes,
1996–2000.

campus was virtually unchanged during that time. We can take the positive
data—the decrease in the number of freshmen who smoked from 1996 to
2000—and plot it on a graph to show a positive trend in smoking cessation
(Fig. 6–12).

However, the same statement provides a negative picture, that is, the overall
number of people smoking on the campus remains about the same. This one
statement could be graphed in two different ways: The positive graph illustrates
that the number of freshmen smoking has decreased, and the negative graph
shows that the total percentage of people smoking remains unchanged.

Bar and Line Graphs. *Bar* and *line graphs,* also known as *charts,* relate information along the horizontal (*x* axis) and the vertical (*y* axis). In a bar graph,
one axis is used to represent the group or indicator, and the other axis is used
to plot the data for the group. For example, Figure 6–12 is a bar graph showing
the categories (1996, 1997, 1998, 1999, 2000) along the *x* axis that are the years
in which freshmen smoking was measured. The data plotted along the *y* axis are
the percentage of freshmen (smoking) for each year. If we change the bar graph
to a line graph we could follow the percentage of people smoking over the
course of the 5-year period. In Figure 6–13 the bars have been replaced with
points that are connected by lines. Line graphs are used to plot data over time.
This graph easily depicts the trend of the same data as it is measured continuously, month to month or year to year.

Note the labels and headings used in Figures 6–12 to 6–14 and in Table 6–6.
The headings describe the graph or chart, giving the reader an idea of what information is included. On bar and line graphs, the labels on the axes identify
what is being measured and how it is being measured. On the pie chart, we

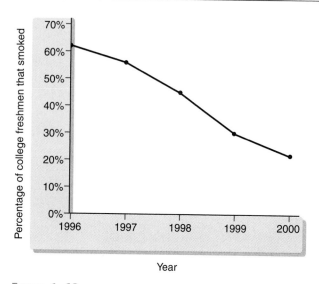

FIGURE 6–13.

Line graph of same data as in Figure 6–12.

could use a key to indicate which color is associated with each group. The following is a list of reminders for creating graphs:

- Include information about the time frame of the data or the date the data were collected.
- Make sure your graph is legible, especially if you plan to present the information on an overhead projector to a large group.
- Choose the best graph for the data that you are presenting, for example, percentages relate well on a pie chart, but the total of the percentages must equal 100% for the pie chart to be accurate.
- Be prepared to explain your graph if questioned by the audience.

Pie Chart. A *pie chart* is a graphical illustration of information as it relates to a whole. For example, we can illustrate the percentage of people on campus who smoke as a pie chart. When you think about this type of chart, imagine a pie. The pieces of the pie represent percentages. If the pie is cut into even slices, all of the pieces will be equal. However, when we show all of the people on campus who smoke, we can easily determine which group smokes the most (Fig. 6–14).

Decision Matrix. A **decision matrix** can help a group to organize information. This tool is used when the quality improvement team must narrow its focus or choose among several categories or issues. For example, if a performance improvement team is organized to decrease smoking on the college campus, the members may begin by brainstorming and determining all of the issues that influence a person's choice to smoke. Once the team has identified the things on campus that influence the choice to smoke, the team will need to decide which

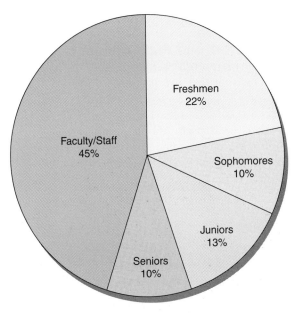

FIGURE 6–14.

Pie chart of the percentage of people on campus who smoke
(see Figure 6–12).

influences they can change. A decision matrix can be used to analyze which of
the influences when taken away would cause a decrease in the number of smokers. Table 6–6 shows a decision matrix in which each group of smokers is analyzed to determine which issue has the greatest influence on that group's choice
to smoke.

First note that we have set up a table, with the first row identifying the
groups of smokers and the first column identifying the issues that may influence a person's choice to smoke. To complete the decision matrix, the performance improvement team analyzes each group according to the influences
they found. Team members can write their comments in the squares or they
can assign a value, in this case, *1* for least likely to influence the person to
smoke, *2* for moderate influence, and *3* for most likely to influence the person
to smoke. The final column on the right is a total or decision column. The influence with the highest rating or the influence that occurred in each of the
categories would be the team's target. In this case, the first and decidedly easi-

TABLE 6–6. Decision Matrix						
	Freshmen	**Sophomores**	**Juniors**	**Seniors**	**Faculty-Staff**	**Total**
Commercials	2	2	2	2	1	9
Smoking areas	3	3	3	3	3	15
Peer pressure	3	3	2	2	1	11

est way to decrease smoking on campus is to eliminate some of the smoking areas.

Flowchart. A *flowchart* is a tool used to organize the steps involved in a process. Because the performance improvement team is interdisciplinary, some of the team members may not understand the process that they are intended to improve. The flowchart provides an illustration of how the process works within the facility. For an example, refer to the advance directive flowchart shown in Figure 6–7. The figure shows how the facility informs the patient about the advance directive and how the health care professional obtains the patient's signature on the acknowledgment form. Flowcharts help the team streamline a process and eliminate unnecessary steps.

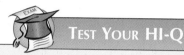

TEST YOUR HI-Q

Which graph would you use to show that the overall percentage of people smoking on campus has remained unchanged?

Health Care Facility Committees

Committees are a formal organizational tool that facilities use to conduct business. The committee structure of the health care facility is outlined in the medical staff bylaws, rules, and regulations. Some committees are a requirement of an accreditation agency. Although all health care facilities have committees, the roles and functions of committees in each facility vary. Examples of committees within a health care facility are medical staff departments, infection control, safety, surgical case review, pharmacy and therapeutics, and HIM. The following discussion briefly explains how these committees use health information.

Medical Staff Committees

The medical staff of a health care facility is a self-governed group of physicians divided into departments based on their practice, such as the department of medicine, department of surgery, department of obstetrics, and department of pediatrics. The medical staff structure is directed by an elected group of physicians; such positions include chief or president of the medical staff, president-elect (incoming chief of staff), and chairperson of each department. Each medical staff department has a committee meeting in which business directly related to that field of medicine is discussed. The committee reviews patient cases, determines appropriate documentation, and discusses standards of care, as necessary. The medical staff departments also use statistics acquired from health information to make decisions regarding physician membership, privileges, and compliance with accreditation standards.

Accreditation by JCAHO requires that a facility review specific cases of patient care in the areas of surgery, medication usage, and blood and tissue usage. For example, the department of surgery will perform *surgical case review* as an accreditation requirement. The facility reviews statistics related to surgeries and the health records of surgical cases with unexpected outcomes, for example, a patient who goes into cardiac arrest during an appendectomy or a case in which the wrong operation was performed. *Medication usage* is typically reviewed by the pharmacy and therapeutics (P&T) committee. The P&T committee is composed of members of the medical staff, with nursing, administration, and hospital pharmacist also represented. The committee reviews medications administered to patients, specifically targeting any adverse reactions that a patient has had as a result of medication. The P&T committee also oversees the hospital formulary, which is a listing of the drugs used and approved within the facility. *Blood usage* is also a review that requires participation from the medical staff. This review analyzes the appropriate protocol, method, and effects for patients receiving blood transfusions (or blood products).

The business and decisions of the departments of the medical staff are reported to the Medical Executive committee for action, recommendation, or correspondence to the governing board. The "med exec committee," as it is commonly called, acts as a liaison to the governing board of the facility. This committee is composed of the chief of staff and elected positions, with a representative from each of the medical staff departments.

HIM Committee

The HIM committee, commonly referred to as the medical record committee, serves as a consultant to the director of the HIM department. At a minimum, the HIM committee acts as the forms committee, as discussed in Chapter 3. However, in some facilities, the HIM committee is also responsible for reviewing the documentation in patient health records and assisting in compliance with accreditation standards. There are many important health information issues that can be addressed by this committee. Figure 6–15 is a sample agenda for the HIM committee; the committee can review the findings of the record review teams, the percentage of delinquent medical records, and quality assurance and quality improvement activities. Members of the HIM committee are the director of HIM, physicians from each department of the medical staff, nursing staff, and quality management personnel.

Infection Control Committee

The infection control committee is organized to analyze the rate of infection of the patients within a facility. This committee meets regularly to determine whether patients are entering the facility with unwanted infections that can harm the staff or other patients, or if they are acquiring infections within the facility that affect their care, treatment, and length of stay.

AGENDA FOR HIM COMMITTEE

Health Information Management Committee
Meeting: October 19, 2000

Agenda
  I.   Call to order
  II. Review of minutes
  III. Old business
  IV. Record review
  V.   New business
  VI. Reports
          Delinquent record count
          Quality audit of HIM functions
  VII. Adjourn

Next Meeting: November 16, 2000

FIGURE 6–15.

Agenda for HIM committee.

HIT BIT

Nosocomial infections are those infections acquired by patients while they are in a health care facility.

The infection control committee is also involved in preventing and investigating infections. Members of the infection control committee include physicians, nurses, quality management personnel, and HIM personnel. To evaluate infection control rates within a facility, the committee must analyze information from patient health records.

Safety Committee

The safety committee is organized to assist the safety officer, who is responsible for providing a program to create a safe environment for patients, visitors, the community, and staff. Health care facilities must adhere to numerous requirements from the Occupational Safety and Health Administration (OSHA), JCAHO, state licensing boards, and federal agencies. The safety committee evaluates the information presented by the safety officer, ensures safety of the environment, and performs disaster planning. Occasionally the safety committee also reviews the incident reports of cases related to the facility's environment. Members of the safety committee are appointed and may include clinical and non-clinical employees.

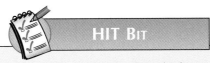

HIT BIT

The safety officer is typically a member of the facility's administration.

References

Abdelhak M, Grostick S, Hanken MA, Jacobs E: Health Information: Management of a Strategic Resource, 2nd ed. Philadelphia, WB Saunders, 2001.

Rudman WJ: Performance Improvement in Health Information Sciences. Philadelphia, WB Saunders, 1997.

Suggested Reading

Cofer JI, Greely HP: Quality Improvement Techniques for Medical Records. Marblehead, MA, Opus Communications, 1996.

Merriam-Webster's Collegiate Dictionary, 10th ed. Springfield, Mass, Merriam-Webster, Inc., 1993.

Random House Webster's College Dictionary. New York, Random House, 1991.

Web Sites

ACS on line: Available at **www.facs.org.** What is the American College of Surgeons?, February 8, 1999.

AHA on line: Available at **www.aha.org/about/history.html,** August 31, 2000.

CDC on line: Available at **http://www.cdc.gov/aboutcdc.htm,** August 2000.

CHAPTER SUMMARY

Health information is widely accepted as an important part of the health care industry. Often the acceptance factor takes for granted that the health information will be timely, complete, accurate, and valid. This chapter reflects the importance of continued efforts to ensure quality health information so that it may be used effectively to make decisions about patient care. We recognize the importance of standardized information on all patients as first required by the ACS minimum standards. With standardized information, health care professionals are able to compare one patient's care with another's and determine the quality of each. Standardized information allows for similar information to be shared as well as compared.

Perhaps the most eye-opening issue surrounding the uses of health information is that outsiders do not recognize its importance until an HIM professional points it out or, more pointedly, until what is needed is not available, as was recognized by the ACS in 1917.

Quality health information allows others to use this vital information for the benefit of patients, communities, payers, and providers.

REVIEW QUESTIONS

1. List and describe 10 uses of health information.
2. How is health information used to measure quality of patient care?
3. Explain the PDCA method for quality improvement.
4. Identify three committees and how they use health information.

PROFESSIONAL PROFILE
Assistant Director, HIM

My name is Kim, and I am the assistant director of the HIM department. I am responsible for coordinating review of health records to ensure compliance with JCAHO standards. Record review is performed on a monthly basis at Parker Hospital, a 500-bed acute care facility. According to standards, my staff and I review 50 records each month. I make sure that all of the records are pulled before the meeting and prepare enough forms for review of the 50 records. During the multidisciplinary review meeting I help the team members when they have a problem interpreting a standard or locating information in the health record. When all 50 records are reviewed, I collect the forms and tabulate the scores to determine the compliance with each standard. I then present the results of this review to the HIM committee for recommendation and action, as necessary. If the committee suggests a corrective action to improve compliance with a standard, I coordinate that effort. Following the implementation of the corrective action, I report back to the HIM committee to show whether compliance has improved.

APPLICATION

Record Review

As a member of the record review team, use the health record forms provided on the Introduction to Health Information Technology Companion Website and the generic record review form (see Fig. 6–8) to identify where the information should be found in the record.

7

Retrieval and Reporting of Health Information

Chapter Outline

Organized Collection of Data
Primary and Secondary Data
Data Set
Creation of a Database

Data Review and Abstracting
Data Quality Check

Data Retrieval
Retrieval of Aggregate Data
Indices
Identification of a Population
Optimum Source of Data

Reporting of Data
Reporting to Individual Departments
Reporting to Outside Agencies
    Registries
    Vital Statistics

Statistical Analysis of Patient Information
Analysis and Interpretation
Presentation

Routine Institutional Statistics
Admissions
Discharges
    Transfers
Census
Hospital Rates and Percentages

Reference

Suggested Reading

Chapter Summary

Review Questions

Professional Profile

Application

In Chapters 2 and 3 we discussed collection of health data for documentation in the health record. The health record is used to gather health data (data sets) for storage in a physical location and/or database to provide a meaningful method for retrieval of the information for future use. Organizing specific data elements for each patient allows reporting of health information as it is mandated by law, accreditation, policy, or necessity.

Other important reasons to collect specific health data are statistical analysis, outcome analysis, and quality improvement. Data analysis is a critical function in all health care facilities. To analyze data within one record or between two or more records, the data elements must be collected in the same way. An important function of the health information management (HIM) department is the organized retrieval and reporting of these data. In Chapter 3, we discussed the collection of health data based on providing proper patient care and for following health care professional guidelines. The data were categorized into reports, such as the history and physical (H&P), laboratory reports, and nurses' notes. In this chapter, we discuss the importance of collecting specific data in an organized format—such as a database—so that the health information can be analyzed and reported as necessary.

Organized Collection of Data

Primary and Secondary Data

Health data can be categorized as primary or secondary. **Primary data** are those data taken directly from the patient or the original source. Primary data also describe the information obtained by a caregiver after observation of the patient. Examples of primary data are the history given by the patient to the nurse (Fig. 7–1) and the patient's blood pressure or temperature reading as recorded by the monitor or the nurse. These data elements are documented in the patient's health record in a format that transforms the raw data into usable information. Therefore, the patient's health record contains primary data.

When information is taken from the primary-source document for use elsewhere, those data become **secondary data** (Fig. 7–2). When the patient is discharged, the HIM department coding employee determines the appropriate International Classification of Disease, Ninth Revision—Clinical Modification (ICD-9-CM) code to describe the diagnosis. Diagnosis codes are entered into the patient's abstract (discussed later in this chapter), facilitating the diagnosis index and billing process. The diagnosis, procedure, and physician indices are examples of secondary data. One purpose of this chapter is to explain the collection of primary data for use in secondary data documents.

HIT BIT

Remember the difference between data and information: The *data* collected during patient care become health *information* only after careful organization and compilation. Data are raw elements. Information is (human) interpretation of data.

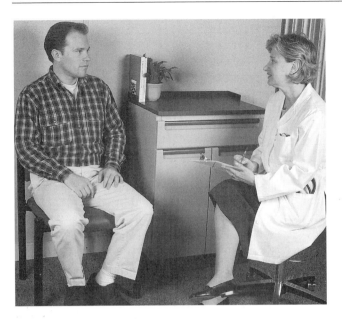

FIGURE 7–1.

Primary data are collected when the nurse talks to the patient to
obtain his health history. (From Jarvis C: Physical Examination
and Health Assessment, 3rd ed. Philadelphia, WB Saunders, 2000,
p 642.)

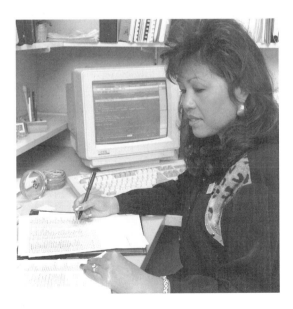

FIGURE 7–2.

As an HIM clerk reviews a health record and enters data
into the abstract, she is creating secondary data. (From
Clark MA, Mazza VS: Health Unit Coordinating: Expanding the Scope of Practice. Philadelphia, WB Saunders,
1999, p 60.)

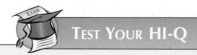

TEST YOUR HI-Q

List an example of primary data found in the health record.

Data Set

A **data set** is a group of elements collected for a specific purpose. A data set requires a standard method for collecting data elements so that they can be compared. To compare data we must be sure that everyone is collecting the information the same way. For example, we collect certain information on all patients regardless of the health care services needed—name, address, phone number, and age. This information is a data set for the patient's personal identification. It is the information that allows the facility to identify one patient separately from other patients, male from female, mother from baby. Each facility must make sure that its data sets are designed to comply with federal requirements as well as the internal needs of the facility.

As discussed in Chapters 2 and 3, there are specific requirements that mandate data sets for various health care organizations according to their service. Table 7–1 shows the data sets required by the type of facility. For example, the Uniform Ambulatory Care Data Set (UACDS) is required in all ambulatory care facilities. The federal government, as a payer, is very interested in the services that are provided to its beneficiaries. Collection of specific data, as required by the Uniform Hospital Discharge Data Set (UHDDS) for acute care, allows the Health Care Financing Administration (HCFA) to analyze patients, the health care provider, and services. The analysis is possible because each data element is being collected the same way for every patient in the United States. Table 7–2 provides a summary of the data elements required by UHDDS.

Notice that HCFA has requested information to identify the patient, provider, and services. The specific manner in which this information is collected allows HCFA to compare Medicare patients regardless of where they receive health care services. Each data element has been defined; for example, the attending physician, according to UHDDS definition, must be the clinician "who is primarily and largely responsible for the care of the patient from the beginning of the hospital episode" (Hanken and Water, 1994, p. 20). The definition provided for each data element specifies what should be captured for that data element.

TABLE 7–1. Data Sets by Facility Type	
Data Set	**Facility Type**
Uniform Hospital Discharge Data Set (UHDDS)	Acute care
Uniform Ambulatory Care Data Set (UACDS)	Ambulatory care
Minimum Data Set (MDS), Resident Assessment Instrument (RAI)	Long-term care
Outcome and Assessment Information Set (OASIS)	Home health
Health Plan Employer Data and Information Set (HEDIS)	Managed care organizations

TABLE 7–2. Required Contents of the Uniform Hospital Discharge Data Set (UHDDS)	
1. Patient identification number	10. Surgeon's identification number
2. Date of birth	11. Principal diagnosis
3. Sex	12. Other diagnoses
4. Race and ethnicity	13. Principal procedure and the date of the procedure
5. Residence	
6. Health care facility identification number	14. Other procedures and the date(s) of the procedure(s)
7. Admission date	
8. Discharge date	15. Disposition of the patient at discharge
9. Attending physician's identification number	16. Expected source of payment
	17. Total charges

Throughout the course of the patient's care, data are collected by many health care professionals. The mandated data set is typically a summary of that information collected in a specific manner. Without a specific requirement for data, some facilities might not include data elements that are helpful to users when performing an analysis. For example, the patient's gender is a data element that is always helpful. However, if there was no specific requirement for how the gender is captured, some facilities might not capture the data, and others might capture the data in different ways. Realistically, without a requirement, the field that captures the patient's gender could read F, 1, or A, for female; and M, 2, or B, for male (Fig. 7–3).

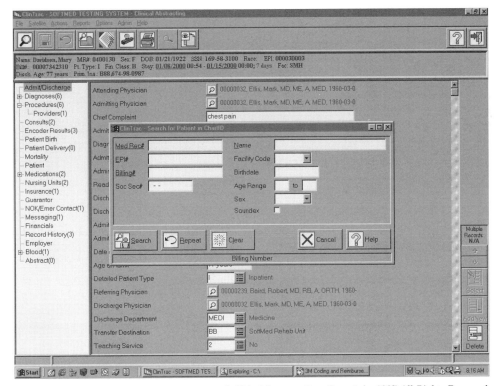

FIGURE 7–3.

Data set for patient gender. (Courtesy of SoftMed Systems, Inc., Bethesda, Md.)

HIT BIT

In rare cases it is necessary to have classification of "unknown" for gender. Some health care applications have an "unknown" category for gender that may be recognized as U, 3, or C.

If each health care facility determined its own method for collecting the patient's gender data, HCFA would have to interpret each facility's method for classifying this information. By defining a specific data set and the method in which the information should be shared with the federal government on the UB-92 form (see Chapter 9), the government has mandated a data set for patients. Ultimately, this information is collected on all patients in an acute care facility regardless of who is paying and therefore allows for the comparison of the information internally and externally.

Creation of a Database

The data collected for each patient create a **database.** This database is a collection of data elements organized in a manner that allows efficient retrieval of information. The data collection can occur on paper or in a computer software program. For our discussion, we will consider the computer-based patient record; however, keep in mind that any collection of data elements can be considered a database.

Computer software is designed for health care facilities to organize patient health information in a systematic, defined format. The program requires collection of data in a special format, alphabetic or numeric, as discussed in our data dictionary explanation (Table 7–3).

HIT BIT

Federal laws and standard-setting organizations exist to ensure that the health information contained in the databases of health care organizations and related entities is maintained in a defined, standardized format that allows comparison and sharing through an electronic or computerized format. They also strive to ensure the confidentiality and security of health information in the electronic and computer-based environment.

The Health Insurance Portability and Accountability Act (HIPAA) is a broad law that includes requirements for electronic health information to be stored in a standard transferable format that is confidential and secure.

Health Level Seven (HL-7) standards allow computer systems to exchange clinical and administrative data.

TABLE 7–3. Data Dictionary with Range of Valid Values					
Name	**Definition**	**Size**	**Type**	**Example**	**Valid**
Day	Day of the month	2 characters	Numeric	15	1–31
Month	Month of the year	2 characters	Numeric	08	1–12
Temperature	Patient's temperature	5 characters	Numeric	98.6	85–110

Because each data element is defined before it is collected, the database is a useful source of information. For example, "attending physician" is one of the data elements that is collected. This datum can be collected in the admission record by entering the identification number for the physician who matches the description of the attending physician (see Table 3–1). This information (which is contained in the physician index) is collected for each patient discharged. The collection of this data element on all patients in the database makes it possible to **query** or ask the database for information specific to the attending physician. For example, facilities should review records on a representative sample of all physicians on the medical staff at the facility (see Chapter 6). To do so, one must be able to run a **report** that lists records for each physician. The physician identification data element allows one to query the database for a report and sort the information by physician. Then one can be sure that a good sample of physicians is reviewed during the record review process.

We know that some data are required by the federal government. However, other data elements are retrieved only as specified by the facility. These types of data must be collected in the way they are going to be useful in the future. For example, in some cases, the type and frequency of a patient's consulting services, such as physical therapy, occupational therapy, or respiratory therapy, may influence the patient's outcomes. To collect this type of information, each consulting discipline may be given a number (1, physical therapy; 2, occupational therapy; 3, respiratory therapy; 0, no therapy), and then as each patient record is abstracted, consulting services are identified and the corresponding numbers for the services provided to that patient are entered into the abstract. Later we can access that information in the database in any way that we want; for example, we can look at consulting services associated with a specific diagnosis or procedure or with a physician. An example of other data that may be collected is advance directive acknowledgments (see Chapter 6). Facilities can include a field to capture whether a patient has signed the advance directive acknowledgement statement.

HIT Bit

Query is the term used to describe the searching of a database for specific elements.

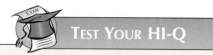

Data Review and Abstracting

Patient health data are gathered at admission and throughout the course of the patient's care. In a computer-based patient record most of the data are captured, and the health information employee verifies the abstract. In the paper environment, once the patient is discharged the health information employee must correlate the information in the computer system with the patient record. The employee verifies the information to be sure an abstract is created for the correct patient. Verification of the abstract is a detective control. Fixing any noted errors is a corrective control (see Chapter 4). The **abstract** can be defined as a summary of the patient's encounter. It provides a brief synopsis of the patient's care that would otherwise require a thorough review of the entire patient record. The abstract is a set of data elements, including those previously discussed in this chapter. At a minimum, each facility collects those data elements required by HCFA; it determines additional data elements for internal analysis of patient information.

The process of summarizing the patient's information in a database by data entry of specific data elements is called *abstracting*. To complete an abstract, the HIM clerk must review the health record. The review is necessary to determine the appropriate data element for each field. As we discussed, the health information coder must review the record to determine the accurate code (ICD-9-CM or Current Procedural Terminology [CPT]) to represent the patient's diagnosis and procedures. To make this determination, the coder relies on the documentation in the record and his or her knowledge of coding. The other information that is captured as part of the abstract is the patient's disposition, the place the patient goes to after discharge from the facility—home, nursing home, or another acute care facility. This information is usually entered in the form of a code, for example, 1 for home, 2 for nursing home, 3 for home with home health, 8 for death. If you look at Table 7–2, you can see that in an acute care facility this is the minimum information that must be collected. Examples of additional information that is typically captured are type of anesthesia, length of surgery, and consent. By collecting this information in the abstract, the facility is able to query the system (run reports) for information related to these topics.

The patient's abstract is a common source of secondary data, and its creation or validation is a major function of the health information management department. Figure 7–4 is an example of a patient abstract screen. Figure 7–5 contains the forms that were used to retrieve the data elements for this abstract. Note the information required in the abstract: patient's name, address, diagnosis, procedure, date, and length of procedure. As you review Figures 7–4 and

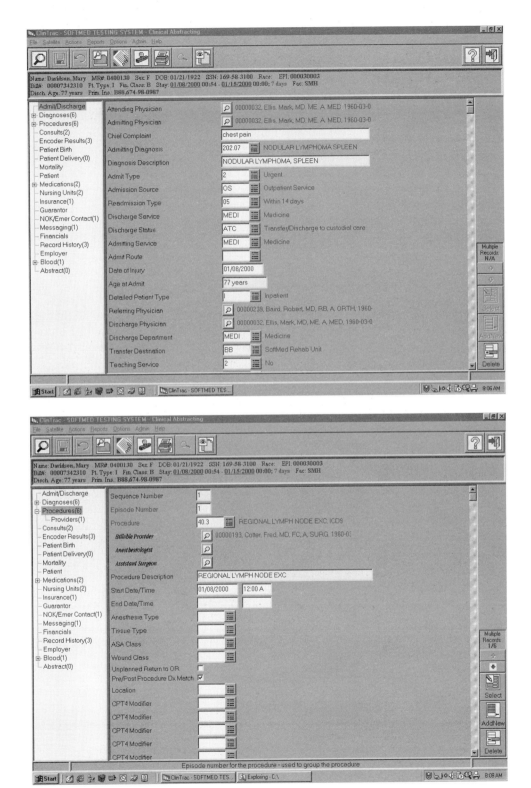

FIGURE 7–4.

Patient abstract screens. (Courtesy of SoftMed Systems, Inc., Bethesda, Md.)

Illustration continued on following page

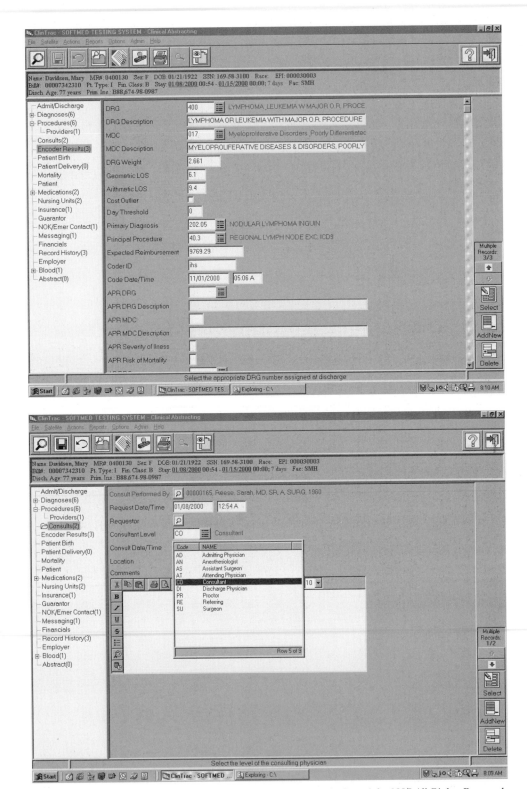

FIGURE 7–4.

Continued

OPERATIVE REPORT

Patient's name: Mary Davidson

Hospital no.: 400130

Date of surgery: 01/07/2000

Admitting Physician: Mark Ellis, MD

Surgeon: Fred Cotter, MD

Preoperative diagnosis: Nodular lymphoma
Postoperative diagnosis: Nodular lymphoma
Operative procedure: Regional lymph node excision

PROCEDURE AND GROSS FINDINGS: Under general anesthesia,
after usual sterile preparation and draping, the patient was . . .

The patient tolerated the procedure well.
Approximate blood loss 200 mL.

Fred Cotter, MD

DD: 01/07/2000
DT: 01/07/2000

FIGURE 7–5.

The operative report from the patient's record was used to retrieve the data elements required in
the patient abstract shown in Figure 7–4.

7–5, you can see how the clerk was able to determine the correct data to enter in this abstract.

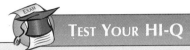

TEST YOUR HI-Q

The type of anesthesia used during the surgery is a required data element in the abstract. Using the operative report in Figure 7–5, can you determine what type of anesthesia this patient received?

When all required elements of the patient's data have been captured, the abstract is considered complete. All patient records must be abstracted as required to satisfy payer and facility guidelines for specific information. Each patient receiving services in a health care setting has an abstract. However, the abstract differs according to the setting, for example, ambulatory care or long-term care.

Some of the typical queries of the abstract database include

- List of patients for a physician
- List of patients by diagnosis, diagnosis related group (DRG), or procedure
- List of patients by patient financial class
- List of patients by age
- List of patients with consulting physicians

HIT BIT

Historically, abstracting was done manually by completing the required elements on a data form (Fig. 7–6). The form would then be fed into a computer system or organized for analysis.

Today, this function is typically automated in a computer system.

Data Quality Check

It is always necessary to ensure the quality of the abstract information. The concepts of data quality that we have already discussed are validity, accuracy, completeness, and timeliness. Likewise, quality checks of the database are necessary to determine and ensure its quality.

For the purpose of maintaining a quality database, the first step is to check the accuracy of the data. To do so, someone other than the initial clerk, usually a supervisor, routinely checks the abstracts. This means that the patient health record is pulled, the abstract is retrieved from the database, and the data elements are verified. In general, only a sample of the abstracts is reviewed. However, the supervisor must be sure to choose a random sample of abstracts that includes all of the employee's work. Errors noted are corrected, documented,

HEALTH INFORMATION MANAGEMENT ABSTRACT

1. Last name ☐☐☐☐☐☐☐☐☐☐☐☐ First name ☐☐☐☐☐☐☐☐ M.I. ☐
2. Medical record number ☐☐☐☐☐☐
3. Birth date ☐☐☐☐☐☐☐
4. Age ☐☐☐
5. Race ☐ (W–White, B–Black)
6. Sex ☐ (M–Male, F–Female)
7. Street address ☐☐☐☐☐☐☐☐☐☐☐☐☐☐☐☐☐☐☐☐☐☐☐☐☐☐☐☐☐☐☐
8. City ☐☐☐☐☐☐☐☐☐☐☐☐☐☐☐☐☐☐☐ State ☐☐ Zip code ☐☐☐☐☐
9. Admission date ☐☐☐☐☐☐☐
10. Discharge date ☐☐☐☐☐☐☐ Disposition ☐ (1–Home, 2–Nursing home, 3–Rehab
    4–Home w/home health
    5–Transfer to other acute care facility)
11. Attending physician number ☐☐☐☐
12. Service ☐☐☐
13. Principal diagnosis ☐☐☐☐☐☐
14. Other diagnosis ☐☐☐☐☐☐
15. Principal procedure ☐☐☐☐ Procedure date ☐☐☐☐☐☐☐☐
16. Surgeon\Operating physician number ☐☐☐☐
17. Other procedures ☐☐☐☐
18. Procedure dates ☐☐☐☐☐☐☐☐
19. Operating physician number ☐☐☐☐
20. Death ☐ (1–Died, 2–Discharged alive)
21. Autopsy ☐ (1–Yes, 2–No)
22. DRG ☐☐☐
23. MDC ☐☐
24. Emergency room ☐ (1–Yes, 2–No)
25. Physical therapy ☐ (1–Yes, 2–No)
26. Consultation ☐ (1–Yes, 2–No)

FIGURE 7–6.

Paper abstract data collection form. (Adapted from Abdelhak M, Grostick S, Hanken MA, Jacobs E: Health Information: Management of a Strategic Resource, 2nd ed. Philadelphia, WB Saunders, 2001, p 219.)

analyzed, and tracked to improve the quality of the database. The quality of the data is extremely important because of the high volume of information that the database provides for the health care facility.

The quality of the database enables performance improvement activities and appropriate decisions about the facility or about individual patients.

HIT BIT

Remember that data quality audits must be recorded for future comparison. It is important to document compliance or noncompliance with a set standard of quality for data. This information, over a period of time, provides support for improvement efforts, indicates a need for improvement, or demonstrates quality.

Data Retrieval

We have discussed collecting the data, developing the database, and all of the various elements that data contain, and storing it in the paper- or computer-based record. Once a database exists, it is possible to use the data for analysis or comparison. When health information is needed for utilization review, quality assurance, performance improvement, routine compilation, or patient care, the HIM department is asked to retrieve that data. Through the abstract function, health information personnel have stored this information in a systematic method for this type of retrieval. Therefore, with the right instructions on what information is needed and how it is intended to be used, the HIM personnel can provide quality health information. Compilation of all or part of health data for groups of patients is called aggregate data.

Retrieval of Aggregate Data

Aggregate data comprise a group of like data elements compiled to provide information about a group. For example, a collection of the length of stay (LOS) for all patients with the diagnosis of congestive heart failure (CHF) would be aggregate data (Fig. 7–7). Further review of the report shows that the LOS data element for each patient has been retrieved. This report can be analyzed to determine average LOS and most common LOS. Sorting by any single data element for each of these patients produces a meaningful list of aggregate data.

TEST YOUR HI-Q

What is the average length of stay (ALOS) for the group of CHF patients described in Figure 7–7?

Report of patients w/DRG 127

MR #	Patient	D/C Date	LOS	Physician	DRG
056023	Austin, Dallas	02/27/2000	5	Angel, M.	127
197808	Bixby, Helena	02/12/2000	3	Kobob, L.	127
945780	China, Dollie	02/14/2000	6	Chow, A.	127
348477	Combeaux, Plato	02/02/2000	4	Thomas, B.	127
403385	Dimaro, Cheri	02/28/2000	5	Angel, M.	127
471416	Dondi, Mac	02/04/2000	3	Thomas, B.	127
362156	Foster, Dan	02/22/2000	4	Chow, A.	127
483443	Lates, Ricky	02/10/2000	6	Kobob, L.	127
483441	Smeadow, Shane	02/01/2000	5	Thomas, B.	127
201801	Titan, Tami	02/14/2000	4	Thomas, B.	127

FIGURE 7–7.
List of congestive heart failure patients shows aggregate data retrieval.

A health information professional needs the following information to identify the appropriate information needed by the person requesting the report: the name and contact phone number of the person making the request; the date of the request as well as the date parameters for the information requested; the specific information requested; and the reason for the request. This information will aid the person querying the database to ensure that the most appropriate information is retrieved from the database.

Indices

The abstracting process has enabled facilities to create indices for diagnoses, procedures, and physicians. The database can also provide information about any group of patients according to the instructions given by the requestor to the health information personnel and further refined by health information personnel queries to the database. For example, it is common to identify all of a physician's patients for a particular time period. The easiest way to access (obtain a list of) all of a physician's patients is to have already systematically identified on each patient record during the abstract process who the attending physician is, as we have already described. This listing of patients by physician creates what we have historically called the *physician index.*

The **indices** in the HIM department are vital in the organized collection of patient data according to the patient's diagnosis, any procedures performed, and the physicians who cared for them. The indices are used to obtain patient information or aggregate data according to the diagnosis treated, procedure performed, or physician.

Historically, manual indices were maintained on index cards (Fig. 7–8A) or ledger books. Health information personnel recorded the patient's information on index cards according to the diagnosis, procedure, and attending physician. For example, each diagnosis would have an index card, and the health information employee would record each patient with that diagnosis on the card. There-

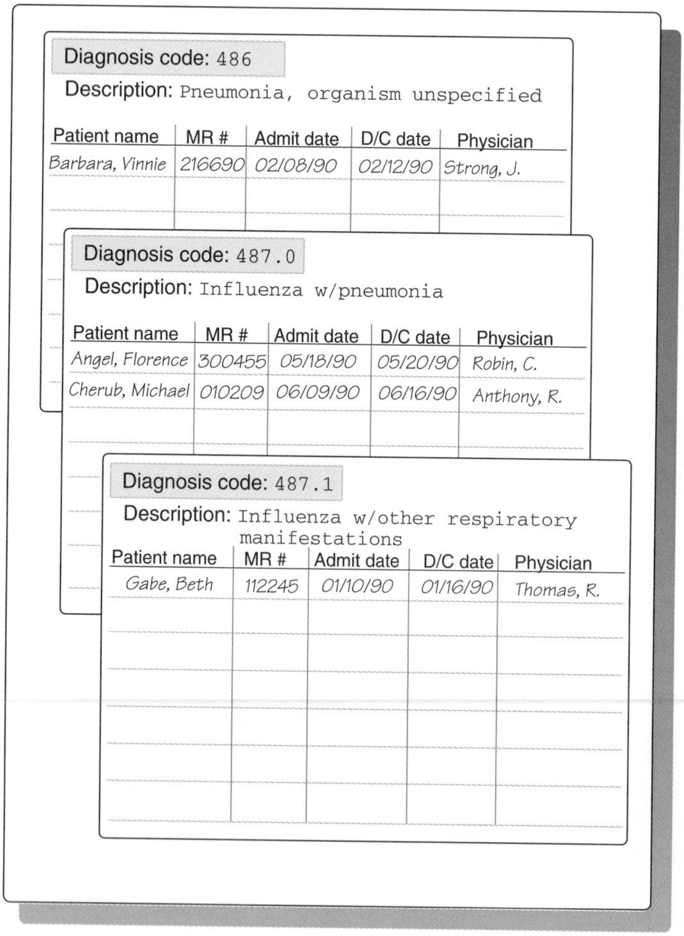

Diagnosis code: 486

Description: Pneumonia, organism unspecified

Patient name	MR #	Admit date	D/C date	Physician
Barbara, Vinnie	216690	02/08/90	02/12/90	Strong, J.

Diagnosis code: 487.0

Description: Influenza w/pneumonia

Patient name	MR #	Admit date	D/C date	Physician
Angel, Florence	300455	05/18/90	05/20/90	Robin, C.
Cherub, Michael	010209	06/09/90	06/16/90	Anthony, R.

Diagnosis code: 487.1

Description: Influenza w/other respiratory manifestations

Patient name	MR #	Admit date	D/C date	Physician
Gabe, Beth	112245	01/10/90	01/16/90	Thomas, R.

A

FIGURE 7–8.

Diagnosis index shown in a manual format *(A)* and a computerized format *(B).*

Diagnosis Index		Discharges: 01/01/01 – 03/31/01				06/16/2001
Diagnosis Code	Description	Medical Record #	Admit Date	D/C Date	LOS	Physician
650		010111	12/30/00	01/01/01	2	Oscar, D.
		125544	12/31/00	01/01/01	1	Jons, J.
		098805	01/02/01	01/04/01	2	Vida, E.
		112096	01/05/01	01/06/01	1	Oscar, D.
		113095	01/09/01	01/12/01	3	Jons, J.

B

FIGURE 7–8.
Continued

fore, if a list of all patients with a particular diagnosis was needed, the health information employee would pull the appropriate diagnosis card.

The automation of health information now allows health information personnel to capture this information during the abstracting process because computer software can identify fields of information and create reports accordingly. Figure 7–8B shows a diagnosis index in computerized format.

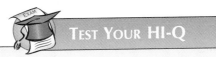

TEST YOUR HI-Q

What other type of report or information could you obtain from the indices?

Identification of a Population

In order to retrieve appropriate useful information, you must be able to identify the population of patients. Identifying the population and being able to retrieve that population efficiently is an extremely important characteristic of data retrieval. How is the population identified? For example, in health care a **population** can be defined as a group of people aggregated according to their race, age, gender, diagnosis, procedure, service, or financial class. A **sample** is a small representation of the entire population. A sample is often used when the population is too large to study in its entirety.

Another common example of pulling information through the identification of a population is for surgical case review or utilization review. For these studies, the population of patients is based on a diagnosis or the operation they had. The clinical data are recorded in the process of caring for the patient. Therefore, when abstracting the patient health record, it is easy to determine and enter the diagnosis and procedure codes. In a paper record, the diagnoses and procedures are typically found on the face sheet after coding, and this information is also entered into the computer database.

Therefore, identifying a group or population of patients for analysis is assisted by good database structure, which is supported by creating the proper data dictionaries that we discussed earlier (see Chapters 2 and 3).

Optimum Source of Data

The next thing to discuss in terms of data retrieval is how to ascertain the optimum source of the data. In a well-constructed database, with unique data dictionary definitions, the computer program will have stored the data in only one place. Therefore, the data will always be recorded at the best time by the best person. For example, if you want to retrieve a population of all of the pneumonia patients, the computer knows that there is only one place that the patient's diagnosis is recorded, and it will go to that location to review each patient record and determine which patients have the diagnosis of pneumonia, and then it will retrieve all the appropriate records for a report.

However, in a paper record, understanding what is an optimum source of data becomes critical. In many paper environments, the same information is recorded multiple times. The patient's admitting diagnosis, for example, is recorded on the face sheet by the admitting clerk; it is recorded on the nursing assessment by the nurse; and it is recorded on the admitting notes by the physician. What is the optimum, most reliable place to determine the patient's admitting diagnosis? It depends on why you want the information. If you want to know what the patient thought he or she was admitted for, then the admitting record is probably the most important place to look. However, if you want to know clinically what the physician thought the patient was admitted for, then you are going to retrieve the admitting notes.

Another example of how important it is to identify the optimum source of data is during a Joint Commission on Accreditation of Healthcare Organizations (JCAHO) survey. JCAHO surveyors may ask to review specific records, for example, records of restraint patients. This information is not normally identified in the patient abstract. From the health information point of view, several different data elements in the database can indicate that a patient may have been restrained. In a computerized system, a special data field can be added to indicate (yes or no) whether a patient was restrained. If a special data field does not exist, other information in the abstract may help identify restraint patients. For example, certain diagnoses indicate that a patient may have required restraints, for example, patients with organic brain syndrome or delirium.

Trying to find the optimum source of data requires knowing your database and knowing how to query it and relate the data elements, as well as being a bit of a detective. Sometimes you have to begin with data that you know you did not collect and work backward. For instance, if the Chief Financial Officer wants to know how many fertility treatments your facility did, where would you go to get that information? Would you query physicians, diagnoses, or procedures? You would look up procedure codes for fertility treatments and then query your system for all of those procedures. The result should be a list of patients, their health record numbers, and the fertility procedures performed.

Reporting of Data

Reporting to Individual Departments

The health data collected in the HIM department is used by various departments in the health care facility (see Chapter 6). The quality management department uses the database to retrieve specific cases and to review the documentation found in the health records in order to determine compliance with accreditation standards, perform quality improvement studies, or study patients outcomes. The finance department may use the information in the HIM department to verify or prepare financial reports and budgets.

Reporting to Outside Agencies

There are various agencies associated with health care facilities that routinely require information. Some states gather information from facilities to create a state health information network. The information in the database is shared (without patient identifiers) so that facilities can compare themselves to other facilities. Organ procurement agencies may request information on deaths for a certain period to assess the facility's compliance with state regulations for organ procurement. In Chapter 6 we discussed the need to report certain statistics to the Centers for Disease Control and Prevention so that they can study disease prevalence, incidence, morbidity, and mortality.

REGISTRIES

A **registry** is a collection of data specific to a disease, diagnosis, or implant. Common registries are Tumor or Cancer Registry, Trauma Registry, AIDS Registry, Birth Defect Registry, and Implant Registry. The purpose of a registry is to study or improve patient care. The data are collected specific to the diagnosis, disease, or implant, so that the users can compare, analyze, or study these groups of patients.

VITAL STATISTICS

Vital statistics refer to the number of births, deaths, and marriages, and statistics on health and disease. In the health care facility we report specific information regarding patient births and deaths to the state's Department of Vital Statistics, also known as Vital Records. Newborns must be registered with the Department of Vital Statistics within a specific time frame after birth. Within the health care facility, the HIM department is sometimes responsible for recording newborns' demographics, parents, and clinical information to submit to Vital Records.

Death certificates must also be submitted to Vital Records following a person's death. The death certificate records the person's demographics and the cause and place of death. In some states this information is initiated by the nursing staff and completed by the funeral home; in others, the HIM staff may be required to participate in the submission of this information to the Department of Vital Statistics.

Statistical Analysis of Patient Information

Determining what report to run is sometimes only the first step in providing information to a user or committee. Once a report has been run, further review of that report may be necessary to provide truly useful information for decision making or interpretation. For example, refer to Figure 7–7, which we used for patient LOS in the aggregate data explanation. That report could be useful in determining ALOS. Facilities typically review the ALOS for specific patient diagnoses. The facility's average is then compared to a national, corporate, or local average. This further analysis can determine whether a facility is within the acceptable limits (LOS) for that diagnosis. The utilization review department analyzes patient LOS for each diagnosis related group (DRG) and diagnosis. In order to provide this information, a report must be run and then formatted in an appropriate list or graph to represent the information for presentation at a meeting.

Analysis and Interpretation

Once patient data have been collected and stored in a database, reports can be run and the data can be analyzed, interpreted, or presented with various tools. The simplest methods for analyzing patient data involve the statistical evaluations of mean, median, and mode. Interpretation is an explanation of the data.

Mean. The statistical mean describes the average of a group of numbers. It is common to analyze patient data to determine various averages: length of stay, cost per case, or patient age. For example, to determine the average age of patients receiving a coronary artery bypass graft (CABG), we would sum the ages of the group of patients and then divide by the total number of patients in the group. Figure 7–9 provides a list of seven patients who had a CABG. To find the

Report of CABG patients

MR #	Patient	D/C Date	LOS	Physician	Age
560230	Bianco, Helena	02/07/2000	7	Angelo, R.	45
978081	Chowski, Shane	02/10/2000	8	Kobob, L.	53
045780	Gombeaux, Glenn	02/04/2000	12	Chi, A.	55
748473	Phoster, Dodi	02/12/2000	14	Houmas, C.	42
005338	Sondi, Mac	02/08/2000	8	Angelo, R.	69
671414	Stephens, Henri	02/14/2000	9	Houmas, C.	68
062150	White, Jean	02/20/2000	8	Chi, A.	59

FIGURE 7–9.
A list of coronary artery bypass graft (CABG) patients can provide data to find the mean age of this group. We sum all the ages in column 6 and divide by 7: The mean age of this group is 56 years.

mean age, we sum all of the ages (45 + 53 + 55 + 42 + 69 + 68 + 59 = 391), then divide by 7 (391/7 = 55.85, or 56). The average or mean age of patients in this group is 56 years.

Median. The median describes the midpoint. Simply arranging a group of numbers in order from lowest to highest and then counting toward the midpoint gives the median of a group of data. The median is used to study groups of data that contain values that are significantly different from the rest of the group. For example, the median of 1, 2, 3, 3, 5, 6, and 20 is 3. This is more representative of the group than the mean, which is 5.7, or 6. Using the same group of data from Figure 7–9, we can analyze the median. To begin this analysis, first arrange the data in order: 42, 45, 53, 55, 59, 68, 69. Because there are seven numbers, it is easy to determine the midpoint. Which number is halfway between 1 and 7? The answer is 4. So beginning with the first patient's age—42—count to the fourth patient's age—55. Fifty-five is the median age in this group of patients.

Mode. Mode describes the number that occurs most often in a group of data. We use the mode to study the most common or high-frequency data element. In the list of CABG patients in Figure 7–9, each age occurs only once. However, if we analyze the LOS for these patients we notice that there is a common LOS that occurs frequently in this group of patients. The LOSs for the patients in Figure 7–9 are as follows: 7, 8, 12, 14, 8, 9, and 8. The LOS that occurs most often is 8. Therefore the mode LOS in this group of patients is 8 days.

TABLE 7–4. Presentation Tools and Their Uses	
Presentation Tool	**Explanation**
Bar graph	Used to group data; information is plotted along *x* and *y* axes.
Line graph	Used to represent data over a period of time; information is plotted along the *x* and *y* axes
Pie chart	Used to represent data in relation to the whole group; illustrates percentages
Decision matrix	Used to narrow the focus of the group or to make decisions between categories or issues

Presentation

Following analysis and interpretation, the data can be presented as information. To present data in a meaningful yet simple manner, tools are used to illustrate the information. Although there are many tools, the most commonly used are the bar graph, pie chart, and line graph. We discussed these tools in Chapter 6; Table 7–4 provides an explanation of how these presentation tools are used.

Routine Institutional Statistics

As we discussed in Chapter 1, there are a number of ways to describe and distinguish among health care facilities. Analysis, interpretation, and presentation of data provide **statistics** that further identify a facility and its activities. Figure 7–10 contains a list of important statistics for Community Hospital for the year 2000.

Admissions

Health care organizations always maintain statistics on the number of patients who are admitted to the facility. Review Figure 7–10 to identify the number of patients admitted to Community Hospital during 2000. There were 14,400 adults and children admitted. The number of adults and children (14,400) does not include the number of newborn (NB) patients admitted (960). Unless otherwise specified, newborn statistics are recorded separately from adults and children, because the newborn is admitted to the facility for the purpose of being born. Even though the newborn may be ill, that is not the reason for his or her admission. A birth is an admission, and a health record is created for each newborn at birth.

Discharges

Health care facilities also maintain statistics on the number of patients leaving the facility. The second item in Figure 7–10 is discharges. Once again, we separate the newborns from the adults and children. Note that the discharges in-

2000 Year-end Statistics for Community Hospital		Description
ADMISSIONS		
Adults & children	14,400	Total number of adults and children admitted during the year
Newborns	960	Total number of babies born in the hospital during the year
DISCHARGES (including deaths)		
Adults & children	14,545	Total number of adults and children discharged during the year
Newborns	950	Total number of newborns discharged during the year
INPATIENT SERVICE DAYS		Number of days of service rendered by the hospital
Adults & children	75,696	to adults and children
Newborns	1993	to newborns
TOTAL LENGTH OF STAY		Sum of all the individual lengths of stay of
Adults & children	72,107	all adults and children discharged during the year
Newborns	1974	all newborns discharged during the year
BED COUNT		
Adults & children	220	Number of beds staffed, equipped, and available
Bassinets	20	Number of bassinets staffed, equipped, and available
MORTALITY DATA		Deaths (these numbers are included in Discharges, above)
Total adults & children		
Under 48 hours	20	Total adult and child deaths within 48 hours of admission
Over 48 hours	138	Total adult and child deaths 48 hours after admission
Total newborns		
Under 48 hours	3	Total newborn deaths within 48 hours of admission
Over 48 hours	2	Total newborn deaths 48 hours after admission
Anesthesia deaths	1	Number of patients who died after receiving anesthesia
OPERATIONS		
Number of patients operated on	1200	Number of patients on whom operations were performed
Surgical operations performed	1312	Number of individual surgical procedures performed
Anesthesia administered	1200	Number of individual administrations of anesthesia
Postoperative infections	30	Number of patients who developed infections as a result of their surgical procedures
OTHER DATA		
Nosocomial infections	231	Number of patients who developed infections in the hospital
Cesarean sections	303	Number of deliveries performed by cesarean section
Deliveries	1304	Number of women who gave birth in the hospital

FIGURE 7–10.

Community Hospital 2000 year-end statistics.

clude deaths, because death is, effectively, a discharge. We still need to know the number of deaths for statistical purposes, so we also list them separately. Other discharges include the patient's release by discharge order from the physician, leaving against medical advice (AMA), and transfer to another facility.

TRANSFERS

Patients can be transferred from one unit to another inside a facility, or they can be "discharged" and transferred to another facility (Fig. 7–11). When a patient is transferred to another facility the discharged disposition may be one of the following:

- Transfer to rehabilitation facility
- Transfer to skilled nursing facility (internal to the facility)
- Transfer to skilled nursing facility (external to the facility)
- Transfer to another acute care facility
- Transfer to long-term acute care facility
- Transfer to nursing home

INTRAHOSPITAL TRANSFERS

	Unit A	Unit B	Total
5/31/00 midnight census	3	2	5
Transfers in	+1	+2	+3
Transfers out	-2	-1	-3
6/1/00 midnight census	2	3	5

Transfers between Units A and B have no impact on census

Here is a table that reflects the same information:

	Unit A	Unit B	Total
6/1/00 midnight census	3	2	5
Admissions	+2	0	+2
Discharges	-2	-1	-3
6/2/00 midnight census	3	1	4

FIGURE 7–11.

Intrahospital transfers.

HIT Bit

The transfer of a patient to another facility requires the transfer of sufficient information to support effective continuity of care. There is usually a special *transfer form,* and copies of all or part of the health record may accompany the patient. The receiving hospital (the hospital to which the patient is transferred) counts the patient as an admission. Interhospital transfer describes this movement of a patient from one facility to another. Intrahospital transfer reflects movement of a patient between nursing units and therefore has no overall impact on census. Figure 7–11 shows the transfer of patients between two nursing units on May 31, 2000.

Census

The total number of patients in the hospital is called the **census.** Census-taking is an activity that counts the number of patients in beds at any given time. Admissions increase the census; discharges decrease the census (Fig. 7–12).

The census is taken at the same time every day, usually midnight, so that the facility can compare the census from day to day, over time. This census number is also called the *midnight census.* For practical purposes a computer database allows the patient registration department to view the census at any time.

In Chapter 1 we learned that hospitals are licensed for a specific number of beds. This means that the hospital is not able to physically care for more patients than the number of beds allowed by the state license. Because of this, the facility must always know how many patients are occupying beds. The patient registration department, also known as the admissions department, is responsible for assigning a patient to a room.

CENSUS

	Total
6/1/00 midnight census	5
Admissions	+2
Discharges	-3
6/2/00 midnight census	4

Because the number of discharges (decrease) was more than the number of admissions (increase), the inpatient census decreased.

FIGURE 7–12.

Census.

Hospital administrators like to review the census by nursing unit, wing, or floor. This view enables administrators to identify underutilized areas for planning purposes. It also allows nurse management to plan and control staffing. The impact of the two admissions and three discharges on the census taken between June 1 and June 2, 2000 (shown in Fig. 7–12), is detailed by nursing unit (see Table 7–6).

For statistical purposes, we record the midnight census for comparison over time. A census, however, does not measure all of the services provided by the hospital. What about the patient who is admitted at 10:40 AM and dies before midnight? That patient would not be present for the counting of the midnight census. The facility counts these patients in the service days for the facility called *inpatient service days (IPSD)*.

Can you tell from the census report in Figure 7–12 how many patients received services on June 2, 2001? Actually, we do not have enough information. Table 7–5 shows the admission and discharge detailed by patient. We can see that the two patients who were admitted on June 2 were also discharged the same day. Table 7–6 analyzes the service days received by those patients. From our analysis, we can see that there were actually 6 days of service (IPSD) rendered by the hospital.

TABLE 7–5. Number of Patients Who Received Services Detailed by Patient

	Inpatients	Total
6/1/00 midnight census	M. Brown	5
	S. Crevecoeur	
	F. Perez	
	P. Smith	
	R. Wooley	
Admissions	C. Estevez	+2
	B. Mooney	
Discharges	S. Crevecoeur	−3
	C. Estevez	
	B. Mooney	
6/2/00 midnight census	M. Brown	4
	F. Perez	

P. Smith
R. Wooley

TABLE 7–6. Analysis of Patients Who Received a Day of Service on June 2, 2000		
Inpatients	Analysis	6/2 Day of Service
M. Brown	Inpatient on 6/1 and 6/2	1
S. Crevecoeur	Discharged 6/2	0
C. Estevez	Admitted and discharged 6/2	1
B. Mooney	Admitted and discharged 6/2	1
F. Perez	Inpatient on 6/1 and 6/2	1
P. Smith	Inpatient on 6/1 and 6/2	1
R. Wooley	Inpatient on 6/1 and 6/2	1
Total days of service		6

At the end of 1999, there were 325 patients in Community Hospital. At the end of 2000, the adults and children census was 180 (see Fig. 7–13). There were 145 fewer adults and children in the hospital at the end of the year 2000 than there were at the beginning. How did that happen? Look at the admissions and discharges. There were more discharges than admissions during the year: 145, to be exact.

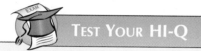

TEST YOUR HI-Q

What was the number of average monthly discharges at Community Hospital for the year 2000?

Understanding the relationship among the statistics helps us to use these data effectively. For example, in Chapter 1 we learned about LOS and ALOS. Looking at Figure 7–10, we know that there were 14,545 adults and children discharged in 2000. The total LOS for all of those patients, added together, was 72,107 days. Therefore, the ALOS for adults and children in 2000 was 4.9 days (72,107 ÷ 14,545 = 4.9).

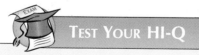

TEST YOUR HI-Q

What was the newborn ALOS for 2000?

All health care facilities keep track of their statistics according to the fiscal year, which is a 12-month reporting period. A facility's reporting period can be the calendar year January 1 through December 31, or it can be July 1 through June 30, or October 1 through September 30. Figure 7–13 is organized into fiscal periods. To understand this, think of how a year is organized into days, weeks, and months. When we calculate and report statistics, we do so by the relevant fiscal period. In addition to days, weeks, and months, we also group the months into quarters. Each quarter represents 3 months, or approximately one fourth of the year. Health care statistics are frequently organized in this manner.

THE FISCAL YEAR

QUARTER	Month	# of Days	Admissions	Discharges	Census	
					325	12/31/99
I	January	31	1125	1148	302	
	February	29	1543	1555	290	
	March	31	1445	1430	305	
II	April	30	1406	1398	313	
	May	31	1242	1247	308	
	June	30	1004	994	318	
III	July	31	1254	1248	324	
	August	31	1145	1148	321	
	September	30	1212	1224	309	
IV	October	31	1478	1502	285	
	November	30	1567	1598	254	
	December	31	1229	1303	180	
Total		**366**	**15,650**	**15,795**		**12/31/00**

2000 was a leap year. In non-leap years, February has 28 days, for a total of 365 days in the year. How many weeks are there in a year?

FIGURE 7–13.

The fiscal year.

In Chapter 1, we also discussed occupancy. We calculated occupancy by dividing the number of days that patients used beds by the number of beds available. The number of days that patients used beds is called the inpatient service days. IPSD are calculated daily by adding the admissions to the census, subtracting the discharges, then adding back the patients who were admitted and discharged on the same day. Patients who were admitted and discharged on the same day used beds, but they do not appear in the midnight census.

HIT BIT

In counting days of service, like length of stay, we count the day of admission but not the day of discharge. This makes sense because if the hospital counted the day of discharge as well, it would conceivably charge twice for the same bed on the same day. The same principle allows us to count one day of service for a patient who is admitted and discharged on the same day.

TABLE 7–7, Inpatient Service Days Calculated from Census	
	Total
6/1/00 midnight census	5
Admissions	+2
Discharges	−3
6/2/00 midnight census	4
Patients admitted and discharged on 6/2	+2
6/2/00 inpatient service days	6

The census need not be analyzed patient by patient to calculate IPSD. We can obtain the total number of patients admitted and discharged on the same day from census reports (Table 7–7). Once IPSD have been calculated, the data can be added, averaged, graphed, and trended over time. It is also a means to calculate occupancy, as mentioned, because it includes all patients who were admitted and discharged the same day. Because the census counts only patients in beds at a point in time, IPSD is a better measure of the use of hospital facilities. Figure 7–14 illustrates all the IPSD concepts we have discussed.

CENSUS STATISTICS

A&C = Adults and children   Adm. = Admissions
N/B = Newborn   D/C = Discharges
NICU = Neonatal ICU   IPSD = Inpatient service days

	Adults & Children			Newborns		
	UNIT A	UNIT B	TOTAL A&C	N/B nursery	NICU	TOTAL N/B
6/1/00 midnight census	15	17	32	3	1	4
Admissions/births	+4	+2	+6	2	0	2
Discharges/deaths	-5	-4	-9	0	0	0
Transfers in	+2	+1	+3	0	+1	+1
Transfers out	-1	-2	-3	-1	0	-1
6/2/00 midnight census	15	14	29	4	2	6
Adm. & D/C 6/2/00	+2	+1	+3	0	0	0
6/2/00 IPSD	17	15	32	4	2	6

In the past, spreadsheets like this were prepared daily, by hand. Imagine how complicated that could get with 500 patients spread over 16 nursing units! Fortunately, computers do the majority of work for us. Even if the main system doesn't present the information the way we want to see it, computerized spreadsheet programs help us to reorganize it. However, there is a very important rule you need to learn about computer reports: "Just because something comes from a computer doesn't mean it's correct!"

FIGURE 7–14.
Census statistics.

RATES AND PERCENTAGES

RATE:

$$\frac{67 \text{ female patients}}{134 \text{ total patients}} = \frac{1}{2}$$

One out of every two patients is female

PERCENTAGE:

$$\frac{67 \text{ female patients}}{134 \text{ total patients}} = .50 \,(\times 100) = 50\%$$

Fifty percent of patients are female

FIGURE 7–15.

Rates and percentages.

Hospital Rates and Percentages

There are many ways to look at hospital statistics. One very common method is to look at the number of times something occurred, compared to (divided by) the number of times it could have occurred:

$$\frac{\text{No. of occurrences}}{\text{No. of times something } could \text{ have occured}}$$

This basic calculation provides a rate of occurrence. Multiplied by 100, the rate is expressed as a percentage. See Figure 7–15 for an example of rates versus percentages.

Once we know how to calculate percentages, we can look at occurrences in a facility as rates and percentages. For example, we may want to know the percentage of hospital patients who acquired nosocomial infections. (Nosocomial infections are infections that patients acquired while in the hospital, as opposed to infections that were present on admission.) In Figure 7–10, we see that there were 231 occurrences of nosocomial infections at Community Hospital in 2000. Because 15,495 (14,545 + 950) patients were treated (discharged), 15,495 is the number of possible occurrences of nosocomial infections. The percentage of nosocomial infections is 1.5%:

$$\frac{\text{No. of occurrences}}{\text{No. of times something } could \text{ have occured}} \times 100$$

$$\frac{231 \text{ nosocomial infections}}{15,495 \text{ discharges}} \times 100 = 1.5\%$$

HEALTH CARE STATISTICS FORMULAS

Average Inpatient Service Days:

$$\frac{\text{Total inpatient service days for a period (excluding newborns)}}{\text{Total number of days in the period}}$$

Average Newborn Inpatient Service Days:

$$\frac{\text{Total newborn inpatient service days for a period}}{\text{Total number of days in the period}}$$

Average Length of Stay:

$$\frac{\text{Total length of stay (discharge days)}}{\text{Total discharges (including deaths)}}$$

Bed Occupancy Rate:

$$\frac{\text{Total inpatient service days in a period} \times 100}{\text{Total bed count days in the period}}$$
$$(\text{bed count} \times \text{number of days in the period})$$

Newborn Bassinet Occupancy Ratio Formula:

$$\frac{\text{Total newborn inpatient service days for a period} \times 100}{\text{Total newborn bassinet count} \times \text{number of days in the period}}$$

Other Rates Formula:

$$\frac{\text{Number of times something occurred} \times 100}{\text{Number of times something could have occurred}}$$

FIGURE 7–16.

Health care statistics formulas.

The key to understanding hospital rates and percentages is to understand the underlying data and how those data elements relate to each other. Some of the most common types of calculations are shown in Figure 7–16.

Thus, there are many ways to report data. How data are reported depends on the needs of the user. It is important for the health information professional to understand the needs of the user in order to help identify the data for meaningful reporting and presentation.

Reference

Hanken MA, Water KA (eds): Glossary of Healthcare Terms. Chicago, American Health Information Management Association, 1994.

Suggested Reading

Abdelhak M, Grostick S, Hanken MA, Jacobs E: Health Information: Management of a Strategic Resource, 2nd ed. Philadelphia, WB Saunders, 2001.

Quinn J: An HL7 overview. Journal of AHIMA 70(7), 1999. www.ahima.org/journal/cutting.edge/9907.html.

CHAPTER SUMMARY

Health information must be collected in a systematic, defined format known as data sets. This collection of data is then stored in a database for future use. The data sets and database must comply with law, accreditation, policy, and the needs of the organization. The database is then a source of information for departments within the organization as well as agencies external to the facility.

The data can be analyzed, interpreted, and presented to appropriate users by using the following tools: statistical mean, median, and mode, as well as bar graphs, pie charts, and line graphs. The analysis of a facility's data is also referred to as the facility's statistics, which describes the services and activities of the facility.

REVIEW QUESTIONS

1. Identify the minimum required data elements of a patient health information abstract.

2. Identify appropriate methods for capturing useful patient data.

3. List individual departments and outside agencies to which you might report information.

4. List the statistical tools and explain their use.

5. What is the formula for computing the average length of stay?

PROFESSIONAL PROFILE
Coding Supervisor

My name is Maggie, and I am the coding supervisor in Woodlawn Memorial Hospital, a medium-sized hospital. Woodlawn has 250 inpatient beds, 30 bassinets, a skilled nursing unit with 25 beds, a rehabilitation unit with 20 beds, and one unit leased to a long-term acute care facility. In addition, we have a same-day surgery wing, a pain management clinic, and a physician's clinic located within our facility. I am responsible for the daily operations of the coding staff in the facility: I supervise six coders, four full-time and two part-time employees.

My supervision of the daily routine includes

- Ensuring that accounts are coded within 72 hours of the patient's discharge
- Assisting case management with questions regarding patient DRGs
- Handling business office issues
- Coordinating questions to physicians regarding their documentation

I also oversee the quality of the data contained in the HIM database.

During a recent conversion of our software I participated on the team that developed a data dictionary. In this process I became the contact person for all matters concerning the HIM database. In this new role, I am the person who processes all requests for reports from the HIM database. When the quality management, administration, physician, or case management staff needs information from our database, they come to me. I make sure I know

- What information they want
- Why they need it
- The time frame for the information
- When they need the report

This information helps me run the correct report so that the person may use the information as necessary in their presentation, decision making, or investigation.

I find this part of my job very rewarding. I enjoy receiving a request that people think is impossible and knowing that our HIM database contains the information that they are looking for. Providing those reports is really exciting.

APPLICATION

Making Data Informative

Health information professionals are commonly asked to analyze data for presentation. The presentation may be a simple table or report, or it may include graphs.

Using the Internet, locate a database of patient information for query of a DRG assigned by your instructor. Prepare a report with a graph for presentation to your instructor.

Using the CABG report in Figure 7–9, prepare a presentation for your instructor demonstrating the average length of stay for patients of each physician.

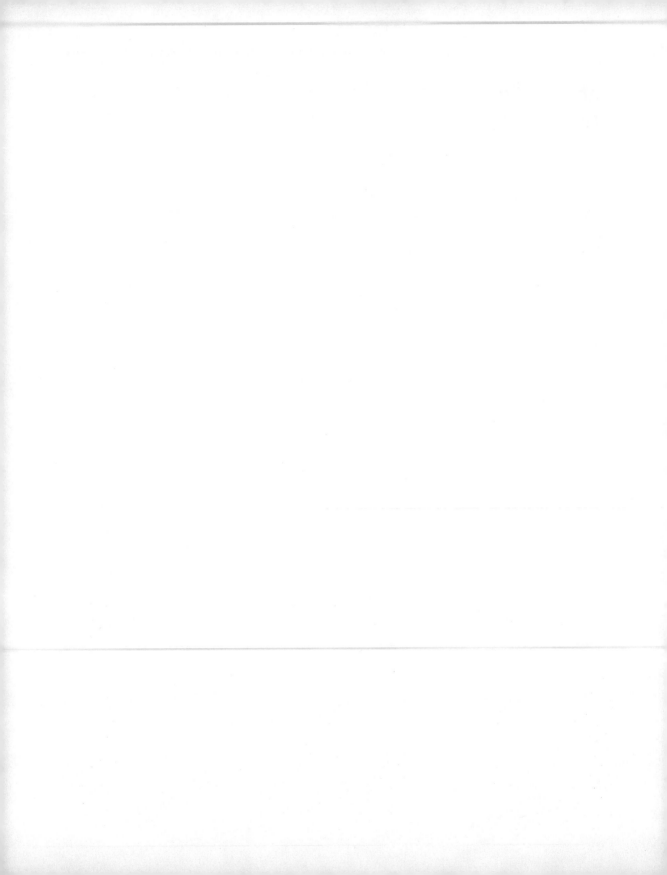

Unit Three

REIMBURSEMENT
and LEGAL ISSUES

8

Confidentiality and Compliance

Chapter Outline

Confidentiality
Definition
Legal Foundation
Scope

Access
Continuing Patient Care
Reimbursement
Litigation
Access by Patient

Consent
Informed Consent
Admission
Medical Procedures
Release of Information
    With Consent
    Without Consent
    Emergencies
    Special Consents

Preparing a Record for Release
Validation and Tracking
Retrieval
Reproduction
Certification

Compensation
Distribution

Internal Requests for Information
Sensitive Records
    Employee Patients
    Legal Files

Compliance
Licensure
Accreditation
    Joint Commission on Accreditation of
        Healthcare Organizations
Corporate Compliance
Professional Standards

Suggested Reading

Chapter Summary

Review Questions

Professional Profile

Application

By the end of this chapter, the student should be able to

- List and describe the types of subpoenas.

- Define jurisdiction.

- Prepare information for copying; photocopy it; and send it out.

- Differentiate between release of patient information with and without consent.

- Develop and implement departmental policies and procedures regarding release of information to patients.

- Develop and implement departmental policies and procedures regarding release of information to care providers.

Vocabulary

access

business record rule

compliance

Conditions of Admission

confidentiality

consent

defendant

hearsay rule

informed consent

Joint Commission on Accreditation of Healthcare Organizations (JCAHO)

jurisdiction

litigation

outsourced

physician-patient privilege

plaintiff

prospective consent

retrospective consent

subpoena

subpoena ad testificandum

subpoena duces tecum

The topic of confidentiality was touched on briefly in Chapter 4 as we discussed the function of release of information. In this chapter, we explain release of information and discuss confidentiality as it relates to the actions of health care workers and outside parties. The function of release of information is generally the responsibility of the health information management (HIM) department, but a number of other individuals also become involved. We also discuss the importance of confidentiality, the rules that are critical to ensuring the confidentiality of a health record, and problems that can occur when requests for release of records are received.

Confidentiality

Definition

Confidentiality is discretion regarding disclosure of information. In very simple terms, it's like keeping a secret. When a patient is receiving medical care, no matter what the facility, no matter who the provider, that information is confidential—it is secret. It may not be released to a person who is not authorized to receive it.

Legal Foundation

The foundation for confidentiality is **physician-patient privilege.** This concept refers to communication between the patient and his or her physician. In order to promote complete and honest communication between a physician and his or her patient, no such communication can be disclosed to other parties. Only the patient can waive the right to keep that communication confidential. Although not a universally accepted tenet, it implies that the facility owns the physical or electronic record, but the patient owns the information in the record.

Although physician-patient privilege has been upheld in court, there are very few statutes governing confidentiality at this time. A statute is a law that has been passed by the legislative branch of government. Currently, the vast majority of legal rules regarding confidentiality are found at the state level. Because each state may pass its own laws and corresponding enforcing regulations, the rules vary from state to state. On the federal level, there are two notable regulations: one concerns alcohol and drug records and the other has to do with records in federal facilities (see discussion of these at the end of the chapter).

Scope

The scope of confidentiality is very broad. It includes not only the confidentiality of the written or computer-based record but also spoken information. For example, for employees of a health care facility to stand in a crowded elevator discussing a patient by name is a very clear violation of confidentiality. Sometimes, even putting a patient's picture on the wall, or putting a patient's name and diagnosis on a blackboard in a public hallway, can be considered violations of patient confidentiality.

There are some very basic guidelines that a health care professional can follow when he or she works in a health care facility. First, patients should never be discussed among employees or among health care professionals in a public venue. In the cafeteria, elevators, stairwells, hallways, even in the patient's room, health care professionals need to understand that others may be able to hear their conversations. Therefore, patient-specific conversations should not take place where they can be overhead.

If the necessity arises to discuss a patient in a public place, the patient can sometimes be discussed without reference to personal identification. You can refer to the patient by diagnosis or in some other nonidentifying manner. However, care should be taken even in this regard. For example, discussing a patient by room number can be revealing if that conversation takes place in front of someone who knows what room the patient is in, for example, a family member. This may seem like common sense to you, but it is one of the most frequently committed violations of a patient's right to confidentiality. All employees should sign a confidentiality agreement upon hiring. Annual re-signing of that document, along with in-service training about the necessity for confidentiality and facility policies and procedures, is recommended. Figure 8–1 is a sample Confidentiality Statement.

A second issue in confidentiality is the physical maintenance of the patient's health record. Physical documents should be kept in a binder or folder at all times. Binders or folders containing a specific patient's documents should be identified only with the patient's name, health record number, and room number (if applicable). The outside of the folder or three-ring binder, no matter how the record is maintained, should not contain any diagnostic information or anything of significance that could be read by a casual passerby. On the nursing unit, only the bed number should be visible on the patient's binder. An important exception to this is a warning about allergies. Patient allergies should be clearly noted on the front of the binder. There is a strong temptation to mark the binder with clinically significant information, such as HIV POSITIVE. Such sensitive information should not be visible. Some facilities get around this by placing color-coded stickers or other symbols on the outside of the binder.

Another issue is that confidentiality procedures extend to the hallways and the patient's room itself. The patient's actual diagnosis, procedures, and appointments should not be displayed where the casual observer can see them. This is a common failing in facilities where multiple individuals need to know the activities of a patient. For example, in an inpatient rehabilitation facility, patients do not tend to remain in their rooms. They are transported to other parts of the facility for therapy, or they may be sent out of the facility for a procedure. The temptation is to write this information in a common area where all health care providers can see it. The public hallway is not the place for that. Such postings should be confined to restricted areas.

In a computer-based environment, there are some special considerations as well. A health care professional sitting at a computer terminal accessing a patient's record, either for information purposes or for data entry purposes, may

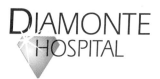

Diamonte, Arizona 89104 • TEL. 602-484-9991

CONFIDENTIALITY STATEMENT

I, _____ , understand that in the course of my activities/business at or for Diamonte Hospital, I am required to have access to and am involved in the viewing, reviewing, and/or processing of patient care data and/or health information.

I understand that I am obligated by State Law, Federal Law, and Diamonte Hospital to maintain the confidentiality of these data and information at all times.

I understand that a violation of these confidentiality considerations may result in punitive legal action against me.

I certify by my signature below that this Confidentiality Statement has been explained to me, and I agree to the principles contained herein as a condition of my activity/business at or for Diamonte Hospital.

_____
Signature/date

_____
Witness/date

FIGURE 8–1.

Confidentiality statement.

be called away from the terminal. It is very important for the person to log off the terminal before leaving, because anything on the computer screen can be seen by anyone walking by.

Even health care professionals have no right or need to access a patient's record unless he or she is actually working with the patient. Computer-based systems should always provide an automatic log-off if activity is not taking place after a certain period of time. For maintenance of confidentiality, a typical computer screen saver is not sufficient. The entire record should be logged off and made inaccessible without special security codes.

Access

Health care professionals must continuously weigh the need for confidentiality versus access to patient information. **Access** refers to the ability to learn the contents of a health record, by obtaining it and/or having the contents revealed. There are many reasons why individuals would want access to a record—for example, continuing patient care, reimbursement, and litigation (see Chapter 6). Control over that access is critical, because it is inappropriate to release information to individuals without the proper authorization.

Continuing Patient Care

Confidentiality presents some interesting issues for continuing patient care. Theoretically, only the attending physician and the health care workers involved with the patient have access to the patient's health record. However, what if the patient returns to the facility at a later date? If the original attending physician is not available or is no longer associated with the facility, does that mean no one can look at the previous record? Obviously, for the sake of the patient and the patient's continuing care, the new attending physician is authorized to access the record. Thus, within the same facility, when the patient presents for care, access to the previous records can be granted to the health care providers—specifically the attending physician, consultants, and other allied health professionals—with direct patient involvement.

Any other access to a patient's record requires specific patient authorization. An example of inappropriate access is a physician or other facility employee who looks at a friend's or family member's record without the patient's permission. Without the patient's consent, they ordinarily have no right to access the patient's chart.

It is important to convey to employees of the HIM department and to all employees of the facility that inappropriate access to a record is illegal and should be punished. The dismissal (firing) of employees who inappropriately access health records is not excessively harsh.

In addition to review by professionals within the facility, the chart may need to be reviewed by health care professionals outside of the facility in which the patient was originally treated. For example, a pregnant patient is admitted at term to an acute care facility, gives birth, and is released with the baby. Does the baby's pediatrician, if he or she did not attend the baby in the hospital, have the right to see the record? The pediatrician does *not* have the right to see the records. However, the mother has the right to authorize the pediatrician to see them.

Later in this chapter, we discuss how authorization is accomplished. HIM department personnel are frequently called on to release records to a patient's current caregiver. Although this is appropriate and desirable, it cannot be accomplished, in general, without the patient's consent.

Reimbursement

Another reason to access health records is for reimbursement purposes. In the current health care environment, various payers (discussed in Chapter 9) may need to review the record. In general, the payer, the person who is financially responsible for the bill, has the right to access the records. This is accomplished in several ways:

- Authorization through the insurance company
- Authorization through the Conditions of Admission
- Retrospective authorization

When the patient originally obtains health insurance, the insurance company asks the patient to sign a document stating that the insurance company can access the health record whenever the insurance company deems it necessary. If any question arises as to whether that consent exists, the health care facility has the right to ask for a copy of the signed statement, and the insurance company should provide it with no problem.

The Conditions of Admission form that the patient signs on entry to the hospital also contains a statement that health records may be released to the party who is financially responsible. This type of consent constitutes **prospective consent.** In other words, the patient is consenting to release of information before that information has been generated. This is considered acceptable for routine care. Under certain circumstances, patients may preauthorize release of information to family members and health care professionals in the same manner. This is a fairly common practice when multiple parties are involved in the development of the patient's care plan.

In some circumstances, prospective consent is not sufficient. In other cases, the patient may choose to have more control over the release of information about his or her condition. In those cases, **retrospective consent** is necessary. Retrospective consent means that the patient authorizes access to the health record after the care has been rendered. In general, the patient does have the right to refuse to consent to the release of information. There are, however, consequences to refusing to allow the payer, for example, to have access to the record. The payer may, in turn, refuse to pay for the patient's care. If that happens, the patient would become responsible for the bill. Therefore, there is a financial incentive for the patient to allow the payer access to the record.

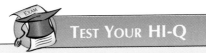

TEST YOUR HI-Q

Why would an insurance company want a copy of a patient's record?

Litigation

Litigation is another area in which consent to release information is vital. **Litigation** is the process by which one party sues another in a court of law. This occurs quite often when a patient has been injured, either accidentally or intentionally. The party who is suing is the **plaintiff.** The party who is being sued is the **defendant.**

The legal aspects of health information and health care in general are too broad to discuss in this book. However, a general understanding of how a trial works is helpful knowledge for the HIM professional.

Most lawsuits that involve access to medical records are based on some injury to the patient. A shopper slips and falls in the grocery store and sues the store. A physician amputates the wrong foot, and the patient sues the physician and the hospital. A pedestrian is hit by a car and sues the driver.

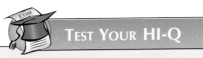

TEST YOUR HI-Q

In each of the three examples just mentioned, who is the plaintiff and who is the defendant?

The plaintiffs in these cases file a complaint with the court, stating the issues, the reason they chose that particular court, and what they want the court to do. In the grocery store example, the plaintiff may file a complaint in a state court stating that the grocery store's floor was wet and posed a hazard, which was the cause of the accident. The complaint is filed in that court because the store is located in that state and the plaintiff lives in that state. The plaintiff wants the court to agree that the store was at fault and to order the store to pay for the plaintiff's medical care and loss of income. The steps in this type of litigation are listed and defined in Table 8–1.

There are two steps in the above-mentioned lawsuit in which health records may be required. The first step is during the discovery process. During discovery, the lawyers may want a copy of the documentation of the plaintiff's treatment in order to verify the extent and timing of the injuries as well as the nature, extent, and cost of care. The record may be needed again in court during the trial, if it is used as evidence. During both of these steps, either the original record or a copy of it may be required.

TABLE 8–1. Steps in a Civil Lawsuit	
Complaint	Plaintiff's written claim, including a description of compensation or other relief and an expression of the court's jurisdiction in the matter. Complaint may be followed by a counterclaim and other communications establishing the position of both parties on the issue.
Discovery	Investigation of the facts of the case, including taking statements, interviewing witnesses, and obtaining and reviewing documentation.
Pretrial conference	Meeting of the parties with the trial judge to resolve or clarify outstanding issues and explore potential settlement.
Trial*	Presentation of both sides of the case in court. Judgment may be rendered by a judge or jury. In some cases, a judge may override the verdict of a jury.
Appeal	The loser of the trial may request a review of the trial proceedings by a higher court. Appeals must be based on perceived errors or problems with the original trial, not purely on dissatisfaction with the outcome.
Satisfying the judgment	The final disposition of the case, such as the collection of damages.

*Trials vary, depending on the type of case, the jurisdiction, and the type of court. Local court rules vary from state to state. HIM professionals are frequently requested to provide documentation at the discovery and trial steps. Data from McWay D: Legal Aspects of Health Information Management, 1st edition. © 1996. Delmar, a division of Thomson Learning. Fax 800-730-2215.

The use of health records as evidence in court is based on the **business record rule.** The business record rule states that health records may be accepted as evidence if they are

- Kept in the normal course of business
- Recorded by individuals who are in a position to be knowledgeable of the events that are being recorded
- Documented contemporaneously with those events

The business record rule is an exception to the **hearsay rule,** which prohibits secondhand accounts of events. If the heresay rule applied to health records, then a nurse's documentation of a patient's statements or a physician's subjective notes would not be admissible evidence.

The choice of a court in which to file the complaint is primarily a matter of **jurisdiction.** Jurisdiction means that the court has authority over the issue and/or the person. There are courts of limited jurisdiction, such as traffic court, which may decide only certain types of cases. Other courts have general jurisdiction, such as state courts, and they may decide a wide variety of cases. In general, these courts have jurisdiction over citizens of the states in which they operate. There are also federal courts, whose jurisdiction extends to issues regarding federal statutes, regulations, and treaties; events that occur on federal land; and citizens of different states.

There are several different avenues through which access to the record can be obtained during litigation. First, the patient can sign a consent to release the information to either the patient's lawyer or the defendant's lawyer. It is presumed that when a patient institutes litigation and uses the medical condition as a foundation for the litigation, he or she is waiving the right to confidentiality.

Special care must be taken in this context to ensure that only information pertinent to the litigation is released to the parties involved.

Another avenue of approach is through the **subpoena** process. A subpoena is a direction from an officer of the court. The direction may be to testify (**subpoena ad testificandum**) (Fig. 8–2) or to provide documentation (**subpoena duces tecum**). The HIM department may receive a subpoena from the patient's lawyer or from the defendant's lawyer. A subpoena is valid for access to health record's only if the subpoena itself is valid and the court through which the subpoena is issued has jurisdiction over the party to whom the subpoena is addressed. Figure 8–3 lists the common elements of a valid subpoena.

Finally, access may be obtained through a *court order*. A court order is the direction of a judge who has made a decision that the direction is necessary. Again, the issue of jurisdiction arises. For example, if an elderly patient's children seek to declare the patient legally incompetent (unable to make decisions about his or her affairs), the judge may issue a court order to obtain the patient's health records. Figure 8–4 gives the components of a valid court order authorizing disclosure.

Access by Patient

Access to the health record is generally provided to the patient, but the patient needs to sign a consent in order to obtain the information. An important role of the HIM professional is to assist the patient in determining what portions of the record are really needed. An appendectomy patient who wants to retain pertinent records about the operation would not, in general, need the entire record. The discharge summary and operative report may provide sufficient information for the patient's purposes.

In order to assist patients in managing their health care throughout the continuum, it is important to encourage them to obtain those portions of the record that are absolutely necessary. For example, patients should maintain in their personal files records of major encounters with health care facilities, such as copies of operative reports, anesthesiology reports, and perhaps discharge summaries of important stays in a health care facility. This helps them document their own health history and facilitates continuing patient care in situations in which much time has passed between encounters. Remember that facilities are permitted to destroy old records. If a patient's appendectomy took place 30 years ago, the paper record may no longer exist. Therefore, it is in the patient's best interests to maintain a personal file of health information.

Whether in a paper-based environment or a computer-based environment, portions of the record that are being accessed need to be duplicated by photocopying the paper record, downloading from a computer, printing from microfiche, or reproduction from other media. In practice, the duplicate is generally provided in paper format, regardless of how it is stored or maintained. The process of providing access to health information is frequently called *release of information or correspondence*. Many large acute care facilities have a number of individuals who are involved in this function. This is also a typical function

AO 88 (Rev.1/94) Subpoena in a Civil Case

Issued by the

UNITED STATES DISTRICT COURT

DISTRICT OF ———————————

V.

SUBPOENA IN A CIVIL CASE

CASE NUMBER: [1]

To:

☐ YOU ARE COMMANDED to appear in the United States District Court at the place, date, and time specified below to testify in the above case.

PLACE OF TESTIMONY	COURTROOM
	DATE AND TIME

☐ YOU ARE COMMANDED to appear in the United States District Court at the place, date, and time specified below to testify at the taking of a deposition in the above case.

PLACE OF TESTIMONY	COURTROOM
	DATE AND TIME

☐ YOU ARE COMMANDED to produce and permit inspection and copying of the following documents or objects at the place, date, and time specified below (list documents or objects):

PLACE	DATE AND TIME

☐ YOU ARE COMMANDED to permit inspection of the following premises at the date and time specified below.

PREMISES	DATE AND TIME

Any organization not a party to this suit that is subpoenaed for the taking of a deposition shall designate one or more officers, directors, or managing agents, or other persons who consent to testify on its behalf, and may set forth, for each person designated, the matters on which the person will testify. Federal rules of Civil Procedure, 30(b) (6).

ISSUING OFFICER SIGNATURE AND TITLE (INDICATE IF ATTORNEY FOR PLAINTIFF OR DEFENDANT)	DATE
ISSUING OFFICERS NAME, ADDRESS AND PHONE NUMBER	

(See Rule 45, Federal Rules of Civil Procedure, Parts C & D on Reverse)

[1] If action is pending in district other than district of issuance, state district under case number.

FIGURE 8–2.

Sample subpoena to testify in a civil case. (From McWay D: Legal Aspects of Health Information Management, 1st edition. © 1996. Reprinted with permission of Delmar, a division of Thomson Learning. Fax 800-730-2215.)

AO 88 (Rev.1/94) Subpoena in a Civil Case

PROOF OF SERVICE

	DATE	PLACE
SERVED		

SERVED ON (PRINT NAME)	MANNER OF SERVICE

SERVED BY (PRINT NAME)	TITLE

DECLARATION OF SERVER

I declare under penalty of perjury under the laws of the United States of America that the foregoing information contained in the Proof of Service is true and correct.

Executed on (date)	SIGNATURE OF SERVER
	ADDRESS OF SERVER

Rule 45, Federal Rules of Civil Procedure, Parts C & D:

(c) PROTECTION OF PERSONS SUBJECT TO SUBPOENAS.

(1) A party or an attorney responsible for the issuance and service of a subpoena shall take reasonable steps to avoid imposing undue burden or expense on a person subject to that subpoena. The court on behalf of which the subpoena was issued shall enforce this duty and impose upon the party or attorney in breach of this duty an appropriate sanction which may include, but is not limited to, lost earnings and reasonable attorney's fee.

(2) (A) A person commanded to produce and permit inspection and copying of designated books, papers, documents or tangible things, or inspection of premises need not appear in person at the place of production or inspection unless commanded to appear for deposition, hearing or trial.

(B) Subject to paragraph (d) (2) of this rule, a person commanded to produce and permit inspection and copying may, within 14 days after service of subpoena or before the time specified for compliance if such time is less than 14 days after service, serve upon the party or attorney designated in the subpoena written objection to inspection or copying of any or all of the designated materials or of the premises. If objection is made, the party serving the subpoena shall not be entitled to inspect and copy materials or inspect the premises except pursuant to an order of the court by which the subpoena was issued. If objection has been made the party may, upon notice to the person commanded to produce, move at any time for an order to compel the production. Such an order to compel production shall protect any person who is not a party or an officer of a party from significant expense resulting from the inspection and copying commanded.

(3) (A) On timely motion, the court by which a subpoena was issued shall quash or modify the subpoena if it

(i) fails to allow reasonable time for compliance:

(ii) requires a person who is not a party or an officer of a party to travel to a place more than 100 miles from the place were that person resides, is employed or regularly transacts business in person, except that, subject to the provisions of clause (c) (3) (3) (iii) of this rule, such a person may, in order to attend trial be commanded to travel from any such place within the state in which the trial is held, or

(iii) requires disclosure of privileged or other protected matter and no exception or waiver applies, or

(iv) subjects a person to undue burden.

(B) If a subpoena

(i) requires disclosure of a trade secret or other confidential research development, or commercial information, or

(ii) requires disclosure of an unretained expert's opinion or information not describing specific events or occurrences in dispute and resulting from the expert's study made not at the request of any party, or

(iii) requires a person who is not a party or an officer of a party to incur substantial expense to travel more than 100 miles to attend trial, the court may, to protect a person subject to or affected by the subpoena, quash or modify the subpoena, or, if the party in whose behalf the subpoena is issued shows a substantial need for the testimony or material that cannot be otherwise met without undue hardship and assures that the person to whom the subpoena is addressed will be reasonably compensated, the court may order appearance or production only upon specified conditions.

(d) DUTIES IN RESPONDING TO A SUBPOENA

(1) A person responding to a subpoena to produce documents shall produce them as they are kept in the usual course of business or shall organize and label them to correspond with the categories in the demand.

(2) When information subject to a subpoena is withheld on a claim that it is privileged or subject to protection as trial preparation materials, the claim shall be made expressly and shall be supported by a description of the nature of the documents, communications, or things not produced that is sufficient to enable the demanding party to contest the claim.

FIGURE 8–2. *Continued*

COMMON ELEMENTS OF A VALID SUBPOENA

1. Name of the court where the lawsuit is brought
2. Names of the parties to the lawsuit
3. Docket number of the case
4. Date, time, and place of the requested appearance
5. Specific documents to be produced, if a subpoena duces tecum is involved
6. Name and telephone number of the attorney who requested the subpoena
7. Signature, stamp, or seal of the official empowered to issue the subpoena
8. Witness fees, where provided by law

FIGURE 8–3.

Common elements of a valid subpoena. (From McWay D: Legal Aspects of Health Information Management, 1st edition. © 1996. Reprinted with permission of Delmar, a division of Thomson Learning. Fax 800-730-2215.)

COMPONENTS OF A VALID COURT ORDER AUTHORIZING DISCLOSURE

1. Name of the court issuing the order authorizing disclosure
2. Names of the parties to the lawsuit
3. Docket number of the case
4. Limitations for disclosure of only those components of the patient's records that are essential to fulfill the objective of the order
5. Limitations for disclosure to those persons whose need for information is the basis for the order
6. Any other limitations on disclosure that serve to protect the patient, the physician-patient relationship, and/or the treatment given, such as sealing the court proceeding from public scrutiny

FIGURE 8–4.

Components of a valid court order authorizing disclosure. (From McWay D: Legal Aspects of Health Information Management, 1st edition. © 1996. Reprinted with permission of Delmar, a division of Thomson Learning. Fax 800-730-2215.)

to be **outsourced,** that is, performed by outside contractors instead of facility personnel.

Consent

In health care, **consent** refers to the agreement of a patient to allow something to occur. Consents underlie virtually all of a patient's contacts with health care professionals.

Informed Consent

In order for a patient to give consent, the patient must be of legal age, competent, and provided with sufficient information to make a reasonable decision about the issue to which he or she is consenting.

Legal age generally refers to having achieved the statutory age, which is determined by state law. Legal age is generally 18 or 21 years old. There are some exceptions, such as married minors, emancipated minors, and minors presenting for psychiatric treatment, substance abuse problems, or prenatal care.

Competency is the patient's ability to make reasonable decisions. A patient who has been declared incompetent by a court has a guardian who can consent on behalf of the patient. In general, a patient is assumed to be competent unless there is evidence to the contrary. When in doubt, the patient's physician should be contacted for guidance.

In the context of consent, health information is an explanation of the process, procedure, or other activity to which the patient is consenting. Sufficient information should be provided to the patient so that he or she can make an informed decision about the matter. This **informed consent** is required before health care can be rendered. Informed consent is obtained on admission to a facility, for certain medical procedures, and for release of information.

Admission

On admission to a health care facility or for a visit at a physician's office, the patient is asked to sign a document consenting to medical treatment. This type of consent is very general and covers routine procedures, such as physical examinations and medical therapies, nutrition counseling, and prescribing medications. In an inpatient facility, this consent is called the **Conditions of Admission** (Fig. 8–5). The Conditions of Admission also include permission for the facility to use patient information for education, research, and reimbursement.

Medical Procedures

The Conditions of Admission form includes only routine procedures and administrative issues. For invasive procedures, such as surgery, a specific consent is required. Anesthesia delivery and human immunodeficiency virus (HIV) testing are examples of other procedures that require specific consent. These consents

Community Hospital
555 Street Drive
Town, NJ 07999
(973) 555-5555

Admission Consent

554879
Green, John
44 Avenue Street
Town, NJ 07999

Dr. Ramundo

1. I understand that I am suffering from a condition requiring diagnosis and medical and/or surgical treatment. I voluntarily consent to such medical treatment deemed necessary or advisable by my treating physician, his associates, or assistants, in the treatment and care rendered to me, while a patient in Community Hospital. I also give permission for the services of any consulting physician that my attending physician deems necessary in his/her treatment of me.

2. I authorize Community Hospital, its medical and surgical staff, and its medical and other employees to furnish the appropriate hospital service and care deemed necessary by my condition.

3. I am aware that the practice of medicine and surgery is not an exact science and I acknowledge that no guarantees have been made to me as to the results of any diagnosis, treatment, or hospital care that I may receive at Community Hospital.

4. I authorize the transfer of medical information to any federal, state, or local government institution, or any agency, nursing home, or extended care facility to which I may be transferred or from which I may require assistance.

5. I certify that the information given by me regarding my health insurance is current and accurate, to the best of my knowledge. I authorize the release of any information needed to act on obtaining reimbursement from the parties so named. I understand that I am responsible for any health insurance deductibles or copayments and I do hereby agree to pay all bills rendered by Community Hospital for my hospital, medical, and nursing care that are not covered by these parties.

6. I authorize Community Hospital to retain, preserve, and use for scientific or teaching purposes, or dispose of at their convenience, any specimens or tissues taken from my body and any x-rays, photographs, or similar data taken during my hospitalization.

7. This form has been fully explained to me and I certify that I understand its contents.

_____   _____   _____
Witness   Signature of patient, agent,   Date
                                                     or legal guardian

FIGURE 8–5.

Conditions of Admission.

are intended, in part, to document the extent to which procedures have been explained to patients, including the known risks of the procedures. Figure 8–6 shows a consent for surgery.

Release of Information

With Consent

There are two types of release of information: with and without the patient's consent. Most of the examples previously mentioned pertain to release of information with the patient's consent. Remember that only the patient can waive the physician-patient privilege. Patient consent is accomplished by an instruction in writing from the patient to the facility.

As with consents for medical procedures, the concept of informed consent applies. The patient must know, in advance, the nature and purpose of the consent. Therefore, consents for release of information should be retrospective. In other words, the patient cannot be fully informed about what is being released until after the information is available. This means that a truly informed consent cannot take place until after the information has been generated.

The issue of informed consent with respect to release of information poses an interesting dilemma. If a patient can only truly consent to the release *after* the information is generated, then how can he or she consent to release of information to a payer *before* to admission to the facility? In fact, patients routinely consent to release of information to a payer at the inception of the insurance contract. The Conditions of Admission frequently includes release of information for reimbursement, education, and research. For most patient care situations, this does not pose a problem. The patient waives his or her right to confidentiality prospectively with respect to the payer because the patient has a strong interest in ensuring that the medical bill is paid. However, there are certain medical conditions that are considered so confidential that prospective consent is not honored. These conditions include HIV testing, drug and alcohol abuse diagnoses, and behavioral health diagnoses. These conditions require special, retrospective consent in most cases. Because state laws vary on these issues, it is imperative that HIM professionals be knowledgeable about the laws in the states in which they practice.

There are 10 elements that are necessary for a valid consent for release of patient information in the normal course of events. Those elements are summarized in Figure 8–7.

- *Date.* This is the date on which the patient makes the consent, usually the date that the form is signed or the letter is written.
- *Patient identification*
  - ❑ The patient's *name* is the primary identifier. However, because many individuals have the same or similar names, additional identifiers should be required.
  - ❑ Patient's *date of birth* (DOB) is helpful, and the social security number (SSN) and/or address also aid in the proper identification of the patient. The *UPIN* (unique patient identification

Community Hospital
555 Street Drive
Town, NJ 07999
(973) 555-5555

| Consent to Operation |
| or Other Procedure(s) |

554879
Green, John
44 Avenue Street
Town, NJ 07999

Dr. Ramundo

1. I understand that _____ is proposed to be performed by_____ and/or his/her associates and whomever may be designated as assistants.

2. I understand that the nature and purpose of the operation or procedure is to _____
   _____
   _____

3. I understand that possible alternative methods of treatment are _____
   _____
   _____

4. I understand that the risks and possible complications of this operation or procedure are
   _____
   _____

5. I am aware that the practice of medicine and surgery is not an exact science and I acknowledge that no guarantees have been made to me as to the result of this procedure.

6. I consent to the examination and disposition by hospital authorities of any tissue or parts which may be removed during the course of this operation or procedure.

7. I understand the nature of the proposed operation or procedure(s), the risks and possible complications involved, and the expected results, as described above, and hereby request that such operation or procedure(s) be performed.

_____   _____   _____
Witness (may not be a   Signature of patient, agent,   Date
member of operating team)   or legal guardian

I have discussed with the above patient the nature of the proposed operation or procedure(s), the risks and possible complications involved, and the expected results, as described above.

_____
Signature of
counseling physician

FIGURE 8–6.
Consent for surgery.

> ## SUMMARY OF ELEMENTS REQUIRED FOR A GENERAL CONSENT FOR RELEASE OF INFORMATION
>
> - Date
> - Patient's name
> - Patient's identifier, such as UPIN, DOB, or SSN
> - Specific information to be released
> - Identification of the party being asked to release the information
> - Identification of the party to whom the information is being released
> - Authorization to release the information
> - Method of distribution
> - Time period for which the authorization is valid
> - Signature of the patient or authorized agent
> - Patient's right to revoke the authorization

FIGURE 8–7.

Elements required for a general consent for release of information.

number, generally the health record number) is also very useful, if known.

- *Specific information to be released.* The consent must specify the time period and specific document or details that are to be released. A request for "any and all records" is not acceptable, because it does not convey awareness of the information to be released. This is particularly important with respect to subpoenas, as discussed later.
- *Identification of the party being asked to release the information.* The owner of the actual documents is named. This is the name of the facility or health care provider who has custody of the documents.
- *Identification of the party to whom the information is to be released.* This may be the name of a facility, a health care provider, or any other party to whom the information is to be released. In other words, to whom does the patient want the information to be sent? It is also very important to include the accurate location of this party.
- *Authorization to release the information.* This refers to a specific statement within the consent. Using the words "authorize" and "release" are helpful. A simple statement suffices, such as "I, Peter Jones, authorize General Hospital to release the specified information to Dr. Sanchez."
- *Method of distribution.* The patient should specify the method by which the record is to be distributed; for example, in person or by regular mail, certified mail, or fax. A consent form may specify a default method, such as regular mail.

- *Time period for which the authorization is valid.* The time period is usually less than a year. Individual state law may specify a default time period, if one is not specified on the consent.
- *Signature of the patient or authorized agent.* The signature of the patient is not always obtainable. For example, the patient may be deceased. In that case, proof of agency, such as power of attorney, should be obtained. If the patient's signature is not on file or is illegible, which may be the case if the patient was admitted to the facility unconscious or the patient is otherwise incapacitated, then the consent document should be notarized or other proof of identification should be provided.
- *Patient's right to revoke the authorization.* The patient or authorized agent has the right to revoke the consent for release of information at any time prior to the actual distribution of the information. This should be explicitly stated on the consent document.

It is not necessary for a patient to complete a special form in order to consent to release of information. A letter addressed to the facility suffices, if it contains all of the elements of a valid consent. Complying with an incomplete consent becomes a matter of professional judgment, within the context of the policies and procedures of the facility. Sometimes, delay in compliance with a request is not warranted just to follow the rules. For example, if a patient writes a letter requesting release of information but he or she does not specifically state what portions of the record are required, a phone call to the patient could clear up that particular issue without further delay. If the patient is going to pick up the record in person, the consent can be completed at that time. The facility's policies and procedures should be clear as to the acceptable forms and methods of requests and distribution. The timing of requests and the order in which they should be filled are important issues. Designating HIM staff for releasing information is a variable.

WITHOUT CONSENT

Another aspect of release of information is release without consent. There are a number of circumstances in which this is perfectly appropriate. For example, many states require reporting of conditions of public health interest. Some of these conditions include cancers, birth defects, and infectious diseases. In these cases, patient consent is not required in order to file reports with the appropriate governmental agency. Suspected child abuse is another instance in which reporting may occur without patient consent. In addition to reporting, representatives of certain special interest groups may have access to patient information without patient consent. For example, as a student, you may be granted access to patient records for educational purposes.

EMERGENCIES

The HIM department may encounter the need to provide information on an emergency basis. A patient may be brought to the emergency department (ED) unconscious, and there may be no appropriate individual available to grant consent to access the patient's existing health record. However, if the patient can be identified and if he or she is known to have previously received health care in the facility, obtaining the health record from the HIM department is merely a matter of a phone call from the ED.

However, what if the patient is in the emergency room of a different facility? In this case, the ED of General Hospital may call the HIM department of Community Hospital in another town asking for an emergency release of information regarding a patient.

The HIM department should have very specific policies and procedures in place to comply with these emergency requests. When the patient is being treated in an emergency situation, no consent is required. Obtaining consent from a family member or from the patient is optimum but not always possible.

In an emergency, there are some simple steps that the HIM professional can take to ensure that, in fact, the call is valid and the necessity to release the information is legitimate. A simple procedure is to obtain the telephone number of the caller, hang up, and call him or her back. For a request from a hospital or physician's office, the telephone number can be quickly verified while the chart is being obtained.

Another procedure that can be implemented, particularly if there is doubt as to the authenticity of the request, is to contact the HIM department at the requester's facility and transmit the information through the department, giving it the responsibility of ensuring that the request is legitimate. A summary of emergency alternative procedures is shown in Figure 8–8.

The procedures we have described are examples. The point is that the HIM professional should never obstruct the access to health information in an emergency situation. However, it is not unheard of for requesters to make nonemergency or nonlegitimate requests. An emergency is a life-threatening situation in which information is needed immediately. Situations that are frequently presented as emergencies but are not true emergencies include the request for immediate information while the patient is in the physician's office. This is not an emergency. In that particular situation, the recipient of the request should always require a formal consent. If the facility accepts facsimile (fax) requests, that may be an alternative to forcing the patient and the physician to wait for the in-

SUMMARY OF EMERGENCY ALTERNATIVE PROCEDURES

- Obtain consent from a family member or caregiver present with the patient
- Obtain telephone number to return call to the requestor
- Confirm location and identity of the requestor
- Contact Health Information Management department at the requesting facility

FIGURE 8–8.
Summary of alternative emergency procedures.

formation. However, some facilities do not comply with these types of requests on an urgent basis, either because they do not accept fax requests or because they have taken the position that timely requests should be given priority.

This is not to say that patients should be denied access to their health records. The only legitimate reason to deny access is if the patient's physician decides that the information in the record would be harmful to the patient. This is an unusual circumstance that pertains primarily to behavioral health cases. In cases in which knowledge of the information in the record would be harmful, as documented by the physican, the record may be released to the patient's agent, frequently legal counsel or another health care professional.

SPECIAL CONSENTS

In terms of special consents, we get a tremendous amount of guidance from federal regulations, specifically the Code of Federal Regulations, Section 42, commonly referred to as 42CFR. This section specifically addresses the requirements for consenting to release information in the case of drug and alcohol abuse. This foundation and its requirements are sometimes mirrored in state regulations for release of HIV/acquired immunodeficiency syndrome (AIDS) and behavioral health records. Figure 8–9 lists the consent requirements for special records.

ELEMENTS OF SPECIAL CONSENTS FOR RELEASE OF INFORMATION

- Date
- Patient's name
- Patient's identifier, such as UPIN, DOB, or SSN
- Specific information to be released, including acknowledgement of the special nature of the information, such as HIV testing, AIDS status, behavioral health diagnosis, or drug/alcohol diagnosis
- Identification of the party being asked to release the information
- Identification of the party to whom the information is being released
- The reason for the release; how the information will be used
- Authorization to release the information
- Method of distribution
- Time period for which the authorization is valid
- Signature of the patient or authorized agent
- Patient's right to revoke the authorization

Differences between this special consent and the consent in Figure 8–7 are highlighted.

FIGURE 8–9.

Elements of special consent for release of information.

With respect to records with health information that includes HIV/AIDS, mental health, and drug and alcohol abuse, the need for a special consent enables us to view these records as a whole. The consent for release of information form differs from a regular consent form in two specific ways: identification of the special nature of the health record and citation of the purpose for the release of information.

The consent form must specifically identify the type of health record that is being requested. For example, using a regular consent form (see Table 8–3) for a record with HIV health information would not be appropriate, because a normal consent form does not indicate that the patient is aware that there is HIV, mental health, or drug or alcohol health information in that particular chart. Prospective consent for release of information is insufficient for release of these types of records.

The other element in the special consent needed for the release of HIV, drug and alcohol, and mental health information in a record is that the purpose of the release must be specified. In a normal consent for release of information, the purpose of the release does not have to be specified, although it frequently is.

It should be noted that the consent for HIV, mental health, and drug and alcohol records is not always satisfied by taking general consents and inserting language addressing the particular special issues. To ensure that the client, specifically the patient, fully appreciates the nature of the consent that is being given, it is desirable that the facility use a special consent form in order to release these records.

Preparing a Record for Release

There are several steps to take in order to properly release health care information. Each facility should have formal, written policies and procedures regarding these steps. The specific policies and procedures vary from facility to facility; however, we can discuss the issues in general. Care should also be taken to train and continually remind personnel of the confidential nature of health information.

Validation and Tracking

On receipt of any request for release of information, the request should be recorded. This may be done in a manual log or in a computerized system. The purpose of recording the request is to track the status and disposition of the request. Many state regulations require that facilities fulfill such requests within a specific time frame, and a tracking log serves to demonstrate compliance.

Every request should be studied to determine whether it is a valid consent. Written procedures should contain a list of the facility's required elements for informed consent. In addition to the completeness of the consent, the authorizing signature should be validated in an appropriate manner. This may be as simple as comparing the signature on the consent with the signature on file in the record. If such validation cannot be accomplished or is not clear, notarization of

Date Request Received	Patient Name	UPIN	Admission Date	D/C Date	Requestor	Information Requested	Date Request Completed	Charge
			TABLE 8–2. Sample Release of Information Log					
6/5/00	Gomez, Maria	576849	3/15/00	3/18/00	Patient	D/C summary	6/10/00	NC
6/5/00	Thomas, Frank	254678	5/12/85	5/27/85	Patient's MD	Complete record	7/4/00	NC

A Release of Information Log can contain many more fields if needed to capture a level of detail that will be useful to the facility. In a paper log, such as this, it is best to keep the form as simple as possible so that all fields will be completed. Unless the information is computerized, it is unlikely that large amounts of data can be usefully compiled because doing so is very labor-intensive. In a computerized system, choices for each field can be menu-based, allowing more detail that can be easily sorted and reported.

D/C, discharge; NC, no charge; UPIN, unique patient identifying number.

the signature or additional proof of identity may be required. A sample release log is shown in Table 8–2.

Retrieval

Retrieval of the patient's information is based on the specific information requested. Care should be taken to ensure that the information retrieved is complete. This may be complicated by the decentralization of records among facility clinics or by incomplete processing of the record. Incomplete records should not, as a general rule, be released. If an incomplete record is released, for example, for a patient still in treatment, the status of the record should be clearly stated in a cover sheet.

Reproduction

A complete copy is made of the specific information requested. Every effort should be made to ensure that the reproduction is clear. When photocopying, personnel must compare the reproduction with the original to ensure completeness and clarity.

Certification

When a copy of a record is required as evidence in a trial, a certified copy may take the place of the original, at the discretion of the lawyer. If the original is required, the director of the HIM department, or his or her designee, accompanies the record to court and may be required to testify on the facility's procedures regarding development and retention of the record. Such testimony may also be required when a certified copy is used.

A certified copy contains a cover sheet, signed by the director of the HIM department or his or her designee, stating that the copy is a complete reproduction of the original record that is on file at the facility. With a paper record, this can be verified by numbering all of the pages in the original record before copying it. The copies will then contain a sequential numbering of the pages. In a computer-based environment, the verification of completeness is different. The facility's procedures should include the process by which verification of completeness can be obtained.

Compensation

Most states permit facilities to charge a fee for providing copies of health records. Some states place a cap, or maximum, on the fees that may be charged. The fee covers the actual services performed: retrieval of the record (search fee), reproduction of the record, and delivery charges (postage). Therefore, an important component of the release of information process is the preparation of the invoice. Some facilities may require that requesters pay the fee, or a portion of the fee, in advance, particularly for large records. As a professional courtesy, health care providers do not charge each other for copies of records. In many cases, insurance companies and other payers have established set amounts that they will pay for copies of records. These fees may differ from the fees charged by the facility to other parties.

TEST YOUR HI-Q

Your facility charges a $5.00 search fee plus $0.75 per page for copying a record. How much will the patient pay for a 125-page record?

Distribution

When a record is released, it should contain a notice that the information may not be re-released. A typical notice might say: "This information is confidential and may not be used for other than the intended purpose and may not be re-released." This is to remind the recipient that the information belongs to the patient not the recipient. Table 8–3 lists the general steps in release of information.

TABLE 8–3. Steps in Release of Information	
Procedure	**Comments**
Log in request	Into a computer tracking system or onto a paper form.
Validate request	Check signature, review the request for completeness.
	Obtain missing information, if possible.
	Verify the validity of a subpoena or court order.
Obtain record	Retrieve the record from storage.
	Incomplete records should be completed before release.
Copy record	Photocopy or print from computer system.
	Copy only the required sections, as specified in the request.
Prepare invoice	Calculate charges and prepare an invoice.
Distribute copy	Obtain signed receipt if picked up in person.

> This facsimile message and the document(s) accompanying this telefax transmission may contain confidential information which is legally privileged and intended only for the use of the addressee named above. If the reader is not the intended recipient or the employee of the intended recipient, you are hereby notified that any dissemination, copying, or distribution of this communication is strictly prohibited. If you received this communication in error, please notify us immediately by telefax or telephone and return the original documents to us via the U.S. Postal Service at the above address. Thank you for your help.

FIGURE 8–10.

Sample confidentiality notice for faxed information. (From Andress AA: Saunders Manual of Medical Office Management. Philadelphia, WB Saunders, 1996, p 150.)

The patient or the individual to whom the record is being released may arrive in person to pick up the record. Policies and procedures should define how the patient or individual should be identified, and the individual picking up the record should sign a receipt. Often the record is mailed. Care must be taken to ensure that the address is correct and legible on the envelope so that the record is not misdirected. Records may also be sent electronically, by fax machine or Internet connection, such as e-mail.

Records sent by fax machine should be accompanied by a cover sheet. The cover sheet should contain a confidentiality statement (Fig. 8–10). Internet transmission of confidential information is becoming more common, particularly in the physician's office setting. Consideration should be given to the security of the Internet and whether the recipient is able to handle the information confidentially. For example, many employers automatically monitor their employees' e-mails. Therefore, sending medical information to a patient at his or her place of business inherently breaches confidentiality. The patient must be made aware of the issues before authorizing transmittal in this manner.

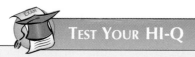

TEST YOUR HI-Q

If reproduction fees (copy costs) are based on photocopying paper records, how do you think these fees should be affected by reproduction of computer-based records and electronic transmission of information?

Internal Requests for Information

Now that we have obtained an understanding of the nature of consents and the nature of confidentiality, we address some of the issues that arise in everyday practice within a health care facility. Routinely, there are numerous instances in which patient information is requested by facility personnel. Some of these requests include utilization review, performance improvement, and a variety of ongoing clinical reviews, such as surgical case review and infection control. These requests should be documented in writing both for internal control purposes (chart tracking) and to ensure that the request is valid.

The routine release of information for patient care should be handled with some caution. Even within a facility, there are many attempts to obtain information inappropriately. The reasons vary dramatically, from family and friends' overstepping their curiosity about a patient's condition, to health care professionals' spying on each other's practices. In the case of a physician's request, authorization is easily determined by checking the record to ensure that the physician requesting the chart is listed as an attending or consulting physician on that particular case. HIM departmental policies and procedures should be clear and specific regarding release of information internally as well as regarding steps to be taken by personnel when there is doubt as to the legitimacy of the request.

Sensitive Records

There are two major types of sensitive records: employee patients and legal files. Although there may be no statutory or regulatory requirement to handle these records differently from others, there are practical considerations in handling them.

EMPLOYEE PATIENTS

Maintaining the confidentiality of employee records is particularly difficult. In a small facility, a paper record can be maintained in a secure file. In a large facility, this may be impractical. Therefore, facility policies and procedures should include specific language regarding the sensitivity of health information pertaining to fellow employees. In a computer-based environment, knowledge that an audit trail of access to the record will be monitored may provide a deterrent to inappropriate access. The confidentiality statement shown in Figure 8–1 includes this language.

LEGAL FILES

Special attention should be paid to records that have been requested for litigation involving the hospital, hospital personnel, or a physician. Every effort should be made to obtain control of those records immediately on receipt of the notification, and special care should be taken to safeguard these records in a special area inaccessible to all but authorized personnel. If possible, the records should be locked in a file used exclusively for that purpose. Photocopies of the records can be circulated for review and discussion; however, the original records should not be out of the safekeeping of HIM personnel. The temptation to alter records becomes extremely strong under these circumstances. Safeguarding the records in the above-mentioned manner removes that temptation and ensures the safety and availability of the records for legal proceedings.

Compliance

A role of increasing importance in HIM is that of ensuring **compliance** with the many statutes, regulations, and other rules imposed on the facility and the professionals who work there. Part of the compliance function is monitoring data quality. Another function is ensuring the completeness and timeliness of records. The following sections discuss the most common areas of concern to HIM professionals.

Licensure

As we stated in Chapter 1, individual states license facilities for operation within that state. A state's licensure requirements, which can be found in the state's administrative code, may contain very specific provisions for the content and retention of specific clinical documentation. These provisions may take the form of a listing of elements to be maintained in a health record. They may also be included in statements about a facility's medical staff. The provisions for health records may be as detailed as specifying which documents need to be included or which types of data need to be collected. Whatever provisions are listed for a specific type of facility, HIM personnel need to be aware of these rules and ensure that any activities under their span of control are in compliance with those rules.

The first step in ensuring compliance with any rule is to review the rule and to obtain an understanding of what the rule really means. Therefore, every health information technology professional should have access to a copy of the specific portions of the licensure regulations that apply to his or her activities. Although it is not necessary in terms of everyday practice for each person to have a copy of the document, it is certainly appropriate for such a document to be available to personnel in the facility.

In practice, each individual person in the facility is responsible for a small portion of the compliance with the specific regulations. The responsibility for the overall compliance with the particular regulations rests with the director of the particular department. In the case of the HIM department, the director typically is responsible for compliance.

One of the best ways to convey to employees in the HIM department how to comply with various regulations is to ensure that there are written policies and procedures in the department that address these particular issues. Employees should be trained with these issues in mind. It is also important to cross-reference the policies and procedures to the specific regulations for compliance.

HIM professionals often become involved in researching regulations and assisting in the interpretation of regulations and development of policies and procedures to comply with those regulations. Frequently, HIM professionals become involved in facilitywide compliance issues. This happens because of the pervasive nature of the documentation that is handled after a patient's discharge. For example, if a regulation dictates that physician telephone orders need to be signed within a certain time frame after being ordered, HIM personnel are frequently involved in the development of the procedures and controls to ensure the monitoring of that activity, because in their reviewing of the chart after the patient's discharge they are in a position to note noncompliance with this procedure.

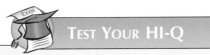

TEST YOUR HI-Q

If your state licensure regulations stated that all records in an acute care facility must be completed within 30 days of discharge, or that all requests for records be filled within 30 days of the original request, how would the health information professional be involved in ensuring compliance with these rules?

Accreditation

State licensure of a facility is mandatory. Accreditation is optional. Remember that accreditation is the process by which independent organizations verify that a facility complies with standards of practice developed by that organization. There are accrediting bodies that deal with a specific type of health care facility, and there are accrediting bodies that deal with many different types of health care facilities. The **Joint Commission on Accreditation of Healthcare Organizations (JCAHO),** known primarily for accrediting acute care facilities, also accredits other facilities such as rehabilitation, long-term care, and ambulatory care networks. Because JCAHO is so important, we use it as our example of how accreditation works. The accreditation process is very similar, regardless of the accrediting body.

JOINT COMMISSION ON ACCREDITATION OF HEALTHCARE ORGANIZATIONS

JCAHO publishes its standards annually in several formats, including a *Comprehensive Guide* that pertains to each setting. The standards are updated annually to reflect changes in health care delivery, organizational philosophy, and environment. In order to become accredited, a facility applies to the JCAHO, completes a detailed questionnaire, and undergoes an intensive site visit called a survey. JCAHO surveys facilities routinely every 3 years; however, special surveys may take place more frequently.

Routine JCAHO surveys are planned well in advance. Ideally, a facility should be in continuous compliance with the standards; however, because the standards change annually, it may take facilities a little time each year to adjust their operations accordingly. Because the achievement of accreditation is so very important, many facilities spend a great deal of time preparing for a survey, ensuring that documentation and various procedures are in compliance. Although it is important to discuss the preparation for a JCAHO survey, we feel obliged to point out that if a facility is in continuous compliance with JCAHO standards, continually updates its procedures to ensure compliance, and structures its reporting to document that compliance, then very little preparation is needed prior to a JCAHO survey. Nevertheless, we must also point out that in reality, the day-to-day operations of a facility do tend to take precedence over the continuous compliance issue. Therefore, most facilities scrutinize their compliance documentation and procedures on more of a periodic basis than a continuous basis.

The preparation for a routine JCAHO survey frequently begins with the appointment of a JCAHO steering committee. It is very important that the HIM department be represented on the steering committee. In some cases, the director of the HIM department chairs or co-chairs that committee. Other members of the committee may include a variety of department directors and managers. The director of nursing or his or her designee and a physician's representative are critical participants. There are a number of management-level individuals on the committee, and they divide the responsibilities for reviewing compliance among themselves.

Some of the activities of the JCAHO steering committee are to review current JCAHO standards and compare them to current policies and procedures, to ensure that the policies and procedures are updated, to conduct mock surveys, to prepare staff for the JCAHO visit, to review reports that will be required, and to assemble large quantities of documentation that are required by the JCAHO surveyors. These activities are largely delegated to the appropriate departmental management, but many employees become involved in the procedures for preparing for the JCAHO survey.

Corporate Compliance

As a result of increasing pressure from the federal government, health care organizations have spent a great deal of time and effort in recent years to demonstrate their commitment to data quality, particularly in terms of accurate billing. Some of this pressure comes from the federal Department of Health and Human Services' (DHHS) Office of the Inspector General (OIG), which has received increased funding in recent years for enforcing accurate billing through audits and penalties. In addition, the Health Insurance Portability and Accountability Act (HIPAA) of 1996 and the Balanced Budget Act of 1997 increased the penalties for failure to comply with regulations.

A *corporate compliance* program is a facilitywide system of policies, procedures, and guidelines that help to ensure ethical business practices. These policies, procedures, and guidelines should include, for example, ethics statements, strong leadership policy, commitment to compliance with regulations, and ways for employees to report unethical or noncompliant activities and behaviors. Part of a corporate compliance effort is a *coding compliance* program. A coding compliance program ensures accurate coding and billing through training, continuing education, quality assurance, and performance improvement activities. An excellent beginning reference for learning about corporate compliance is the American Health Information Management Association's practice brief, *Seven Steps to Corporate Compliance: The HIM Role.*

As we are writing this book, the DHHS is in the process of publishing its final rules regarding various aspects of HIPAA. HIM professionals should ensure that they are fully aware of the rules and their impact on the facilities in which they are employed.

Professional Standards

Finally, there are professional standards with which health care professionals must comply. As we mentioned in Chapter 1, each profession has a code of ethics and a set of standards that are imposed by the credentialing body and/or the licensing agency for that profession. HIM professionals comply with the code of ethics of the American Health Information Management Association (AHIMA). In addition, AHIMA supports the profession through its issuance of a variety of publications designed to guide and promote excellence in professional practice. AHIMA regularly issues practice briefs, stating best practices in areas of interest to HIM professionals.

Suggested Reading

Abdelhak M, Grostick S, Hanken MA, Jacobs E: Health Information: Management of a Strategic Resource. Philadelphia, WB Saunders, 2001.

McWay D: Legal Aspects of Health Information Management. Albany, NY, Delmar, 1997.

E-mail Security (Updated). AHIMA Practice Brief. Published in the Journal of AHIMA, 71-2, February 2000.

Facsimile Transmission of Health Information. AHIMA Practice Brief. Published in the Journal of AHIMA, 72-6, June 2001.

Release of Information Laws and Regulations. AHIMA Practice Brief. Published in the Journal of AHIMA, 70-1, January 1999.

Seven Steps to Corporate Compliance. The HIM Role. AHIMA Practice Brief. Published in the Journal of AHIMA, 70-9, October 1999.

CHAPTER SUMMARY

In this chapter, we discussed the legal and regulatory issues governing the development and retention of health information. Informed consent underlies patient admission, treatment, and release of information. Health information is confidential. Patient-physician privilege dictates confidentiality and that records be released only with the consent of the patient. A valid consent for release of information comprises 10 elements: date, patient's name, patient's identifier, addressee, recipient, information to be released, method of release, authorizing language, effective period, and patient/agent signature. However, in an emergency, records may be released without patient consent. Other important issues include compliance with regulatory, accrediting, and professional standards. Health care facilities should make every effort to ensure continuous compliance with the standards imposed by authoritative bodies.

REVIEW QUESTIONS

1. Discuss the steps to release patient information.

2. List and describe the elements of a valid consent for release of information.

3. Describe the documentation that is required within an organization to ensure that a record is kept on everything that is sent out.

4. Describe how to ensure proper billing for the reproduction of records.

5. Compare and contrast the procedures for preparing a record for release to the patient versus a certified copy for court.

6. Locate the licensure regulations for your state.

   a. What are the provisions for the content of a health record?

   b. Are there any references to the cost of photocopying?

   c. What are the rules regarding the timeliness of completion of a record?

7. Describe the accreditation process.

PROFESSIONAL PROFILE
Customer Service Representative

My name is Zak, and I am a customer service representative with a company that performs release of information services for acute care facilities. The company, and others like it, are often referred to as copy services, because our employees spend a lot of time making photocopies!

I am a Registered Health Information Technician. While I was in school, I was hired by the copy service to work as a copy representative. At the facility at which I was placed, HIM department employees logged in the requests, validated the requests, and retrieved the records. Then I would copy the required sections, prepare an invoice, log the completion of the request, and send out the copies. Eventually, the facility turned over the entire function to me.

As a copy representative, I need to know the release of information laws in my state as well as the hospital's policies and procedures. I need to know the contents of the record, how to retrieve it, and how to ensure that the record is complete. In addition, I had to learn the copy service's computer logging and invoicing system. Most importantly, I'm required to maintain a professional attitude at all times and employ good communication skills to ensure a cordial and professional relationship with my clients.

After I graduated from my HIT program, I was promoted to customer service representative. Now I am responsible for training new employees, scheduling and managing their assignments, solving problems that arise, and occasionally substituting for someone who is ill or on vacation. Sometimes, I accompany the marketing manager when she makes presentations to potential new clients. I like to travel to different hospitals and meet new people, and I enjoy the responsibilities, so I'm very happy in this new position.

APPLICATION

Is It Confidential?

You are the Director of Health Information Management in a small community hospital. One day, an employee in the incomplete file area comes to you with a coat. One of the physicians left it in the dictation room, but the employee does not know to whom it belongs. You decide to look in the pockets of the coat to see if there is any identification. In one of the pockets is a prescription bottle of Antabuse. Antabuse is a medication given to alcoholics to help them stop drinking. The patient named on the bottle is a physician at your facility. What should you do with this information? What are the confidentiality issues? Should you have handled this situation differently?

9

Health Care Reimbursement

Chapter Outline

Reimbursement
Types of Reimbursement
  Fee for Service
  Discounted Fee for Service
  Prospective Payment
  Capitation
Comparison of Reimbursement Methods

Insurance
History
Assumption of Risk
Types of Insurance
  Indemnity
  Managed Care
  Self-Insurance

Government Intervention
Medicare
Medicaid
Tax Equity and Fiscal Responsibity Act of
  1982 (TEFRA)
Medicare Prospective Payment System

Prospective Payment Systems
Diagnosis Related Groups
Ambulatory Patient Classifications

Resource Utilization Groups
Other Prospective Payment Systems

Billing
Patient Accounts
Chargemaster
Charge Capture
Uniform Bill (UB-92)
HCFA-1500

Impact of Coding
Coding Quality
Chargemaster Review

Reference

Suggested Reading

Chapter Summary

Review Questions

Professional Profile

Application

By the end of this chapter, the student should be able to

- Identify and explain major reimbursement methods.

- Describe APCs, RUGs, and DRGs.

- Identify and explain the major components of the HCFA-1500.

- Identify and explain the major components of the UB-92.

- Identify and describe the players in reimbursement.

- Identify unethical billing practices.

Vocabulary

Ambulatory Patient Classifications (APCs)

billing

capitation

case mix

charge capture

Chargemaster

charges

claim

coding compliance plan

Cooperating Parties

deductible

Diagnosis Related Groups (DRGs)

discounted fee for service

encounter form

fee for service

fiscal intermediaries

flexible benefit account

grouper

health maintenance organization (HMO)

indemnity insurance

insurer

Major Diagnostic Categories (MDCs)

managed care

maximization

Medicaid

Medicare

Minimum Data Set (MDS)

National Center for Health Statistics (NCHS)

optimization

patient accounts

per diem

preferred provider organization (PPO)

premiums

prospective payment

prospective payment system (PPS)

reciprocal services

Resource Utilization Groups (RUGs)

risk

Tax Equity and Fiscal Responsibility Act of 1982 (TEFRA)

Title XVIII

Title XIX

usual and customary fees

working DRG

wraparound policies

In Chapter 2, we introduced the concept that physicians would eventually send a patient's insurance company an invoice for services provided. In Chapter 3, we mentioned that the coding of an inpatient chart would initiate billing. In this chapter, we explore in general how reimbursement is accomplished in the health care industry, who is involved in the reimbursement process, what methodologies are used to calculate reimbursement, and how health information technology professionals are involved in the process. One of the most visible roles that health information professionals play is enacting their part in the reimbursement process. Therefore, we have devoted an entire chapter to the issues on various types of reimbursement.

Reimbursement

The term reimbursement is something of a misnomer. We use it today to refer to the payment to a physician or other health care provider for services rendered. Actually, the term reimbursement means to be repaid, in the sense that we have paid something out of our own pockets and we are being repaid. For example, a traveler on a business trip may pay for the hotel with a personal credit card. On returning from the trip, the traveler's company repays, or reimburses, the traveler the amount of the hotel charges. With respect to reimbursement in health care, the same sequence of events occurs when a patient pays a physician directly and then requests reimbursement from an insurance company. However, in general, the health care industry has come to call the direct payment to a physician or a health care facility *reimbursement,* regardless of who is actually remitting the funds and when.

Reimbursement takes many different forms. Historically, it was not uncommon for a physician to be paid in kind. For example, a physician went to a person's house, treated his or her illness, and received chickens as compensation. Reimbursement today is generally monetary. However, in many parts of the world, including some areas of the United States, chickens and other in-kind reimbursement are acceptable.

It is interesting to note that historically, a physician did not necessarily receive the payment that he or she charged, but rather the payment that the patient thought the physician's services were worth. In the early 20th century, the focus changed to paying what the physician charged for the service. More recently, the amount of compensation given to a physician or other health care provider has been decided by neither the patient nor the physician, but by the insurance company. In the following discussion of types of reimbursement, we have categorized reimbursement by the control that the health care provider has over the fees that are charged.

Types of Reimbursement

Fee for Service

As previously mentioned, a physician or other health care provider does not necessarily need to receive money as compensation. Perhaps chickens, bread, or other food is appropriate under certain circumstances. In other circumstances, services might be traded: "You treat my pneumonia, and I will take care of your plumbing." Therefore, exchange of services, or **reciprocal services,** is certainly a basis for reimbursement, with the valuation of those services left to the parties involved. Monetary compensation can also be rendered and is the generally accepted reimbursement method in the United States.

Fee for service is the term assigned to the payment for services rendered by the health care provider, whether it is a physician, a facility, or another clinician. For example, a patient goes to the physician's office with the chief complaint of a runny nose. The physician performs a problem-focused history and physical examination. The office visit costs $40.00. That is the fee. The service provided was an office visit. Say the patient needs an allergy shot. The office visit costs $40.00, and the allergy shot costs $20.00. The total cost of the visit is $60.00. In this example, we can see that there is a fee that corresponds to the service rendered: fee for service.

If we compared the fees charged by physicians in a particular geographic area, we would find that the fees for services are similar. Ignoring the very high and very low fees in our comparison, we would be able to determine the **usual and customary fees** charged by physicians in that area. To determine usual and customary fees, we compare not only the service but also the specialty of the health care professional providing the service.

DISCOUNTED FEE FOR SERVICE

Now imagine that there is a group of 100 patients who get together and decide that they are going to take all of their business to a certain physician, if he or she will give them a discount. This would bring a good deal of business to the physician. If every patient went once a year, that would be an average of two additional patients a week. So, the physician might be inclined to give a discount to that particular group if they promise to give all of their business to him or her. When a physician or other health care provider offers services at a discounted rate, that is, at a fee that is lower than what they would ordinarily charge to a person walking in off the street, that arrangement is called **discounted fee for service.** The fee that the physician or the health care provider ordinarily charges for that individual service is the fee for service. The discounted fee for service is lower than the usual and customary fee.

Within this category of reimbursement are other negotiated fees. Some insurers reimburse at flat rates for services, such as per diem rates. Particularly for inpatient health care providers, such per diem rates may represent a significant discount from the accumulated fees for the various services performed.

PROSPECTIVE PAYMENT

Prospective payment is a method of determining the reimbursement to a health care provider based on predetermined factors, not on individual services. There are a number of insurance companies and government agencies that use prospective payment systems for reimbursement. Prospective payment system

(PPS) is the term used to describe Medicare's reimbursement to hospitals, which we will discuss later in this chapter. Prospective payment is a statistically developed method that identifies the amount of resources that are directed toward a group of diagnoses or procedures, on average, and reimburses on that basis. For example, after reviewing 10,000 inpatient pneumonia cases, it may be determined that patients tend to be hospitalized for 3 to 5 days, in the absence of any significant co-morbidities (additional diagnoses) or complications (additional diagnoses or procedures that result from the original diagnosis or treatment of the diagnosis). Based on the amount of resources that a pneumonia patient would consume under these circumstances, a fixed amount is assigned to that case. Prospective payment may be based on diagnosis, procedure, or a combination of both.

CAPITATION

Another type of payment is **capitation.** Capitation involves the payment to a health care provider regardless of whether the patient comes into the facility for a visit or how frequently the patient visits the provider. For example, the insurance company may pay the primary care physician $5.00 a month for every patient that he or she treats, whether the patients come in or not. Table 9–1 summarizes the four methods of reimbursement.

Comparison of Reimbursement Methods

Let's compare these four different types of reimbursement—fee for service, discounted fee for service, prospective payment, and capitation. Remember our earlier example of the patient's office visit for an allergy shot. We have already determined that the total cost of the visit is $60.00. Under discounted fee for service, the physician charges only the discounted fee. If the discount is 10%, then the visit costs $54.00. Under a prospective payment system, the insurance company pays for the visit based on the reimbursement allowable for the allergy shot, after determining that the diagnosis justified the treatment; perhaps the insurance company pays $30.00 for allergy shot visits. Under capitation, the insur-

TABLE 9–1. Comparison of Reimbursement Methods	
Method*	**Description**
Fee for service	Pay for services rendered
Discounted fee for service	Pay for services rendered, but at a rate lower than the usual fee for service
Prospective payment	Pay a flat rate, based on diagnoses, procedures, or a combination of the two
Capitation	Pay a regular, flat rate to the provider, whether or not services are rendered

*There are numerous variations on these methods, and exceptions to a normal method of payment are made under certain circumstances. For example, under prospective payment, additional compensation can sometimes be obtained if it is medically necessary for the patient to be hospitalized far in excess of the average length of stay for the diagnosis or procedure.

ance company pays the physician $5.00 per month for the patient. That's $60.00 per year. If the patient doesn't return, the physician has been paid the full fee ($60.00) for the services provided. If the patient returns three more times for the same services ($240.00 for the year), then the physician has performed services at a 75% discount.

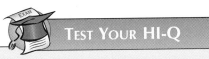

TEST YOUR HI-Q

What incentive do physicians have to operate under each of the four methods of reimbursement discussed?

Insurance

History

Insurance companies have existed for centuries. Notably, Lloyds of London insured cargoes on merchant ships, which were frequently subject to loss from piracy, weather, and other types of catastrophes. The beginnings of insurance in health care date back only to the mid-19th century, when companies insured railroad and paddleboat employees in the event of catastrophic injury or death. A lump sum was paid to the employee or the employee's family for these events.

The origins of modern health care insurance as we know it today began after the Great Depression of 1929. The decline in health care industry income prompted the development of hospital-based insurance plans. For example, for a payment of a small sum, the hospital guaranteed a specific number of days of hospital care at no additional charge. The most successful of these plans was developed at Baylor University (Sultz and Young, p 28), which eventually became the model for what we know today as Blue Cross Hospital Insurance. As we continue our discussion of health insurance, we use a number of terms that are defined collectively in Table 9–2.

Early health care insurance was paid for by the person, sometimes through the employer, union, or other organization. In the original Baylor University scheme, teachers were paying $0.50 a month, which entitled them to 21 days of hospital care (Sultz and Young, p 28). The insurance company became a third party in the relationship between the physician and the patient.

After World War II, employers began offering benefits to employees, including health insurance. Benefits packages became useful in enabling employers to hire and retain employees. Employees benefited because they did not need to spend the money on premiums anymore, and employers benefited because health insurance benefits were relatively low cost. Insurance companies benefited because they increased their client base. However, this thrust a fourth party into the physician-patient relationship: the employer.

Originally, the focus of insurance was on the coverage of services at the health care provider's fee. If the provider raised the fee, the insurance company raised

TABLE 9–2. Terminology Common to Health Insurance Policies	
Benefit	Amount of money paid for specific health care services or, in managed care, the health care services that will be provided or for which the provider will be paid
Beneficiary	One who is eligible to receive or is receiving benefits from an insurance policy or a managed care program
Benefit period	Time frame in which the insurance benefits are covered; varies from insurance policy to policy
Claim	Request for payment by the insured or the provider for services covered
Co-payment	Type of cost-sharing in which the insured (subscriber) pays out-of-pocket a fixed amount for health care service
Coverage	Types of diseases, conditions, and diagnostic and therapeutic procedures for which the insurance policy will pay
Deductible	Amount of cost that the beneficiary must incur before the insurance will assume liability for the remaining cost
Exclusion	Specific conditions or hazards for which a health care policy will not grant benefit payments; often includes preexisting conditions and experimental therapy
Fiscal intermediary	Contractor that manages the health care claims
Insurance	Purchased contract (policy) in which the purchaser (insured) is protected from loss by the insurer's agreeing to reimburse for such loss
Out-of-pocket costs	Moneys that the patient pays directly to the health care provider
Payer	Party who is financially responsible for reimbursement of health care cost
Premium	Payment required to maintain policy coverage; usually paid periodically
Preexisting condition	Disease, injury, or condition identified as having occurred before a specific date
Reimbursement	Payment by a third party to a provider of health care
Rider	Policy amendment that either increases or decreases benefits
Policy	Written contract between insurance company and subscriber (insured) that specifies the coverage, benefits, exclusions, co-payments, deductibles, benefit period, and so on
Subscriber	Person who elects to enroll or participate in managed care or purchase health care insurance
Third party payer	Party (insurance company, state or federal government, other) that is responsible for paying the provider on behalf of the insured (subscriber, patient, member) for health care services rendered

From Abdelhak M, Grostick S, Hanken MA, Jacobs E: Health Information: Management of a Strategic Resource. Philadelphia, WB Saunders, 1996, p 37.

its **premiums** in order to cover these costs. As health care costs increased, the premiums began to increase dramatically. Currently, many employers pay only a part of the premiums, with employees bearing the rest of the cost.

Assumption of Risk

Our previous example of the patient's visit for an allergy shot in the comparison of reimbursement methods serves to illustrate the different financial outcomes of the methods for the physician and to emphasize the concept of **risk**. Risk, in this case, refers to the financial impact of the reimbursement method: Which party is most likely to lose financially, and under what circumstances will it lose? Health care providers render services, for which they expect to be compensated. Patients need these services, but they would like someone else to pay for them. Insurance companies are willing to assume the risk of having to pay for expensive services, but they would like to balance that risk by insuring a large number of patients, many of whom will not need health care services. The assumption of risk is the foundation of the concept of insurance.

Insurance companies serve the public by assuming the risk of financial loss. If you own an automobile, you probably have auto insurance. You pay periodic premiums to the insurance company, which in turn bears all or part of the cost of an accident or other adverse event. The auto insurance company, although assuming the risk of financial loss in the event of an accident, is gambling that you won't have one. In fact, it goes to great lengths to predict the likelihood of accidents in certain populations, geographic areas, and vehicles. If you pay $1000.00 per year in auto insurance for 40 years and never have an accident, then the insurance company keeps the $40,000.00 (plus interest). If the insurance company insures a very large number of drivers, only a small percentage of them will ever have a serious accident. In some states, insurance companies are permitted to choose which drivers they wish to insure. Obviously, they would prefer to choose drivers with good driving records and no accidents. In other states, insurers may not choose and must offer insurance to anyone who requests it. This requirement raises the risk that the insurer will be required to pay out settlements, which in turn raises the cost of auto insurance.

Health insurance is similar. The **insurer** wants to cover large numbers of individuals so that the risk that someone will require expensive care is offset by large numbers of individuals who require little care (Fig. 9–1). In an environment of spiraling health care costs, increases in reimbursements trigger increases in premiums. The insertion of the employer into the relationship has at least two effects: loss of control over the choice of individuals to cover and loss of total freedom to raise premiums. The insurer is pressured to accept all employees, reducing the insurer's ability to control risk by choosing individuals to cover. If one individual cancels a policy, the impact on the insurer is far less dramatic than if an employer cancels a group policy. Therefore, the insurer is pressured to keep premiums low if it doesn't want to lose the employer's account.

Types of Insurance

There are many different insurance plans, with an almost endless variety of combinations of benefits and reimbursement rules. Plans may set dollar limits or visit limits on the benefits in given time periods. Nevertheless, plans fall into one of two basic categories: indemnity and managed care. Managed care is further divided into two major types: preferred provider organizations and health maintenance organizations. We discuss the major features of these plans later in the chapter. The plans differ in the relationships among the physician, patient, and insurer. In addition, some plans are more likely than others to use certain reimbursement methods.

INDEMNITY

Originally, the patient payed the physician or other health care provider and then submitted the bills to the insurance company for reimbursement. If it were a covered service, the insurance company would reimburse the patient. Some insurance companies paid 100% of the cost of certain services and a lower

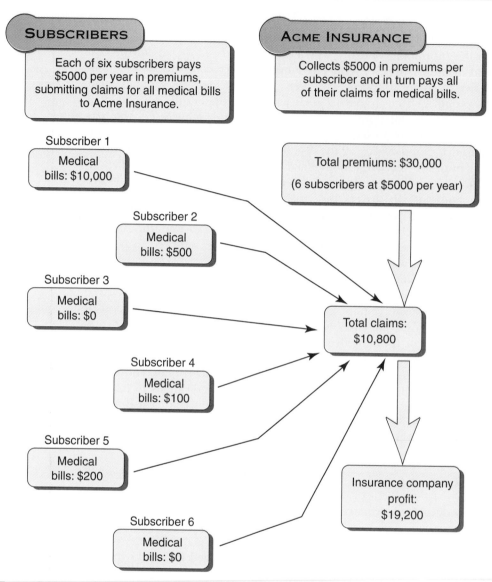

SUBSCRIBERS

Each of six subscribers pays $5000 per year in premiums, submitting claims for all medical bills to Acme Insurance.

ACME INSURANCE

Collects $5000 in premiums per subscriber and in turn pays all of their claims for medical bills.

Subscriber 1
Medical bills: $10,000

Subscriber 2
Medical bills: $500

Subscriber 3
Medical bills: $0

Subscriber 4
Medical bills: $100

Subscriber 5
Medical bills: $200

Subscriber 6
Medical bills: $0

Total premiums: $30,000
(6 subscribers at $5000 per year)

Total claims: $10,800

Insurance company profit: $19,200

FIGURE 9–1.

How insurance companies reduce risk.

percentage of the cost of other services. This type of insurance is called **indemnity insurance,** and it was the predominant type of health insurance for many years. Indemnity plans are still in existence, but managed care has become more important.

An important feature of indemnity insurance is the **deductible.** A deductible is the amount of health care services for which the patient is personally responsible and must be spent before any insurance benefits are paid. For example, a patient with medical expenses of $5000.00 and a deductible of $300.00 pays the first $300.00 out of pocket. Then, the insurer pays whatever portion of the remaining $4700 is covered by the policy. The patient is responsible for any non-covered expenses.

Depending on the insurance company, a deductible could apply for every encounter, for every visit, or for every hospitalization or it could be applied on an annual basis. If you have a family, your deductible could be per person or it could be per family. One effect of the deductible is that routine health care costs often do not exceed the deductible. Therefore, the patient's insurance ultimately covers only unusual or extraordinary expenses.

One of the impacts that indemnity insurance had was to contribute to the increase in the dollars being spent on health care. In the physician-patient relationship, the patient bears the cost of the care and therefore has some influence on the fees. The individual may choose not to go to the doctor in the first place because it is too expensive or might refuse certain services. Indemnity insurance reduces the out-of-pocket expense to the patient, increasing the likelihood that the services of the provider will be used. Consequently, the number of people actually using health care under indemnity insurance plans may increase. In addition, if the insurance company reimburses for health care without reviewing the necessity for the expenditure, then physicians have no incentive to be conservative either in diagnosing or in treating the patient. Combine this with new and greater advances in health care—for example, consider computed tomography (CT) scans, magnetic resonance imaging (MRI), ultrasonography, computer-guided procedures, transplants, and laser procedures. These are tremendous, and often expensive, improvements in the ability to diagnose and treat disease. As more and more services become available and used, the cost of health care rises.

TEST YOUR HI-Q

Based on your knowledge of health records, if an insurance company wanted to check to see whether excessive testing was performed on a patient, where would it look in the chart and why?

In addition to the technology-driven expenses, health care costs increased because a small portion of the health care community provided an excessive number of services to patients. Two x-ray films were taken, when one would have sufficed. A CT scan or MRI was used, when a simple x-ray would have been enough. Frequent blood tests were given, when fewer blood tests would have told the same story.

Health care premiums rose so much that many employers could no longer afford to offer health insurance as a benefit. Many employers solved the problem by hiring more part-time employees, who were not eligible for benefits, as opposed to full-time employees. Other employers hired outside contractors to perform noncritical functions.

Some of the repercussions of rising health care costs were an attempt by the insurance companies to control the amount of dollars that were actually being spent on health care. Insurance companies attempt to control costs in a number of different ways. First, as we have already discussed, they can impose deductibles. They can strictly limit the number of covered services. But insurance becomes less attractive under these circumstances. So what has developed in the insurance industry in the past decade or so is the rise of what is called managed care.

HIT BIT

You may think, from the previous description, that physicians have been the driving force behind the development of managed care in the insurance industry. This is far from the case. In fact, the American Medical Association (AMA) was always in vocal opposition to health insurance, which it stated and reinforced many times. The AMA's position is that third parties should not come between the physician and the patient (Sultz and Young, p 27). This position becomes clearer as we explore the impact of other types of health insurance.

MANAGED CARE

The term **managed care** is very broad. In general, it refers to the control that an insurance company or other payer exerts over the physician selection and reimbursement process.

Think back to Chapter 2 and the scenario of your visit to a physician's office: You went as a patient to a chosen physician with symptoms, the physician developed a diagnosis and treatment plan, you agreed to the treatment, the physician billed you, and you payed the bill.

Compare that to reimbursement under indemnity insurance: The patient goes to a chosen physician with symptoms, the physician develops a diagnosis and treatment plan, the patient agrees to the treatment, the physician bills the patient, the patient pays the bill, the patient gives the bill to the insurance company, and the insurance company reimburses for covered services, less the deductible. Depending on the physician's and the insurance company's procedures, the physician may bill the insurance company directly and then bill the patient later for the unreimbursed portion.

Under managed care, the insurer and the health care provider are combined into one organization. The patient chooses a physician from among those who participate in the managed care plan. The patient then goes to a physician with symptoms, the physician develops a diagnosis and treatment plan, the patient agrees to the treatment, the patient pays a co-payment, and the physician bills the managed care company directly. The managed care company may refuse to pay the physician's bill if the physician does not obtain preapproval for certain treatments, the physician performs treatments that the managed care company does not consider medically necessary, or the patient has chosen a physician who does not participate in the managed care plan.

The idea of managed care is to reduce health insurance by eliminating unnecessary costs, tests and procedures, visits, and hospitalizations. Managed care seeks to effect this cost reduction by controlling as much of the delivery process as possible. The controversy lies in the definition of what is unnecessary health care. For example, many managed care organizations did not consider preventive care to be necessary. It was only through years of study, investigation, and trial and error that they discovered that preventive care was one of the best ways to reduce health care costs. This is no more obvious than when considering pregnancy care. The cost of treating a pregnant woman through prenatal testing, education, and examinations, with the goal of delivering a healthy newborn, is significantly less than that for caring for a newborn whose mother did not receive good prenatal care.

This same analogy can be drawn for dental care. Theoretically, if you have your teeth examined and cleaned every 6 months, you will not have expensive cavities and expensive root canals and expensive gum surgery, because your dentist will help you prevent or detect and treat problems early.

Beyond preventive care, additional controversy continues over the extent to which managed care organizations control the services provided. By requiring preapproval of procedures, second opinions for surgery, and strict adherence to established standards of medical practice, managed care organizations assert that they are delivering cost-effective, quality care. Low patient out-of-pocket costs and reduced paperwork are further enticements. However, patients are often frustrated by the preapproval process, the seeming incentive of physicians *not* to treat, and the limited choice of physicians.

Individuals changing jobs are often faced with changing health care providers if their providers are not included in the new insurer's plan. Patients who live at the outskirts of a plan's primary service area may be required to travel unacceptable distances to receive covered health care services.

Physicians are sometimes frustrated by the emphasis on standards and the discouragement of alternative approaches. Managed care organizations focus heavily on statistical analysis of outcomes and scrutinize physicians whose practices appear to vary significantly from the norm. Managed care has forced physicians to become more aware of and active in managing their own resources by employing reimbursement methods other than fee for service that shift some financial risk to the physician.

Despite controversy and criticism, managed care has become an important presence in the health care arena. Managed care takes a number of different forms, and there are many variations on the relationship between managed care organizations and physicians and other health care providers who deliver their services. At the heart of managed care is the idea that the insurer can gain better control over cost of health care by delivering the services directly. The U.S. Congress supported this concept with the Health Maintenance Organization (HMO) Act of 1973, which encouraged the development of **health maintenance organizations (HMOs)** and mandated certain employers to offer employees an HMO option for health care delivery.

Health Maintenance Organization. An HMO is an organization that has ownership or employer control over the health care provider. An example of an HMO is Kaiser Permanente. Kaiser Permanente has been providing hospital, physician, and other health care for over 75 years. In this staff model HMO, the organization controls the continuum of care by actually owning the hospitals, employing the physicians, and providing essentially all health care services. In other models of HMOs, the organization may contract with a group or a network of physicians and facilities to provide health services. Finally, in an independent practice association (IPA) model, the HMO contracts with individual physicians, a portion of whose practices are devoted to the HMO. Regardless of the HMO model, an HMO seeks to limit services to approved providers. Out-of-plan care is extremely limited and usually requires preapproval.

Preferred Provider Organization. A **preferred provider organization (PPO)** is another managed care approach, in which the organization contracts with a network of health care providers who agree to certain reimbursement rates. It is from this network that patients must choose their primary care physician and any specialists. If a patient chooses a provider who is not in the network, the PPO reimburses like an indemnity insurer: for specified services, with specific dollar or percentage limits, and after any deductible is paid by the insured.

A PPO is a hybrid plan that gives patients the option of choosing physicians outside the plan without totally forfeiting benefits. In addition, PPOs may offer patients a certain degree of freedom to self-refer to specialists. For example, gynecology, urology, and vision specialists may be visited without referral from the primary care physician.

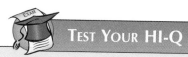

TEST YOUR HI-Q

How do you think a managed care organization controls the utilization of health care resources by all of its subscribers?

SELF-INSURANCE

Although not specifically a type of insurance, self-insurance is an alternative to purchasing an insurance policy. Self-insurance is really a savings plan, with which an individual or an employer seeks to put aside, in advance, funds to cover health care costs. In this way, the individual or the company assumes the financial risk associated with health care. Because the assumption of risk rests with the company or the individual, this is not so much a type of insurance as it is an alternative to shifting the risk to an insurer.

An employer may choose to self-insure for all health care benefits, or it may self-insure in order to provide specific benefits that its primary insurance plan does not cover. For example, an insurance plan may cover preventive care, hospital and physician services, and diagnostic tests. However, it may not cover vision or dental care. The employer may designate a certain dollar amount per

TABLE 9–3. Summary of Payer Types	
Payer	**Major Features**
Self-pay or self-insured	Savings, if any, are used to reimburse health care providers.
Indemnity	Patient has choice of provider; patient pays deductible; many covered services have caps, or maximum reimbursable claims.
HMO	Providers are limited to those in the HMO plan; patient pays a small co-payment; services must be approved as medically necessary; providers are generally employees of the HMO or work for HMO contractors.
PPO	Combination of HMO and indemnity; providers are independent contractors.

employee, with which the employee may then be reimbursed for these other services. Ordinarily, if the annual dollar amount is not spent, it is lost to the employee. Because the issue of confidentiality is so important, employers may choose to contract with an insurer to process health care claims, even if the employer self-insures. Table 9–3 summarizes the four types of insurance that we have discussed.

Individuals may self-insure by saving money on a regular basis, which would be designated for health care expenses. One formal plan that enables individuals to save in this manner is a **flexible benefit account.** A flexible benefit account provides the individual with a savings account, usually through payroll deduction, into which a set amount can be deposited routinely. These funds can then be drawn on to pay out-of-pocket health care and some child care expenses. The advantage to a flexible benefit account is that the funds are withdrawn from the individual's salary on a pretax basis, thereby reducing the individual's income tax liability. The disadvantage is that nondisbursed funds are forfeited at the end of the year.

Government Intervention

The federal government in the United States has historically allocated funds for the benefits of specific populations. In the case of health care, target populations of chronically ill or indigent patients have received low-cost or free health care. Until the 1960s, funding was not entirely predictable, and health care providers were often required to provide a certain amount of unreimbursed charity care. In addition, there were large groups of individuals with limited incomes who were not eligible for federal assistance. The federal government took the plunge in the mid-1960s with the enactment of legislation that made it the largest single payer in the health care industry: Title XVIII and Title XIX of the Social Security Act, which established the Medicare and Medicaid programs. In addition to Medicare and Medicaid, Congress also created the Civilian Health and Medical Program of the Uniformed Services (CHAMPUS), which provides health benefits for military personnel, their families, and military retirees. CHAMPUS is now called TRICARE. The Civilian Health and Medical Program of the Veterans Administration (CHAMPVA) was created in 1973 to provide health services for spouses and children of certain deceased or disabled veterans. Both TRICARE and CHAMPVA are service benefits, not insurance, and are included here to illustrate the extent of the federal government's financial involvement in health care. See also Table 1–5 for a summary of this involvement.

Medicare

Title XVIII of the Social Security Act established the **Medicare** program in 1965. Originally enacted to provide funding for health care for the elderly, Medicare has grown to include patients with disabilities, renal dialysis patients, and transplant patients. For some health care providers, Medicare represents over 50% of their income. Medicare is an extremely important driving force in the insurance industry because where Medicare goes in terms of reimbursement strategies, many insurance companies follow.

The Medicare program, although funded by the federal government and administered by the Health Care Financing Administration (HCFA), does not process its own reimbursements. Reimbursements are processed by **fiscal intermediaries.** The Blue Cross and Blue Shield companies are the most common fiscal intermediaries. These companies are not-for-profit insurance companies that are affiliated with each other through the Blue Cross and Blue Shield Association.

Medicare coverage applies in two categories: Part A and Part B. Part A covers hospital services, and Part B covers physician and other services. Because there are limits to Medicare coverage, many beneficiaries choose to purchase additional insurance, called **wraparound policies,** aimed at absorbing costs not reimbursed by Medicare. Many end-of-life hospital stays generate costs in the hundreds of thousands of dollars. Therefore, wraparound policies can help to preserve estates and save surviving spouses from financial ruin. In recent years, Medicare beneficiaries have also had the option of choosing Medicare HMO plans.

Medicaid

In 1965, Congress enacted **Title XIX,** which created a formal system of providing funding for health care for low-income populations. Also administered by HCFA, **Medicaid** is a shared federal and state program designed to shift resources from higher-income to lower-income individuals. Funds are allocated based on the average income of the residents of the state. Unlike Medicare, which reimburses through fiscal intermediaries, Medicaid reimbursement is handled directly by each individual state. The reimbursement guidelines vary from state to state. Some states have contracted with insurers to offer HMO plans to Medicaid beneficiaries.

Eligibility for Medicaid is determined by the individual states, based on the state's income criteria. The federal government mandates that the following services be included in the program: hospital and physician services, diagnostic services, home health, nursing home, preventive care, family planning, pregnancy care, and child care.

Tax Equity and Fiscal Responsibility Act of 1982 (TEFRA)

With the federal government's firm entry into the reimbursement arena, more individuals have had access to health care services than ever before. The use of health care services rose accordingly, which in turn drove health care costs upward at an alarming rate. Improved access for the elderly meant better care and therefore longer life expectancy, thereby additionally increasing costs. Thus, cost containment became a critical issue. In the early 1970s, professional standards review organizations (PSROs) were established. PSROs conducted local peer reviews of Medicare and Medicaid cases for the purpose of ensuring that only medically necessary services were being rendered. In 1982, PSROs were replaced by peer review organizations (PROs), which is the current designation for this function.

PROs were established through a federal law called the **Tax Equity and Fiscal Responsibility Act of 1982 (TEFRA).** TEFRA included a broad array of provisions, many of which had nothing to do with health care. For example, this act provided the foundation for requiring Social Security numbers when opening brokerage accounts. The following year, Medicare adopted the prospective payment system.

Medicare Prospective Payment System

Also through TEFRA, Medicare was the first payer to universally adopt prospective payment as a method of reimbursement. In 1983, Medicare designated prospective payment through Diagnosis Related Groups as its payment methodology for acute care facilities. This decision was so important that the system itself is called the Medicare Prospective Payment System.

The impact of the prospective payment system on health care was enormous. First of all, a number of states adopted prospective payment systems, so that all payers in those states were required to use prospective payment for reimbursement to acute care facilities. Second, hospitals accepting Medicare patients were paid a flat rate for the patient's entire length of stay. This encouraged facilities to reduce length of stay in order to improve their financial position. Finally, the computerization and data collection activities that are required to support prospective payment systems pushed facilities closer to an electronic patient record.

HIT BIT

When prospective payment systems were first implemented, many hospitals were still maintaining an entirely paper-based record. In order to file the required data with the fiscal intermediary or the private insurer, the data were abstracted from the record and recorded manually on a form. This form was then used to enter the data into a computer for reporting and reimbursement purposes (see Fig. 7–6).

Although prospective payment systems did not have the overwhelming cost-containment impact that was hoped, they have been sufficiently successful that prospective payment methodologies have been developed for other health care settings.

Prospective Payment Systems

Prospective payment systems (PPSs) are based on the statistical analysis of large quantities of health care data for the purpose of evaluating the resources used to treat specific diagnoses and to effect certain treatments. Based on this evaluation, it has been determined that certain diagnoses and/or procedures consume sufficiently similar resources, such that reimbursement to the facility for these patients should be the same.

As we have seen from our previous discussions of clinical data, the focus of treatment, patients' length of stay, and the individuals involved in the care plan differ from setting to setting. Because prospective reimbursement systems are based on just these types of factors, different systems must be developed for each health care setting.

Diagnosis Related Groups

Prospective payment systems, as they apply to acute care, are based on **Diagnosis Related Groups (DRGs).** The statistical foundation of DRGs is based on the assumption that the same diagnosis requires the same type of care for all patients. For example, if a patient is in the hospital with congestive heart failure and nothing else is wrong with him or her, then that patient will probably consume the same amount of resources, have the same procedures performed, require the same number of consultations, and have the same intensity of nursing care as any other patient coming into the hospital with that same diagnosis and no complications. Statistically, based on review of hundreds of thousands of records, this proves to be true. Therefore, it is the patient's diagnoses, or diagnoses combined with certain procedures, that leads to the classification of the patient's stay in a DRG.

It should be noted that there is more than one DRG system in use in the United States or, in fact, the world. Canada, for example, uses Case Mix Groups (CMGs). Medicare DRGs are primarily used for Medicare or for comparison with Medicare rates. However, they contain only diagnoses that pertain to the elderly and a few specific chronic illnesses. Therefore, there are no Medicare DRGs corresponding to pediatrics. To give you an idea of the extent of the difference, the Medicare system has about 500 DRGs; non-Medicare systems have over 700 DRGs.

DRGs are derived from the International Classification of Diseases, Ninth Revision—Clinical Modification (ICD-9-CM) codes that the health information management (HIM) professional assigns, based on the clinical data, usually after the patient has been discharged. DRGs comprise 25 **Major Diagnostic Categories**

(MDCs), divided into medical and surgical partitions, organized primarily by body system. The process of determining the DRG for a patient's stay follows a flowchart very similar to any flowchart created to track a process or procedure. The process of following the flowchart from the principal diagnosis, other diagnoses, and procedures through the MDC to obtain the DRG is called a **grouper.** Because using the grouper manual to determine the DRG is extremely time-consuming and risks human error, grouping is performed by computer.

The purpose of categorizing patients into these groups primarily by diagnosis is to determine the hospital's **case mix.** Case mix refers to the statistical distribution of patients according to their utilization of resources. For example, a patient with tonsillitis consumes far fewer resources than a patient with emphysema and congestive heart failure. It is the tracking of utilization of resources through case mix analysis that helps administrative personnel to do long-range (strategic) planning and to evaluate quality measures, such as mortality and nosocomial infection rates. Originally, DRGs were developed for the purpose of case mix analysis. Using the ICD-9-CM code-based diagnosis index to aggregate specific diagnoses can yield a frequency by diagnosis, but there are thousands of possible diagnoses. With DRGs, there are far fewer items, and they have statistical relevance in terms of length of stay and therefore utilization of resources.

If DRGs are useful for analyzing case mix and utilization of resources, and utilization of resources is the foundation for reimbursement, then it is logical that DRGs can be tied to reimbursement. The dollar calculations of a reimbursement based on a DRG have three components: resource utilization, geography, and other factors. The DRG itself has a certain weight in terms of utilization of resources. Each year, HCFA publishes the DRGs and their assigned weights in the *Federal Register.* The hospital itself has a certain weight, depending on where it is and whether it is in an urban, suburban, or rural area. Hospital weights differ because different areas of the country are more expensive than others in terms of salaries, rent, and other costs. In addition to utilization and geography, there are other mitigating factors in terms of reimbursement, such as graduate medical education and excessive length of stay.

Reimbursement based on DRG is a prospective payment system, because the reimbursement for a DRG has been determined in advance. Hospitals receive a flat rate, with some possible adjustments, per patient, as determined by the DRG. The assignment of the DRG for reimbursement is retrospective. In other words, it takes place after the patient has been discharged. However, the calculation of a **working DRG,** based on the admitting diagnosis, is very useful in managing a facility's utilization of resources. For example, if the working DRG predicts an average length of stay of 4 days, then the clinical staff has a benchmark for monitoring the care of the patient. In addition, hospital administration can monitor the actual lengths of stay versus the DRG benchmarks to evaluate, for example, the hospital's utilization of resources and budgeting.

Although prospective payment has had a huge impact on reimbursement in acute care facilities, it should be noted that fee for service, discounted fee for service, and other negotiated rates are still important reimbursement methodologies in acute care.

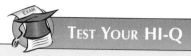

TEST YOUR HI-Q

What impact will incorrect coding have on reimbursement by DRG.

Ambulatory Patient Classifications

In ambulatory health care, a number of different reimbursement methodologies apply: Fee for service and discounted fee for service are most commonly used. A number of insurers are very interested and active in capitation as well. Medicare is the major force behind prospective payment, although more than one PPS is already in place. HCFA recently published its final rules for the outpatient prospective payment system, **Ambulatory Patient Classifications (APCs).**

In ambulatory care, for reimbursement purposes the diagnosis of the patient is secondary to the actual procedures performed. If you think about your trip to a physician's office, this becomes very clear. In an acute care facility, the focus of the stay is the principal diagnosis, either discovering it or treating it. Room and board as well as the services of numerous nursing, allied health professionals, and administrative staff are involved. Statistically, therefore, the utilization of resources can be linked to the diagnosis. However, on an outpatient basis, the diagnosis is not necessarily definitive. Further testing may be needed, and the physician may consider a variety of diagnoses that could possibly apply to the patient, thereby prompting additional visits. The physician's office visit is often separate from diagnostic testing, which is separate from treatment. Activities that, on an inpatient basis, would result in a diagnosis by the end of the stay may be performed in separate events, often by separate health care providers. Therefore, on an ambulatory basis, it is the procedure or the physician's time that becomes the relevant factor in reimbursement. For that reason, it is the Current Procedural Terminology (CPT) codes that drive prospective payment in the ambulatory care environment. The diagnosis stated at the time of the reimbursement claim enables the payer to confirm, or to question, the medical necessity of the procedure. The diagnosis is expressed as an ICD-9-CM code.

As with DRGs, APCs are assigned retrospectively, after the patient has left the facility. Again, a grouper is used to determine the APC, in this case based on the CPT codes. At the time of this writing, HCFA's APCs were intended to reimburse hospital outpatient services and community mental health services. Services performed at the time of the visit are grouped into one or more APCs. Because reimbursement is attached to each APC, a physician's arrival at multiple APCs for one visit requires analysis to determine a single payment.

Resource Utilization Groups

Resource Utilization Groups (RUGs) are the basis for prospective payment in long-term care, specifically skilled nursing facilities (SNFs). Unlike DRGs and APCs, RUGs are not a retrospective reimbursement for an entire stay or visit. Reimbursement based on RUGs is a **per diem** (daily) rate, based on the admission assessment of the patient. In order to understand this, let's review data sets.

As we discussed in Chapters 2 and 3, specific data sets are abstracted and reported retrospectively for both ambulatory and hospital care: the Uniform Ambulatory Care Data Set (UACDS) and the Uniform Hospital Discharge Data Set (UHDDS), respectively. In long-term care, the **Minimum Data Set (MDS)** is collected as part of the Resident Assessment Instrument (RAI). The MDS contains far more data than the UHDDS or the UACDS. It includes the patient's cognitive and medical condition as well as his or her ability to perform self-care and other activities of daily living. As you might imagine, assessment is performed at the beginning of the patient's stay, not at the end. Therefore, reimbursement is based on the patient's care needs, consisting of 1 of 44 groups within 7 broad categories: rehabilitation, extensive services, special care, clinically complex, impaired cognition, behavior problems, or reduced physical function. Although there are other RUG systems in place, Medicare reimbursement must be determined by grouping through the RUG III system.

Another distinguishing characteristic of RUGs is that the nursing staff collects and records the MDS data, including the ICD-9-CM codes, associated with the patient's medical condition. Because nurses complete the MDS and play a large role in the care of these patients, this has seemed to be an efficient process in many long-term care facilities.

Table 9–4 shows a comparison of the prospective payments we have discussed.

Other Prospective Payment Systems

From the payer's perspective, prospective payment can be an extremely effective budgeting tool. Utilization trends can be followed, case mix analysis by health care provider is facilitated, and reimbursement costs can be controlled through rate setting. From the provider's standpoint, however, prospective payment can mean loss of income and loss of some control over the clinical management of the patient.

TABLE 9–4. Comparison of Prospective Payment Systems		
System	Applicable Setting	Reimbursement Based On
DRG	Acute care	Diagnoses and procedures
APC	Ambulatory care (hospitals and community mental health)	Procedures, using diagnoses to verify medical necessity
RUG	Skilled nursing facilities	Minimum Data Set

Nevertheless, Medicare continues to expand its prospective payment systems into additional settings. Prospective payment for home health care has been in place for a year, and for inpatient and rehabilitation it is imminent. It remains to be seen whether private insurance will follow down this road.

Billing

In order to be reimbursed for services rendered to a patient, a facility must alert the payer that payment is due. This is accomplished by **billing.** To the insurer, this bill is a **claim.** In an acute care facility, the billing function is performed in a department that is often called **patient accounts.**

Patient Accounts

The patient accounts department is responsible for ensuring that bills are sent, that they are sent to the correct payers, and that the facility receives the correct payment. Using acute care as an example, there are two key things that have to happen in order to produce (or *drop*) a bill on an inpatient stay: (1) The patient has to have been discharged, so that the bill reflects the patient's entire stay, and (2) the bill has to be coded. Whether or not payers use DRGs as a method of reimbursement, they still will want to see the codes related to the clinical stay. It is through the coding of the diagnoses and the procedures that the payer gets the first impression of what should have actually happened. The list of patients who have been discharged but for whom no bill has yet been drawn is called a variety of things in different facilities. Sometimes it is called the *unbilled list,* sometimes it is called the *discharged no final bill (DNFB)* list. Regardless of the name used, in the absence of proper internal control procedures to track and correct outstanding issues, the DNFB list can run into the millions of dollars. So it behooves the HIM department to become proactively involved in the monitoring of the DNFB list to ensure that whatever is causing the delay in drawing up the bill is not the fault of the coders.

Chargemaster

Whether a facility is reimbursed using prospective payment or some other system, a variety of procedures must be in place to ensure the accurate accumulation of **charges** and the accurate coding of the clinical data. Charges are the facility's individual fees for services provided to a patient. Remember that although Medicare may be reimbursing on a prospective basis, private insurers may be reimbursing by fee for service or discounted fee for service. A facility compares its charges to its actual reimbursements to determine the impact of the various reimbursement methods. In addition, a facility must also keep track of how much it spent in providing the services, that is, its costs. It then compares these costs to the actual reimbursements to help determine whether it is operating profitably (making more money than it spends).

TABLE 9-5. Sample Fields in a Chargemaster	
Field	**Description**
General ledger code	Internal code used by the facility's accounting department to track revenue and expenses
CPT/HCPCS code	Billing code for transmission to the insurer
Cost basis	The cost of the item to the facility
Charge	The amount that the facility charges for the item or service
Description	Definition of description of the item or service
Date	The date of the most recent update of the data for the item or service in the Chargemaster

plus CPT codes

The report of the data fields that contain a facility's charges and costs for individual services is called **Chargemaster.** Table 9-5 illustrates key data fields that usually appear in a Chargemaster. The Chargemaster must be updated on a regular basis, so that fees and associated costs are always current and accurate. At a minimum, it should be updated whenever the applicable billing codes change.

In a physician's office, the process of obtaining reimbursement may rest with the administrative personnel, for example, the medical secretary or medical assistant. In some cases, for example, in a solo practitioner's office, the reimbursement claim may be filed by the physician. Because the insurance industry is so complex and there are many different types of providers all with their own rules, many physicians are turning to billing services to perform the administrative task of claiming reimbursement. The role of medical office personnel or a billing service is to determine what services were performed for which patient, to determine which payer should receive the bill, and to ensure that all services that were provided are billed correctly. In addition, medical office personnel, billing services, or a combination of the two are generally responsible for ensuring that the correct reimbursement is received.

Charge Capture

In Chapter 1, we discussed the roles of certain acute care facility personnel, and in Chapter 3, we described the data collection performed by some of these personnel. Part of the data that are collected is the fee for the service provided. As the patient is receiving these services, the facility should be collecting the data that describe which services are being provided and when. For example, a patient with an intravenous saline drip requires a bag of saline solution, a tube, and a needle, all of which cannot be used again. The charge for these services should be noted. Charges for medications received by the patient, diagnostic tests, and even bandages should be identified and allocated to that patient account. The charges for room, board, and nursing services should be noted daily. Even under prospective payment, the facility should be collecting these data, so that the total charges can be compared to the actual reimbursement.

The process of capturing these data is called **charge capture,** and it can be accomplished in a variety of different ways, which are beyond the scope of this text. Suffice it to say that for every item and every service that the patient receives, a corresponding charge should be recorded in the patient's account. Charge capture is procedurally the responsibility of the individual caregivers in the nursing unit, in the radiology department, or wherever the service is provided. Special data collection devices are designed to capture the charges incurred so that they can be attributed to a specific patient.

In an ambulatory care setting, charges are often captured, by service, on an **encounter form.** An encounter form is usually a single sheet of paper, sometimes double-sided, that contains a list of the most common patient complaints/diagnoses and procedures/services provided by the facility. A comprehensive encounter form includes ICD-9-CM diagnosis codes as well as CPT codes for procedures. Encounter forms facilitate communication between the physician or other health care provider and the administrative personnel who are responsible for coding and billing. Because it is not the encounter form but the health record that supports the reimbursement claim, care must be taken to ensure that the health record evidences all services provided. Figure 9–2 is an example of an encounter form.

HIT Bit

Not all diagnostic testing and other services are billable by the health care facility. For example, a facility may not have an MRI machine. Therefore, the patient is transported to the MRI provider, who bills the payer separately for both the diagnostic test and its interpretation. Additionally, unless the physician is an employee of the hospital, physicians bill separately for their services.

Uniform Bill (UB-92)

The *Uniform Bill (UB-92)* is the primary transmittal format of billing data in acute care facilities (92 stands for the year in which it was revised). The UB-92 was developed by HCFA for use with Medicare reimbursements, but the insurance industry has adopted it as well, so that a UB-92 is generated by the patient accounts department to bill for a facility's services. As part of the UB, the facility generates a detailed bill, listing all of the charges that have been accumulated, as previously discussed. This may or may not be the basis of the invoice, but many insurance companies that are still paying on a fee-for-service or discounted fee-for-service basis require the detailed bill, particularly for audit purposes. Figure 9–3 shows a UB-92.

HCFA-1500

The data collection device that is used for transmittal of billing information in physicians' offices is the HCFA-1500. The HCFA-1500 has fewer fields than the UB-92, but it contains much the same type of information. Figure 9–4 is an HCFA-1500.

	PATIENT VISITS				PROCEDURES cont.					CALCIUM/BONE/KIDNEY			
X	DESCRIPTION	CODE	AMOUNT	X	DESCRIPTION	CODE	ALPHA	AMOUNT	X	DESCRIPTION	CODE	ALPHA	AMOUNT
	NEW PATIENT				Preventive counseling, 15 min.	99401				Calcium, ionized	7190821	ICAL	
	Problem focused Hx	99201			Preventive counseling, 30 min.	99402				Calcium, serum	7190311	CAL	
	Expanded prob/Focused Hx	99202			Preventive counseling, 45 min.	99403				Calcium, urine 24 hr.	7190222	CALU	
	Detailed Hx	99203			Preventive counseling, 60 min.	99404				Creatinine, clearance ht. __	7194754	CRCP	
	Comp Hx/Moderate complex	99204			DIABETES/LIPID					wt. ___			
	Comp Hx/High complex	99205		X	DESCRIPTION	CODE	ALPHA	AMOUNT		Microalbumin, urine 24 hr.	7190335	MLBT	
	ESTABLISHED PATIENT				Cholesterol, HDL	7190053	HDL			Magnesium, serum	7190317	MAG	
	Minimal	99211			C-peptide	7190219	CPEP			Parathyroid hormo	7190387	PTH	
	Problem focused Hx	99212			Glucose serum	7182947	GLU						
	Expanded prob/Focused Hx	99213			HGB A1 C	7190057	HA1			ADRENAL/PITUITARY			
	Detailed Hx	99214			Insulin	7190343	INS		X	DESCRIPTION	CODE	ALPHA	AMOUNT
	Comprehensive Hx	99215			Lipoprotein panel A	7175004				ACTH	7190005	ACTH	
	CONSULTATION				Micral, random	7190335	MLBU			Aldosterone, serum	7190204	ALD	
	Problem focused Hx	99241			Protein, urine 24 hr.	7195011	PROU			Androstenedione	7190336	AND	
	Expanded prob/Focused Hx	99242			GONADAL					Cortisol, serum	7190032	COR	
	Detailed Hx	99243			Estradiol	7190044	ESD			DHEA	7190341	DHEA	
	Comp Hx/Moderate complex	99244			FSH	7190048	FSH			DHEA S serum	7190312	DHES	
	Comp Hx/High complex	99245			LH	7190069	LH			Human growth hormone	7190379	HGH	
	NURSE SPECIALIST				Progesterone	7190078	PROG			Prolactin	7190316	PRL	
	Computer analysis	99090			PSA	7190079	PSA			17OH Progesterone	7190479	HY17	
	Group health ed	99078			SHBG	7190622	SHBG			17OH Pregnagalone	7190480	LONE	
	Skills management (15 min.)	97535			Testosterone	7190086	TEST			Urine catecholimine 24 hr.	7190021	CATU	
	PROCEDURES				Testosterone, Free	7190322	FTES			Urine cortisol 24 hr.	7190033	CORU	
	Accucheck/One Touch	7182948			PSA, Free	7184999				Urine metanephrines 24 hr.	7190475	METU	
	EKG w/interpretation	93000			PROFILES					Urine potassium 24 hr.	7190077	POTU	
	IV infusion, up to 1 hr.	90780			Basic metabolic panel	7180049	CH7			Urine sodium 24 hr.	7190261	SODU	
	IV infusion, each add'l hr.	90781			Comp. metabolic panel	7180054	CMP			Urine VMA 24 hr.	7190534	VMAU	
	Immunization administration	90471			Electrolyte panel	7180051	ELEC						
	Two or more vaccines/toxoids	90472			Hepatic function panel	7180058	HFPA						
	Therapeutic/diagnostic injection	90782			Hepatitis panel	7180059				CHEMISTRY/HEMATOLOGY			
	Specify: med/dose				Lipid profile 2	7190257	LPP2			CBC w/diff & platelets	7190327	CBC1	
	Injection of antibiotic	90788			THYROID					Erthrocyte sed rate	7190330	ESR	
	Specify: med/dose				Antimicrosomal antibody	7190213	TM			Potassium, serum	7184813	POT	
	Occult blood (guaiac)	82270			TSI	7190476	TSIG			Urine culture	7190041	BACTI	
	ANS	95937			Thyroglobulin	7190584	THY			Urinalysis, routine	7190334	URTN	
	24 hour cardiac monitor	93230			T4 - Thyroxine	7190047	FT4			Urinalysis, dipstick	7190384	URCH	
	Pap smear	88150			T3 uptake	7190292	TU			Venipuncture	7190323	VENI	
	Thyroid fine needle asp. (proc.)	7190357			Total T3	7190095	T3 C			GGI	7184773		
	Group counseling, 30 min.	99411			T3-Free	7190595	FT3			HCE	7190329		
	Group counseling, 60 min.	99412			TSH (Thyroid stim hormone)	7190253	TSH						

AUTHORIZATION #		REFERRING MD		Tax ID #	62-1162462
DIAGNOSIS				Previous bal.	
SPECIAL INSTRUCTIONS				Amount paid	
				Today's chrg	
				Amount paid	
Physician signature:		Date:		Total rec'd	

I authorize release of any medical information necessary to process this claim. I also authorize the direct payment of any benefits due me for the described services to _____ I understand I am financially responsible for paying any unpaid balance and will be responsible for the entire bill if this claim is not covered. **Medicare Patients:** The Medicare program requires that all diagnosis be ICD 9 coded. We are unable to provide this service to you at the time of your visit, and therefore, require that you permit us to file an insurance claim with your Medicare carrier.

Patient (Beneficiary) signature: _____ Date: _____

Balance due	
Check one:	
☐ Cash	
☐ Check, M.O.# _____	
☐ MC ☐ VISA	
☐ Care Card # _____	

98381 7/99

FIGURE 9-2.

Ambulatory care encounter form. (From Abdelhak M, Grostick S, Hanken MA, Jacobs E: Health Information: Management of a Strategic Resource, 2nd ed. Philadelphia, WB Saunders, 2001, p 244.)

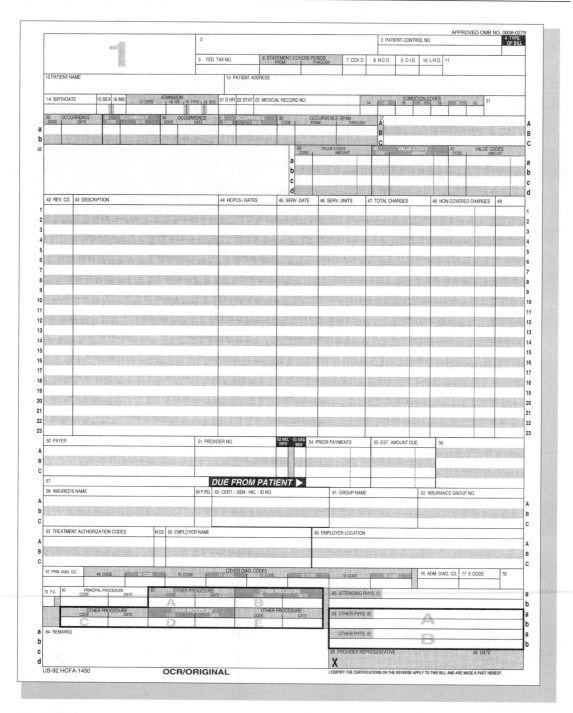

FIGURE 9–3.
UB-92 form. (From Abdelhak M, Grostick S, Hanken MA, Jacobs E: Health Information: Management of a Strategic Resource, 2nd ed. Philadelphia, WB Saunders, 2001, p 242.)

CMS 1450-UB92 hosp inpt & outpt

APPROVED OMB-0938-0008

HEALTH INSURANCE CLAIM FORM

PICA | | |

PICA | |

| 1. MEDICARE | MEDICAID | CHAMPUS | CHAMPVA | GROUP HEALTH PLAN | FECA BLK LUNG | OTHER | 1a. INSURED'S I.D. NUMBER (FOR PROGRAM IN ITEM 1) |

(Medicare #) (Medicaid #) (Sponsor's SSN) (VA File #) (SSN or ID) (SSN) (YD)

2. PATIENT'S NAME (Last Name, First Name, Middle Initial)

3. PATIENT'S BIRTH DATE MM | DD | YY   SEX   M   F

4. INSURED'S NAME (Last Name, First Name, Middle Initial)

5. PATIENT'S ADDRESS (No., Street)

6. PATIENT'S RELATIONSHIP TO INSURED   Self   Spouse   Child   Other

7. INSURED'S ADDRESS (No., Street)

CITY   STATE

8. PATIENT STATUS   Single   Married   Other

CITY   STATE

ZIP CODE   TELEPHONE (Includes Area Code) ( )

Employed   Full-Time Student   Part-Time Student

ZIP CODE   TELEPHONE (Includes Area Code) ( )

9. OTHER INSURED'S NAME (Last Name, First Name, Middle Initial)

10. IS PATIENT CONDITION RELATED TO:

11. INSURED'S POLICY GROUP OR FECA NUMBER

a. OTHER INSURED'S POLICY OR GROUP NUMBER

a. EMPLOYMENT? (CURRENT OR PREVIOUS)   YES   NO

a. INSURED'S DATE OF BIRTH MM | DD | YY   SEX   M   F

b. OTHER INSURED'S DATE OF BIRTH MM | DD | YY   SEX   M   F

b. AUTO ACCIDENT?   PLACE? (State)   YES   NO

b. EMPLOYER'S NAME OR SCHOOL NAME

c. EMPLOYER'S NAME OR SCHOOL NMAE

c. OTHER ACCIDENT?   YES   NO

c. INSURANCE PLAN NAME OR PROGRAM NAME

d. INSURANCE PLAN NAME OR PROGRAM NAME

10d. RESERVED FOR LOCAL USE

d. IS THERE ANOTHER HEALTH BENEFIT PLAN?   YES   NO   *If yes,* return to and complete item 9 a-d.

READ BACK OF FORM BEFORE COMPLETING & SIGNING THIS FORM
12. PATIENT'S OR AUTHORIZED PERSON'S SIGNATURE I authorize the release of any medical or other information necessary to process this claim. I also request payment of government benefits either to myself or to the party who accepts assignment below.

SIGNED _____ DATE _____

13. INSURED'S OR AUTHORIZED PERSON'S SIGNATURE I authorize payment of medical benefits to the undersigned physician or supplier for services described below

SIGNED _____

14. DATE OF CURRENT: MM | DD | YY   ILLNESS (First symptom) OR INJURY (Accident) OR PREGNANCY (LMP)

15. IF PATIENT HAS HAD SAME OR SIMILAR ILLNESS GIVE FIRST DATE MM | DD | YY

16. DATES PATIENT UNABLE TO WORK IN CURRENT OCCUPATION MM | DD | YY   MM | DD | YY   FROM   TO

17. NAME OF REFERRING PHYSICIAN OR OTHER SOURCE

17A. I.D. NUMBER OF REFERRING PHYSICIAN

18. HOSPITALIZATION DATES RELATED TO CURRENT SERVICES MM | DD | YY   MM | DD | YY   FROM   TO

19. RESERVED FOR LOCAL USE

20. OUTSIDE LAB?   YES   NO $ CHARGES

21. DIAGNOSIS OR NATURE OF ILLNESS OR INJURY. (RELATE ITEMS 1,2,3 OR 4 TO ITEM 24E BY LINE)

1. |___ . __   3. |___ . __

2. |___ . __   4. |___ . __

22. MEDICAID RESUBMISSION CODE   ORIGINAL REF. NO.

23. PRIOR AUTHORIZATION NUMBER

24. A DATES OF SERVICES						B Place of Service	C Type of Service	D PROCEDURES, SERVICES, OR SUPPLIES (Explain Unusual Circumstances) CPT/HCPCS	MODIFIER	E DIAGNOSIS CODE	F $ CHARGES	G DAYS OR UNITS	H EPSDT Family Plan	I EMG	J COB	K RESERVED FOR LOCAL USE
From MM	DD	YY	To MM	DD	YY											
1																
2																
3																
4																
5																
6																

25. FEDERAL TAX I.D. NUMBER   SSN EIN

26. PATIENT'S ACCOUNT NO.

27. ACCEPTS ASSIGNMENT? (For govt. claims, see back)   YES   NO

28. TOTAL CHARGE $

29. AMOUNT PAID $

30. BALANCE DUE $

31. SIGNATURE OF PHYSICIAN OR SUPPLIER INCLUDING DEGREES OR CREDENTIALS (I certify that the statements on the reverse apply to this bill and are made a part thereof.)

SIGNED _____ DATE _____

32. NAME AND ADDRESS OF FACILITY WHERE SERVICES WERE RENDERED (If other than home or office)

33. PHYSICIAN'S, SUPPLIER'S BILLING NAME, ADDRESS, ZIP CODE & PHONE #

PIN#   GRP#

(APPROVED BY AMA COUNCIL ON MEDICAL SERVICE 8/88)

PLEASE PRINT OR TYPE

FORM HCFA-1500 (12-90) FORM OWCP-1500   FORM RRB-1500

FIGURE 9–4.
HCFA-1500 form. *physician*

331

Impact of Coding

In our discussion of the various reimbursement methodologies, we have continually reinforced the importance of the ICD-9-CM and/or CPT coding. Because the codes determine the payment and facilitate the claim, the accuracy and timeliness of the codes are critical.

The timing of the postdischarge processing of a record is important. All pertinent data must have been collected in order to assign accurate codes, and the processing cycle must facilitate efficient coding. For example, if a paper-based chart must be assembled and analyzed before it is given to a coder, and if the assembly and analysis sections are 5 or 6 days behind the current discharge date, then records may not get coded until the discharge date plus 7 days. A week is a long time for a facility to go without dropping a bill for a patient's stay. Sometimes, facilities choose to code the record before it is analyzed, in order to drop a bill sooner. Although this sequence speeds payment, it has the potential to cause coding errors when missing elements are not clearly identified.

In addition to timeliness, the codes must be accurate. Accurate coding is necessary for **optimization** of reimbursement, particularly in a prospective payment system. Optimization occurs when the coding results in the DRG that most accurately represents the facility's utilization of resources, based on the diagnoses and procedures. **Maximization,** on the other hand, results in the highest possible DRG. Optimization is highly desirable; maximization is illegal and/or unethical. Under the United States federal government Correct Coding Initiative as well as fraud and abuse audits, maximization could result in criminal prosecution for facility administration. Therefore, strict attention to coding guidelines is critical.

Coding guidelines and the rules for correct ICD-9-CM coding are developed and published by the **Cooperating Parties:** The American Hospital Association (AHA), HCFA, the **National Center for Health Statistics (NCHS),** and the American Health Information Management Association (AHIMA). These groups meet twice annually at a public coordination and maintenance meeting, at which proposals for new codes and changes to ICD-9-CM are discussed. The AHA publishes and maintains authoritative coding guidelines, embodied in *Coding Clinic,* a quarterly booklet containing information about new codes, problematic coding areas, and specific coding questions with the answers. AHIMA offers coding education and two coding credentialing examinations: Certified Coding Specialist (CCS) and Certified Coding Specialist—Physician–Office Based (CCS-P). As previously stated, the AMA publishes CPT codes and guidelines for its own use. These are updated annually for implementation each January. In addition, HCFA publishes CPT reimbursement guidelines, much of which pertains to correct CPT coding.

Coding Quality

Because coding plays such an important role in reimbursement, the quality of coding must be ensured. Both government and private insurers audit charges and coding on a regular basis. Internally, a facility must make every effort to ensure that coding complies with official guidelines. A comprehensive **coding compliance plan** is an important part of a corporate compliance plan (see Chapter 8). In this section, we review some of the coding and coding-related issues of which HIM professionals must be aware.

Chargemaster Review

As previously mentioned, the Chargemaster contains the CPT and other Health Care Financing Administration Common Procedure Coding System (HCPCS) codes applicable to each charge. Because HIM professionals understand CPT coding and its applications, they are often called on to verify the accuracy of the codes in this particular document. The accuracy of the Chargemaster helps to ensure appropriate billing, and it should be reviewed periodically. At a minimum, the Chargemaster should be reviewed whenever new codes are implemented. In an ambulatory care setting, the encounter form should be reviewed for the same reason.

Coding activities also require routine review. Insurers who identify a high percentage of coding errors may increase their audit activities, which in turn places an administrative burden on the HIM department. Therefore, the HIM department should pay particular attention to the supervision, training, and development of its coders, because they play a critical role in reimbursement.

There are a variety of reviews that a coding supervisor can perform in order to ensure that coding is complete, accurate, and correctly abstracted and recorded. Sometimes, for objectivity, outside auditors can be contracted to perform coding reviews. The following discussion pertains to both supervisor and contract reviews, bearing in mind that contract review results should be filtered back to the employees through the supervisor.

There are two fundamentally different approaches to coding audits: general reviews of all records to identify potential problems, and targeted reviews of known or potential problem areas. In *general reviews*, records are selected by a statistical method or by any method that captures a representative sample of records. All coders and all record types should be included in a general review. *Targeted reviews* may be aimed at specific coders, codes, DRGs, or other factors. For example, a coding supervisor knows that inappropriately coding "bacterial pneumonia" instead of the less specific "pneumonia" is fraudulent, because it results in a higher-paying DRG than the facility is entitled to receive. In order to ensure that the coding staff is coding bacterial pneumonia appropriately, the supervisor reviews records with the bacterial pneumonia code. Conversely, the supervisor may review records with the general pneumonia code to determine whether a more severe pneumonia was treated and should have been coded. All errors should be discussed with the coder and training provided to ensure quality improvement.

The training and development of coders is essential. Coding systems and rules change often, and coders must be continuously educated to keep up with these changes. Regular in-service training of coders can greatly reduce the number of errors that occur. Such training should be coordinated with the publication of quarterly issues of *Coding Clinic*. The importance of the CPT coding on outpatient charts should also not be ignored. The guidelines and the individual payers are much more diverse in outpatient coding than they are in inpatient coding; therefore, a watchful eye must be kept on the coders who do the outpatient charts as well.

Reference

Sultz HA, Young KM: Health Care USA: Understanding Its Organization and Delivery. Gaithersburg, Md, Aspen Publishers, 1997.

Suggested Reading

Abdelhak M, Grostick S, Hanken MA, Jacobs E: Health Information: Management of a Strategic Resource, 2nd ed. Philadelphia, WB Saunders, 2001.
Fordney MT: Insurance Handbook for the Medical Office, 6th ed. Philadelphia, WB Saunders, 1999.

CHAPTER SUMMARY

Reimbursement is payment to a health care provider for services. Payment to the provider may be based on fee for service, discounted fee for service, prospective payment, capitation, or a combination of methods. The purpose of insurance is to shift the risk of having to make large reimbursements from the patient to another entity, such as an insurance company. Insurance plans are characterized by the degree of their involvement in the delivery of services. Indemnity plans are not involved in delivery of health services, but managed care plans are heavily involved. Individuals and employers may self-insure to avoid escalating premiums. Federal and state governments fund health insurance for the elderly, the poor, and certain groups of chronically ill patients.

In order to effect reimbursement, billing must take place. The UB-92 is used for acute care facility reimbursement, and the HCFA-1500 is used for physician's offices. Prospective payment is an increasing presence in reimbursement. DRGs, APCs, and RUGs are prospective payment systems currently in use in acute care, ambulatory care, and skilled nursing facilities, respectively. Additional systems are being developed for other health care settings. Regardless of the reimbursement methodology or the billing process, coding is an important function. Facilities must make every effort to ensure that coding is accurate and timely and that coders are properly and continuously trained.

REVIEW QUESTIONS

1. List, compare, and contrast four reimbursement methodologies.
2. Compare and contrast indemnity health insurance plans with managed care plans.
3. Describe government involvement in health insurance.
4. Distinguish between the UB-92 and the HCFA-1500. *328*
5. List three prospective payment systems and describe how reimbursement is derived in each. *DRG, APC, RUG*
6. Discuss the impact of coding on reimbursement. *332*
7. What is the role of the HIM professional in reimbursement?

PROFESSIONAL PROFILE
DRG Audit Specialist

My name is Robin, and I am a DRG audit specialist for a small consulting firm. My firm performs a number of services for hospitals, physicians' offices, and physician group practices. We code records, abstract and enter data, and perform coding quality and compliance audits. My specialty is auditing records to ensure that the optimum DRG was obtained by the coding.

In order to audit records, I needed to have excellent coding skills. I developed these skills as a coder for an acute care facility, coding both outpatient and inpatient records. Later, I went to work for this consulting firm as a coder and now I spend most of my time auditing. In addition to my work experience, I am also a Registered Health Information Technician (RHIT) and a Certified Coding Specialist (CCS).

I can perform several types of audits, depending on what the client needs. Sometimes, I take a random sample of records and review them, just to see if there are any coding problems. I think all facilities should do this on a regular basis, because sometimes coders make mistakes. If you catch the errors quickly, the facility can re-bill with the new codes. Also, the coders need to know if they are doing something wrong. My firm performs these audits periodically, not just on client coders' records but also on our own employees' work.

My favorite audits are DRG audits. To do a DRG audit, I review a computer report of all of the records that have been coded in a time period. I pay particular attention to records that are grouped to an uncomplicated DRG and those that are grouped to a problem DRG. Then, I review some of the records to determine whether I can recommend any coding changes. I discuss my recommendations with the coding supervisor, and she meets with the coders separately to help them prevent future errors. Sometimes, the facility asks me to give training to the coders on particularly difficult issues.

For cases that are reimbursed based on DRGs, this is a really important type of audit, because changes in coding may affect reimbursement. Facilities that routinely code incorrectly, thereby routinely billing the wrong amount for the stay, are subject to penalties from the government or the private insurer. By performing these audits, I really feel as though I'm helping the facility maintain high-quality coding and billing standards. That's a good feeling.

APPLICATION

Implementing ICD-10

For almost 20 years, ICD-9-CM has been the classification system used by health care providers in the United States to collect diagnosis and some procedure data for reporting and, more recently, reimbursement purposes. If and when HCFA adopts ICD-10, the industry will follow. Implementation of ICD-10 will involve a massive effort on the part of health industry professionals throughout the country. Based on your knowledge of health care data, coding, and reimbursement, what do you think will be the impact of ICD-10? Imagine that ICD-10 will be implemented in 1 year. If you were the Director of Health Information Management at an acute care facility, what steps would you take to ensure a smooth transition?

SUPERVISION and PROFESSIONAL DEVELOPMENT

10

Human Resource Management

Chapter Outline

Human Resources

Organization Charts
Facility Organization
  Span of Control
  Unity of Command
  Delegation
Health Information Management Department Organization

Health Information Management Department Workflow
Health Information Management Functions
  Retrospective Processing
  Concurrent Processing
  Computer-Based Processing

Department Planning
Mission
Vision
Goals and Objectives

Prioritization of Department Functions

Evaluation of Department Operations and Services

Department Policies and Procedures
Policy and Procedure Review

Health Information Personnel
Job Analysis
Job Description
  Writing a Job Description

Employee Productivity
Manual Productivity Reports
Computerized Productivity Reports

Employee Evaluations
Poor Evaluations

Hiring Health Information Management Personnel
Advertisement
Application
  Screening Applicants
Interviewing
Assessment

Fair Employment Practices

Department Equipment and Supplies
Supplies
  Filing
  Copy Machines and Printers
  Transcription and Dictation Equipment
  Software
  Miscellaneous Supplies
Monitoring Use of Department Resources

Ergonomics

References

Chapter Summary

Review Questions

Professional Profile

Application

By the end of this chapter, the student should be able to

- Identify and prioritize HIM department functions and services.

- Organize the appropriate workflow of HIM functions and services.

- Perform job analysis.

- Write job descriptions using ADA requirements.

- Develop plans, goals, and objectives for HIM employees.

- Assess and design an ergonomically sound work environment for HIM personnel.

- For a new HIM department, identify file space, ergonomics, dictation/transcription area, and equipment and supply needs for department functions and services.

- Develop HIM department policies for employee operations and conduct.

- Compare work performance of HIM employees to establish new standards.

- Collect data and report on productivity of an HIM employee and on department productivity, and analyze department data for implementation of new productivity standards.

- Evaluate the effectiveness of HIM department operations and services.

- Monitor the use of department resources, including inventory, budget, and planning.

- Establish standards for performance of employees in HIM functions and services.

- Develop department policy and procedures for HIM functions and services.

Vocabulary

delegate	mission	productivity
ergonomic	objectives	span of control
full-time equivalent (FTE)	organization chart	unity of command
goals	performance standards	vision
job analysis	policy	
job description	procedure	

In this chapter we discuss the management of health information management (HIM) employees and their roles and responsibilities. This chapter (and the following chapter on training and development) specifically focuses on issues, tools, and techniques unique to health information management. We explore human resources, organization, planning, policy and procedure, equipment, supplies, education, and training and development.

In previous chapters we focused on the performance of the common functions in an HIM department and the many issues, uses, and requirements surrounding health information. As you read this chapter, you are expected to understand the functions of an HIM department and to have reached a level of competence so that you can perform many of the functions efficiently.

Human Resources

The term *human resources* is most often associated with a department within an organization. The human resource department maintains personnel records, handles employee benefit issues, advertises, interviews, hires, disciplines, and terminates facility employees. The human resource department works with the managers in the health care facility, as necessary, when developing job descriptions and performance standards, conducting employee performance evaluations, and handling employee conduct problems, and manages other technical aspects of employment.

As a supervisor, manager, or director of the HIM department you will be significantly involved in human resource management. Although the human resource department is your consultant on these matters, you will need to know the appropriate methods and tools for managing employees within the HIM department.

Human resources within the HIM department refers to the human beings (employees) who are the source of support needed to accomplish health information functions. Employees are resources that can be defined as "assets." We need humans to perform HIM functions to ensure timely, complete, and accurate health information. Furthermore, the appropriate management of this asset, the employee, has an impact on the entire organization. Management is a skill, because different situations call for different measures to accomplish a task. That is to say, what works in one facility or with one employee may not always work with another.

In the workplace, people are called employees, personnel, or associates. Employees can be classified according to hours worked (full-time or part-time) or by position, that is, management or staff. Employee classifications by hours worked are full-time, part-time, and temporary (also known as PRN [as needed], per diem, pool, etc.) (Table 10–1). A **full-time equivalent (FTE)** is one who by definition works 32 to 40 hours each week excluding overtime (or in some cases 64 to 80 hours every 2 weeks), thereby earning full benefits as offered by the health care facility. Full-time status affects employees' benefits in terms of hours earned in paid time off (PTO), vacation, holiday benefits, and retirement options. For example, an employee who works 40 hours each week is considered a

TABLE 10–1. Employee Classifications		
Classification	**Common Terms**	**Description**
Full-time	FTE	Employee who works 32–40 hours each week, or 64–80 hours every 2 weeks, earning full benefits
Part-time	PT	Employee who typically works 16–20 hours each week, occasionally earning benefits at half of the full-time rate
Temporary	Pool, PRN, per diem	Employees scheduled to work as necessary due to increased workload

full-time employee, and he or she may earn 4 hours of vacation each week. Additionally, the organization might match retirement benefits for the full-time employee at a rate higher than for other classes of employees.

A part-time (PT) employee is one who typically works 16 to 20 hours each week, thereby earning benefits at half the weekly rate of a full-time employee, if benefits are earned at all. For example, a part-time employee may earn 2 hours of vacation, sick leave, or paid time off for every 20 hours of work. Temporary or per diem employees, on the other hand, rarely earn any type of employee benefit. Per diem employees are scheduled to work as needed in the facility when the amount of work exceeds what the normal employees can accomplish. These employees are valuable to the organization when there is an unexpected excess of work. We refer to these categories again when we discuss HIM department structure later in the chapter.

HIT BIT

A full-time equivalent (FTE) works 40 hours per week. Often a department is allowed a number of FTEs that is not even. This fraction typically accounts for the part-time employees. For example: The HIM department is allowed 100 hours each work week for coding. How many FTEs equal 100 hours? The answer is 100 divided by 40 (1 FTE) equals 2.5 FTEs. There are 2.5 FTEs allowed in the coding department each week. We discuss more about FTEs later in the chapter.

The additional employee classification of management or staff can indicate an employee's position and responsibility within the department or organization. Those in management or supervisory positions have responsibility for other employees. Staff employees are responsible for daily tasks and functions, and they report to a supervisor or manager.

Organization Charts

One method used by health care facilities to describe the arrangement of departments and positions is the **organization chart.** The organization chart illustrates the relationship between departments, positions, and functions within the organization. To understand an organization chart, we must understand the symbols used. The traditional structure of an organization chart resembles a pyramid, in which there are more departments and personnel at the bottom than at the top. An organization chart uses boxes and lines to represent departments and positions within the facility. Boxes indicate a department or position. The higher the box within the chart, the higher the authority and responsibility. Boxes on the same level indicate similar levels of authority or responsibility. Lines connecting the boxes indicate a relationship. Solid lines indicate a direct relationship. Broken lines indicate an indirect (or shared) relationship. The lines in the organization chart illustrate who is above and who is below in the chain of command. *Chain of command* refers to the order in which decisions are made within the facility. For decisions that need approval, the organization chart describes who must give that approval.

Facility Organization

The traditional health care facility is composed of departments with specialized personnel or services, related to the health care professions discussed in Chapter 1. Refer to Figure 10–1 as we discuss the organization chart of a medium-sized health care facility. The box at the top of the chart represents the ultimate authority and responsibility within the organization. This authority is called the governing body, board of directors, or board of trustees. Every facility has this type of authority at the top of the organization.

HIT Bit

All health care facilities have a governing board. A for-profit facility is owned by shareholders. A not-for-profit facility is held "in trust" by the community it serves.

There are typically 8 to 25 members on the board, depending on the size of the facility. Members of the board include the chief executive officer (CEO), members of the medical staff, and members of the community (Abdelhak, et al, 1996, p 23). The board meets regularly to review the business of the health care facility, set direction, and monitor progress. The board has two distinct relationships, as shown in Figure 10–1. One is the delegated authority from the board to the CEO (president) for the daily operations of the facility. The other is the relationship with the facility's medical staff.

The medical staff is the organization of the physicians who practice and participate in the operations of the health care facility. The medical staff has a structure governed by the members of the staff and described in the facility's bylaws, rules, and regulations. An example of medical staff structure is shown in Figure 10–2.

The chief executive officer, under the governing board, is given the authority to oversee the daily management of the health care facility. The CEO must

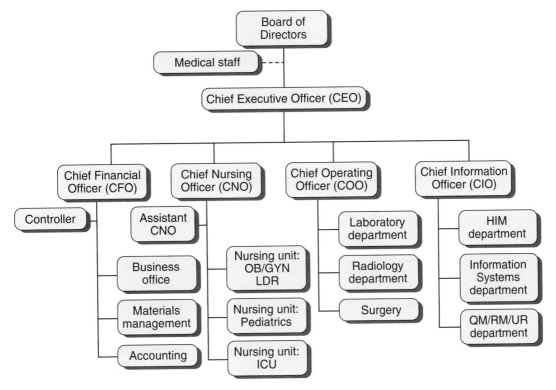

FIGURE 10-1.

Health care facility organization chart.

guide, motivate, and lead the organization under the direction of the governing board.

Below the CEO are several administrative positions. These positions have similar authority and responsibility over specific departments (services) within the organization. These administrators report to the CEO. This level of the administration is also known as the chiefs, assistant administrators, or vice presidents of finance, nursing, information, and quality.

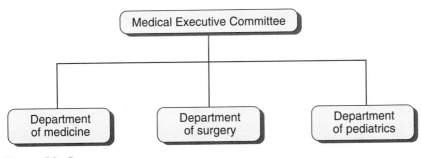

FIGURE 10-2.

Medical staff organization chart.

The personnel responsible for managing specific departments report to the above-mentioned administrators. The managers of the departments are known as directors, department heads, or managers. Below department directors are supervisors and then staff employees. The managers of each department have authority over the supervisors within their departments, and finally the staff employees within each department report to their respective supervisors. Notice how this organization chart indicates the lines of authority and responsibility. The organization chart is a good indicator of appropriate span of control and unity of command.

SPAN OF CONTROL

In an organization chart, the number of positions or employees shown below the box for an administrator, manager, or supervisor indicate the **span of control** for that position. The span of control refers to the number of employees that report to one supervisor, manager, or administrator. The span of control for one supervisor must be appropriate so that management is efficient and effective. Too many varied responsibilities or employees under one supervisor (especially in a large facility) can lead to ineffective management. The appropriate span of control is often determined by the number of employees and their responsibility. A large facility may need more managers than a small facility due to the number of employees needed to accomplish a task or function.

UNITY OF COMMAND

It is also important that one position (employee) report to one manager. This concept is called **unity of command.** Unity of command refers to the sole management of an employee by one manager. If one employee has two supervisors, then the employee can be torn between which manager's authority is higher or which manager's rules and requests take precedence. If both managers have deadlines, which one must be met first? Who decides? If the employee has only one manager, then the employee knows that he or she is accountable to that manager according to the role and responsibility of the position.

DELEGATION

Delegation describes what a manager does when he or she gives a responsibility to an employee for completion of a project or task. When you **delegate** something, you give the employee responsibility and the necessary authority to accomplish the project or task. If you delegate a task to an employee, he or she may need some authority to get the job done, for example, signing forms, making changes in a process, and disciplining employees. Delegation is an important tool that managers use to accomplish multiple tasks. This tool also shows the employee that the manager trusts him or her to do a good job.

Health Information Management Department Organization

Figure 10–3 illustrates the organization of positions within the HIM department. This is an organization chart for a medium-sized HIM department with 30 employees. The box at the top of the chart represents the department director. Ultimately, each HIM department has a top manager responsible for the overall direction of the department. This position may be called director, manager, or department head. The person in this position has the delegated authority from the administration of the facility to act as the custodian of health information. The director also has the responsibility and authority to manage the daily operations of the HIM department. Figure 10–3 shows a department with 1 director, 1 assistant director, 3 supervisors, and 25 staff employees. Keep in mind that job titles for positions within the HIM department vary among facilities.

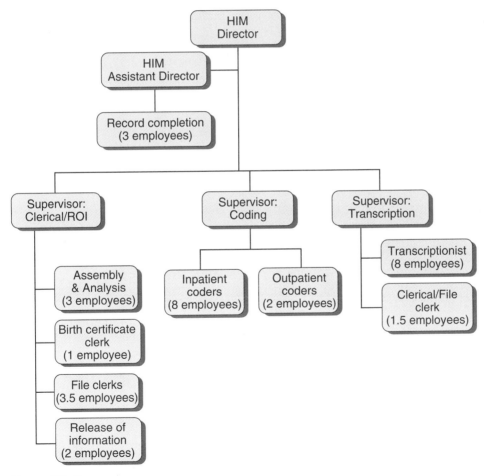

FIGURE 10–3.

HIM department organization chart.

TABLE 10–2. Staff Positions in the HIM Department

Position	Responsibility/Function	Hours	Status
HIM Director	Daily management of the HIM department including	M–F 8 AM–4:30 PM	Full-time
Supervisor	Clerical/ROI/filing	M–F 7AM–3:30 PM	Full-time
HIM Tech I	Assembly and analysis of all patient records	S–Thur, 6:30 AM–3 PM	Full-time
HIM Tech I	Birth certificates Saturday assembly/analysis	Tue–Sat, 8 AM–4:30 PM	Full-time
HIM Tech I	Filing, loose work	M–F, 12:30 PM–9 PM	Full-time
HIM Tech II	Inpatient coding	M–F, 8:30 AM–5 PM	Full-time
HIM Tech II	Outpatient coding	M–Thur, 4 PM–9 PM	Part-time
HIM Tech II	Release of information	M–F, 8:30 AM–5 PM	Full-time
HIM Tech II	Record completion	M–F 7:30 AM–4 PM	Full-time
Transcriptionist	Pathology transcription and coordination of outside transcription	M–F, 8 AM–4:30 PM	Full-time

In addition, the organization chart in Figure 10–3 shows a department that is organized into three supervised sections of health information functions. Each supervisor is responsible for specific functions within the department. There is a supervisor for the assembly, analysis, release of information (ROI), and filing functions, also known as clerical/ROI supervisor. Another supervisor, called the coding supervisor, oversees the coding and abstracting functions. The third supervisor, called the transcription supervisor, is responsible for the transcription function.

Within the HIM department, employees are further identified by the position that they hold or job function(s) performed. HIM departments have clerical and technical staff positions (Table 10–2). The director of the HIM department or the human resource department determines the title for employee positions. Some titles are generic (e.g., HIM Tech I), whereas other titles describe the employee's responsibilities (e.g., assembly and analysis).

Clerical employees are responsible for the functions known as assembly, analysis, and filing. Technical employees perform functions such as coding, transcription, record completion, and release of information (Table 10–2 describes possible job titles). Technical employees' positions are sometimes referred to as HIM Tech II. These staff employees typically report to the first or lowest level of management, known as the HIM supervisor or a team leader. Responsibilities of the supervisor's positions differ in each department, but they may include scheduling, hiring, training, disciplining, and terminating. The supervisor is responsible for ensuring that staff employees are performing their functions timely and according to the policies of the department.

HIT BIT

Exempt employees are salaried; they are not required to punch a time clock. *Nonexempt* employees are paid based on the number of hours worked.

The titles, roles, and responsibilities of positions within the HIM department vary. They are determined by the size, type, and purpose of the health care organization. Smaller facilities with few patient admissions have fewer positions, as well as fewer levels of management. However, larger health care facilities have several employees performing one function, and they require more supervisors and levels of management to oversee daily functions.

HIT BIT

The chain of command refers to the line of authority through which things should be decided. An employee should follow the chain of command for approval or decisions related to his or her job in the department.

Health Information Management Department Workflow

The collection, organization, coding, abstracting, analysis, storage, and retrieval of patient health information are organized into a *workflow* within each health care organization to best suit that facility. Workflow is the order in which the work is organized to progress from one function to the next. Efficient workflow allows department employees to accomplish their functions in a timely, accurate, and complete manner.

It is not possible to discuss every HIM department scenario, so we discuss the general workflow (management and organization of HIM functions) with only a few variations. Variations in the workflow (in different facilities) are necessary to accommodate the type, size, and structure of each health care facility.

HIT BIT

The health information management (HIM) department may also be known as the medical record department or health information services. Names of HIM departments remain diverse across the country.

Health Information Management Functions

Let's review HIM functions and responsibilities as they are commonly described in the health care facility using the paper-based record. *Collection* refers to the retrieval of a health record from the patient care unit for every patient treated by the facility. *Organization* of the record refers to the assembly of the record into a format usable by others, including attaching the record to a file folder labeled appropriately for identification and storage (paper record). *Analysis* involves review of quantitative or qualitative health information to ensure timely, accurate, and complete records. *Coding* is the assignment of alphanumeric or numeric codes to patient diagnoses and procedures for reimbursement and data retrieval. *Abstracting* is the method by which the information within the health record is summarized for future reference. *Record completion* is the processing of an incomplete record as more health data are entered from appropriate health care personnel. *Storage* refers to the filing methods used to maintain records for future use. *Retrieval* describes the function that locates a record for future use following patient care. *Transcription* is the method by which the physician's dictation is turned into a medical report for placement in the patient's record.

These HIM functions occur sequentially and are typically grouped into sections under a supervisor for efficient management (see Fig. 10–2). The need for supervisors within a department, as discussed previously, is determined by the number of employees in the HIM department and their varied functions. The fewer the number of employees, the less need for supervisors. Typically supervisors oversee 6 to 12 employees depending on the functions performed by the group and the employees' need for direct supervision. In other words, if there are 12 transcriptionists, only 1 supervisor may be necessary. However, if you have 12 employees, 6 of whom are clerical workers, 3 of whom are coders, and 3 of whom are transcriptionists, the department may require 3 supervisors, one each for the clerical, coding, and transcription sections.

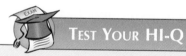

TEST YOUR HI-Q

Congratulations! Your are the new supervisor in the HIM department at General Hospital. Your facility is licensed for 150 beds. Current census is 90. The facility provides general acute care (130 beds), same-day surgery, a 10-bed skilled nursing facility (SNF) unit, and a 10-bed rehabilitation unit. This facility has a paper-based health record and 10 HIM employees, including the director. Table 10–2 provides a list of employees and their responsibilities, hours worked, and employment status (full-time, part-time, or per diem). Which employees report to the clerical/ROI supervisor?

Now that we have an understanding of the organization of the HIM department, let's discuss the workflow.

RETROSPECTIVE PROCESSING

Workflow in the HIM department that performs retrospective processing begins when the patient is discharged from the facility. How does the HIM director decide which functions are performed first? Traditionally, health records were collected, organized, assembled, analyzed, coded, abstracted, completed, and filed (Fig. 10–4). This workflow can be effected by the priorities set within the department. Specifically, the productivity standards for a function may require that one function be performed before another. For instance, if the department is

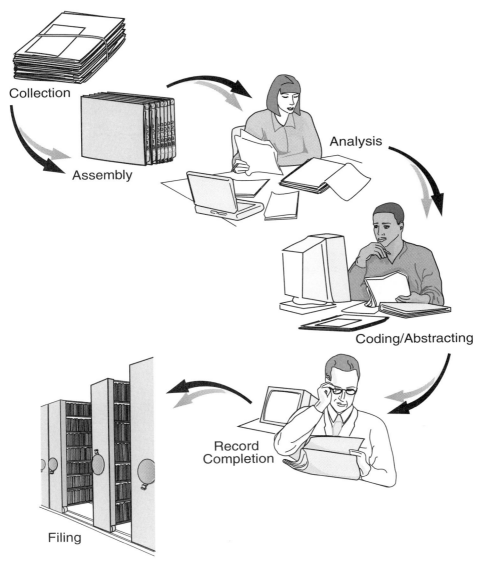

FIGURE 10–4.

Retrospective processing of health information.

motivated to code the health record within 24 hours of the patient's discharge, the coding function may need to take place before the analysis, and coding may be separated from the abstract function to promote coders' productivity.

   Workload and Productivity. Each department must have a method for determining its workload. The amount of work in an HIM department is determined by the number of discharges and by the type and length of stay. The number of patients discharged each day will be the number of records that must be assembled and organized. The type of record determines the detail required in analysis (same-day surgery records require less time to review than inpatient stays). The length of stay (LOS) for those patients discharged affects how long it will take to assemble the patient's charts. If a patient has an LOS in the facility of 2 days, the record is relatively thin (approximately $\frac{1}{4}$ inch). However, if the patient remains in the facility for 3 weeks (LOS of 21 days), the record is relatively thick (approximately 2 to 3 inches) and may require two folders to contain the papers for that one stay. If your facility has many discharges with long lengths of stay, then the assembly process will take longer than in a facility that has few discharges with short lengths of stay.

Supervisors may use *time studies* to determine the appropriate number of personnel for the workload. A time study can be accomplished by monitoring the employee performing the function and the time it takes to complete the task. Actual presence of the supervisor as the employee performs the job may cause the employee to become nervous or irritated. Likewise, a supervisor does not want to waste valuable time watching employees work. Other methods exist to capture this information without physically watching employees. Employees can fill out forms to indicate their performance, productivity, and time (Fig. 10–5).

The standards set for the department must comply with organizational, professional, licensing, and regulatory requirements. These guides determine when many of the functions must be performed, for example, assembly and analysis within 24 hours of discharge and coding within 48 hours of discharge (Table 10–3). Some internal standards may lead the way for new processes, such as

Coding Productivity Report
02/20/2001

Coder	IP Total	IP Mcare	IP Non-Mcare	OP Total	ER	OP Refer	OBS	SDS
JBG	22	20	2	40	0	40	0	0
CRB	15	15	0	55	48	0	7	0
TLM	30	25	5	12	0	0	0	12
SNK	32	20	12	5	0	0	0	5

FIGURE 10–5.

Productivity report of coders in an HIM department.

TABLE 10–3. Typical HIM Department Standards*	
Department Function	**Standard**
Assembly and analysis	Completed within 24 hours of patient discharge
Coding and abstracting	Completed within 48–72 hours of patient discharge
Record completion	Records should be completed within 30 days of discharge
Filing	Completed daily
Release of information	Request should be completed with in 48–72 hours of receipt of an appropriate authorization or request for information
Transcription	
History & physical	Transcribed within 12 hours of dictation
Consults	Transcribed within 12 hours of dictation
Operative reports	Transcribed within 6 hours of dictation
Discharge summary	Transcribed within 24 hours of dictation

* *Note:* These standards are for example only; standards in HIM departments may vary.

concurrent analysis or coding, in order to successfully accomplish department functions within the set time frame.

Workload is also affected by the amount of computerization within the HIM department. Sometimes computerization reduces the complexity of a function and at other times it increases the steps to complete a function.

CONCURRENT PROCESSING

Concurrent health information processing means that the assembly, analysis, coding, and abstracting of the health record is occurring while the patient is in the facility. For example, analysis (review for signatures, forms, content) of the documentation in the health record is performed on the patient care unit. Concurrent analysis of health information is designed to have an impact on the quality of patient care by promoting timely, accurate, and complete documentation of patient health information.

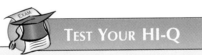

TEST YOUR HI-Q

Identify the reports required on the health record for a patient who has been in the facility for 24 hours.

Which functions occur first during concurrent analysis: coding, abstracting, assembly, analysis, or ROI? Priority is ultimately determined by the goals and objectives of the HIM department (discussed later in the chapter). The performance of concurrent analysis can include several scenarios. One situation may involve employees' being physically relocated to the patient care units. Another scenario may involve sending HIM employees to the patient care unit to perform the function and then reporting back to the department for follow-up or further processing.

TABLE 10-4. Typical Concurrent Processing Standards*	
Function	**Example of Concurrent Processing Standard**
Analysis	Initial analysis for patient signatures, forms, H&P, and physician signatures completed within the first 24 hours of the patient's stay. Routine (daily) analysis performed until the patient's discharge.
Coding and abstracting	Initial coding performed during the first 24–48 hours of the patient's stay. Updated periodically during the patients stay, as the patient's condition warrants. Final coding completed after discharge.
Transcription	
History & physical (H&P)	Transcribed within 12 hours of dictation
Consults	Transcribed within 12 hours of dictation
Operative reports	Transcribed within 6 hours of dictation
Discharge summary	Transcribed within 24 hours of dictation

* *Note:* These standards are for example only; standards may vary depending upon process.

Regardless of the method, productivity standards must also be designed to ensure timely processing. Table 10–4 provides an example of the productivity standards for concurrent processing in an HIM department.

COMPUTER-BASED PROCESSING

Processing of health information in the computer-based patient record (CPR) environment changes the HIM workflow previously mentioned. The CPR system consists of intelligent computer software capable of recognizing and understanding patient record information. A system that knows the requirements of a timely, accurate, and complete health record changes the need to have an employee review the clinical documentation. The system prompts the users when information is contradictory, incomplete, or required. The CPR system negates or limits the need for quantitative analysis, assuming that the computer recognizes pertinent information. However, analysis of the CPR requires the technical skills of the registered health information technician (RHIT). The system maintenance, design, and analysis is a process that requires knowledge of accreditation requirements, coding guidelines, and the clinical aspects of patient care. In fact, the function is likely to resemble that of an auditor or database manager.

Who decides which processing system is best suited for the HIM department? What if a facility would like to change from one processing system to another? These questions are best answered by a discussion on department planning.

Department Planning

Planning is a tool used by the HIM department to prepare for the future. Everyone plans for the future; the difference, however, is that some people plan more than others and some plans are more formal and elaborate than others. Some department plans are formal, written documents; others may be informal, depending on the size, type, or philosophy of the facility. For example, the work-flow in a department is a plan (discussed later under prioritization of department functions). Before employees begin performing the functions of assembly, analysis, and coding, HIM managers want to plan to ensure that the work flows smoothly and that the department achieves maximum productivity.

The HIM department may also plan for changes or improvements. Managers can plan to implement a new procedure—for example, concurrent coding, purging records, or converting the filing method from straight numeric to terminal digit—or they can plan for optimum use of space. Planning involves analyzing the current situation; determining the goal, that is, what is to be achieved or accomplished; and designing a strategy to accomplish the goal.

A plan is a guide for how things are expected to happen in the department. For a more thorough explanation of planning, we discuss a plan to implement the concurrent analysis process.

What type of analysis will be performed concurrently? Will it be quantitative, qualitative, or both? Let's begin with quantitative analysis. What do you hope to accomplish by doing this concurrent analysis? We must analyze how quantitative analysis is presently performed and the effect it has. Ideally, health records are analyzed within 24 hours of discharge. This means that the first day after a patient's discharge, someone from the HIM department retrieves all discharges, checks them into the department, assembles the records according to the facility policy, and attaches the records to a folder marked with the appropriate medical record number for the patient. In concurrent analysis, analysis of patient records begins on the first day of the patient's stay, and then the records are analyzed daily until the patient is discharged.

In health care facilities planning is done on an annual basis. This planning is sometimes called strategic planning because at this time the organization develops a plan of action or strategy for the coming year. Plans are normally guided by the mission or vision of the entire organization.

Mission

A **mission** statement is a declaration of the organization's purpose. Traditionally, the organization's mission statement shows care and concern for those it serves. A mission statement is very important to an organization because it provides a common purpose. This common purpose helps the organization unify to serve its community as a team with specific direction. An example is the mission statement for Diamonte Hospital (our hypothetical acute care facility):

"Diamonte Hospital provides quality health care through dedication and commitment to excellence."

HIM departments may also have a mission. For example, the HIM department of Diamonte Hospital exists to provide efficient quality health information to all customers in order to promote quality health care in the organization. The mission of the department should be in line with the mission for the entire facility.

The following is the mission statement for the HIM department of Diamonte Hospital:

"The Health Information Management Department of Diamonte Hospital exists to provide timely, complete, confidential, and secure health information to all users."

Vision

Another common element to be considered when planning in an organization or department is a **vision.** A vision is a statement of what you expect your organization to become. The vision is a statement above and beyond the mission. For example, the vision may state that while the purpose (mission) is to provide quality patient care and to exceed customers' expectations, the vision is to become the number 1 health care provider in this community. By definition, a vision is unusual foresight or a vivid imaginative conception (Random House, 1995). A vision for an HIM department might be to implement a computer-based patient record; this would be in line with the vision of the organization, if part of the success of quality patient care and becoming number 1 in the community requires a CPR system.

Goals and Objectives

The goals and objectives of the HIM department are typically more recognizable than its mission and vision statements. The department's goals and objectives should complement the organization's mission and vision. In other words, if the organization is committed to quality, then the HIM goals and objectives should address and support quality. The purpose of the goals and objectives is to keep the department focused and provide a guide for improvement.

TABLE 10–5. HIM Department Goals and Objectives*

Goals	Objectives
1. Maintain continuous compliance with JCAHO accreditation standards for timely record completion	1a. The monthly number of delinquent health records will be less than 50% of the average monthly discharges (AMD).
	1b. The number of delinquent H&Ps will not exceed 1%.
	1c. The number of delinquent operative reports will not exceed 1%.
2. Transcription services will facilitate compliance with JCAHO requirement for timeliness of documentation regarding H&P, discharge summary, consults, operative reports	2a. H&P reports will be transcribed within 6 hours of dictation.
	2b. Consultation reports will be transcribed within 12 hours of dictation.
	2c. Operative reports will be transcribed within 12 hours of dictation.
	2d. Discharge summaries will be transcribed within 24 hours of dictation.

* These goals are for example only; they are not all-inclusive.

Managing the daily operations in an HIM department can be an all-consuming task. Therefore, HIM departments annually set **goals** to accomplish new or improved functions. Goals are statements that provide the department with direction or focus. Goals state that the department will strive to achieve something new. Goals can be annual, short term, or long term. Examples of goals for HIM department are listed in Table 10–5.

To reach a goal the department sets **objectives** to direct how the goal will be achieved. Objectives determine what must be accomplished to achieve the goal. Typically, when the objectives are accomplished, the goal is attained. In this text, each chapter has learning objectives. By reading the chapter you should be able to complete the objectives. The objectives also help to keep the authors on track, by knowing what must be accomplished to reach our goal—your understanding of health information technology. Table 10–5 provides some examples of HIM department objectives.

Prioritization of Department Functions

Now that we understand that the facility and the HIM department must plan, we can discuss prioritization of department functions. Prioritizing of health information functions can occur once we have established goals and objectives for the department. Table 10–3 provides a list of potential HIM department standards. Standards for department functions are necessary to keep the information flowing. For example, in this text we have discussed HIM functions in this order: assembly (Chapter 3), analysis, or postdischarge processing (Chapter 4), filing (Chapter 5), and coding (Chapter 9). However, depending on your planning, coding may actually be a function that you want to occur very early in the workflow. Typically, assembly and analysis are the first things you want to accomplish. This organizes the record for future processing, especially coding and record completion. An organized record helps coders find the information they need to assign appropriate codes. The HIM director also wants to make sure that the records are analyzed for deficiencies (quantitative analysis) as quickly as possible, because a record is considered delinquent 30 days after discharge, per JCAHO requirements. The longer it takes for HIM staff to analyze a record, the less time is available to get the record completed by a physician. The department also sets standards for functions such as release of information and transcription. Timely completion of requests for release of information can affect continuity of patient care and possibly reimbursement (if the request is related to payment). The transcription section processes the dictated patient health information into a report that is used in communication and decision making during patient care. Timely completion of this function affects patient care.

Department standards set the framework for efficient and effective management of health information. The standards direct the employees within the department workflow to accomplish their tasks in a timely manner. Sometimes the task directly affects patient care; at other times the task is part of department workflow. Standards can then be used to evaluate the function of the HIM department.

Evaluation of Department Operations and Services

It is important that supervisors and managers continually evaluate their departments based on the department goals, objectives, and standards. In other words, because goals, objectives, and standards create an environment that provides efficient flow of health information, HIM managers use these organizational tools to monitor department progress. If the standard is to assemble and analyze records within 24 hours, then the HIM manager wants to make sure that his or her employees are doing that. Evaluation of goals and objectives takes place annually, but employee-specific productivity should be evaluated at a minimum on a monthly basis to ensure quality in the HIM department. (See discussion on Monitoring the Quality of Health Information in Chapter 6.)

HIM managers and supervisors continually monitor the effectiveness and efficiency of the department through employee productivity reports and through quality assurance monitoring. These measures alert the supervisors to any problems. Significant problems can then be addressed as necessary through employee training, performance improvement, or quality improvement efforts.

Department Policies and Procedures

The policies and procedures of a health care facility are documented in paper or computer format so that the employees, customers, accreditation agencies, licensing bodies, regulatory agencies, and legal authorities recognize the philosophy and methods under which the facility operates. A **policy** is a statement of what the facility does on a routine basis. For example: A health record is maintained for every patient treated in this facility. The **procedure** is the process of how the policy is carried out. For example, the assembly clerk retrieves all discharge records from the nursing units immediately following the patients' discharge. Policies and procedures provide details about

- How, when, and why things are done
- Who performs which tasks, jobs, and functions
- Who is responsible for an activity, an authorization, etc.
- Quality controls and audits
- Historical, routine, and emergency situations

Policies and procedures go together, and indeed they are often documented on the same form. Figure 10–6 shows an example of the previously mentioned policy, that is, a health record is maintained for every patient treated in this facility.

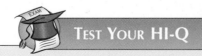

TEST YOUR HI-Q

Identify another issue that could be addressed in a facility's policy statement.

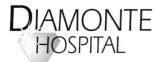

DIAMONTE HOSPITAL

Diamonte, Arizona 89104 ▪ TEL. 602-484-9991

Health Information Management Department
Policy No. 3.01
Health Record Creation and Definition, Unit Medical Record
  Number Assignment

Effective: 01/15/1999	**Reviewed:** 01/2000, 01/2001

Approved:

Policy:

The Health Information Management Department will maintain a health record for all patients receiving treatment at Diamonte Hospital. The record will be kept in accordance with state, federal, accreditation, and professional guidelines. Each patient record will be identified using a unit numbering system.

Procedure:

1. Upon registration at Diamonte Hospital for any service, the patient will be assigned a medical record number and a health record will be initiated.

2. During the patient visit, health information shall be documented in a timely manner on approved facility forms.

3. Following discharge, all patient records will be collected by the Health Information Management Department.

4. The Health Information Management clerk will use the daily ADT (Admission-Discharge-Transfer) reports to verify collection of *all* health records.

5. Records not retrieved the day following discharge will be reported to the Health Information Supervisor immediately, for appropriate action.

Example Policy Only

FIGURE 10-6.
Policy and procedure for maintenance of health records for all patients receiving care in a facility.

The entire health care organization has policies and procedures that have an impact on everyone in the facility. Each department in the health care facility should have specific policies and procedures that outline their processes, responsibilities, and services. It is required that all employees of the facility have access to the Policy and Procedure manual. The HIM department manual contains policies and procedures that relate specifically to health information. Table 10–6 contains a list of contents for an HIM department Policy and Procedure manual.

TABLE 10–6. Contents of an HIM Department Policy and Procedure Manual

Diamonte Health Information Management Department Policy and Procedure Manual

Table of Contents

Section 1		**Introduction**
	1.01	Purpose
	1.02	Responsibility for Policy Development, Update, and Approval
	1.03	Distribution and Access of Policies
	1.04	Diamonte Mission Statement
	1.05	Diamonte Organization Chart
	1.06	Health Information Management Department Mission Statement
Section 2		**General Department Policies**
	2.01	Centralized Health Information Management Department
	2.02	Scope of Service
	2.03	Hours of Operation
	2.04	Confidentiality, Privacy, and Data Security Considerations
	2.05	Confidentiality Statement
	2.06	Department Orientation
	2.07	Training and Education of Department Employees
	2.08	Employee Competency
	2.09	General Policies of the Health Information Management Department
	2.10	Health Information Management Department Organization Chart
Section 3		**The Health Record**
	3.01	Creation and Definition, Unit Medical Record Number Assignment
	3.02	Ownership of the Health Record
	3.03	Guidelines for Entries into the Health Record
	3.04	Abbreviations List
	3.05	Fax Copies in the Health Record
	3.06	Completion of Discharge Summaries
Section 4		**Assembly and Analysis**
	4.01	Health Record Assembly and Chart Order
	4.02	Retrospective Record Analysis
Section 5		**Storage, Access, and Security**
	5.01	Health Record Storage System
	5.02	Security of Health Information
	5.03	Confidentiality and Security of Computerized Information
	5.04	Retention Schedule for Health Records and Related Documents
	5.05	Procedure to Access Health Records
	5.06	Health Record Locations
	5.07	Removal of Health Records from the Health Information Management Department
	5.08	Destruction of Records
Section 6		**Record Completion**
	6.01	Incomplete Chart/Record Completion Process
	6.02	Notification of Incomplete Health Records for Physicians
	6.03	Suspension Process

TABLE **10–6. Contents of an HIM Department Policy and Procedure Manual** *Continued*
Diamonte Health Information Management Department Policy and Procedure Manual

Section 7   **Release of Information**
     7.01   General Policies for Release of Information
     7.02   Consent for Release of Information
     7.03   Notice of Recipient of Information, Disclosure Laws
     7.04   Patient's Right to Health Information, Copies of Health Records
     7.05   Copy and Retrieval Fees
     7.06   Faxing Health Records
     7.07   Release of Information in Case of a Medical Emergency
Section 8   **Quality of Health Information**
     8.01   Monitoring and Evaluation of Quality in the Health Information Management Department
     8.02   Record Review Process/Clinical Pertinence
     8.03   Compliance with Regulations and Standards
Use of Contract Services or Agencies
Job Descriptions
Safety in the Health Information Management Department
     Materials Safety Data Sheets (MSDS)

For example, a policy in the HIM department for coding and abstracting of medical records might state: "The HIM department will maintain accurate diagnosis and procedure indices. The HIM department will maintain appropriate indices by accurately coding all diagnoses and procedures found in the patient's medical records." The procedure then details how coders should go through these records and pull out the primary diagnoses and primary procedures and how they should assign the codes. It should also stipulate or explain how the information is entered into a computer system, for example, how data are collected for compilation of a patient abstract.

The policy manual is a very important tool. The policies and procedures must be accessible to all members of the organization as necessary for the performance of their jobs. Therefore, it is possible to place all policies and procedures on a computerized system, accessible to all employees, allowing them to access the policies on an as-needed basis. This format is attractive to many employees, because policy binders on a shelf are often overlooked or even disregarded. The computer is a new avenue for bringing information to the employee. Increasingly, a facility's policies and procedures are being placed on the facility's Web site. This function allows employees and others to view the policies of the facility from the convenience of their home or office environment.

HIT BIT

Special consideration for a facility's policies in the computerized environment includes securing access to prevent outsiders or unauthorized people from making changes to policies. It is also important to have a paper copy of the policy statements in case the computer is inaccessible.

Policy and Procedure Review

The HIM department director is responsible for ensuring that the departmental policies and procedures are current. This is accomplished by ensuring that policies exist for all necessary functions, responsibilities, and services under his or her control. All policies and procedures should be reviewed annually and as significant changes occur in procedures, regulations, or legislation. Review is as simple as reading through each policy and procedure to verify that the contents are accurate, then initialing and dating the review to authenticate the review.

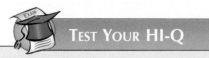

TEST YOUR HI-Q

As the new HIM supervisor, how do you know how your predecessor organized HIM functions? Do you rely on what the employees tell you?

Health Information Personnel

Now that we understand how the workflow is organized in an HIM department, let's discuss how job functions are organized. We discuss organization of the health information functions into job descriptions with performance standards that communicate the manager's expectation of the employee. Then we discuss hiring the appropriate person to perform the job.

Job Analysis

Job analysis is the review of a particular function (e.g., assembly) to determine all of the tasks or components that make up an employee's job. A job analysis is an effective way to assist in the review or creation of an employee job description. When a job analysis is performed, the job tasks are reviewed to ensure that the process works effectively so that employees are not omitting important steps. A job analysis can also ensure that the employee's job fits into the department workflow appropriately. It is important to have the right employee performing the appropriate function at the right time in order to move the work through the HIM department.

Job analysis can be performed by a supervisor or manager working with the employee; together they review and perform the employee's job function. As the supervisor works with the employee, he or she is able to determine the procedures performed by the employee. The supervisor must document the procedures as performed by the employee so that they can be reviewed in total. Following the supervisor's review of the employee's job (which can take a few hours or up to an entire day), the supervisor has actual information to develop a job description and performance standards.

Another effective way to perform a job analysis is to involve the employee by asking the employee to explain how he or she performs the job by using a data collection device. Figure 10–7 is an example of a tool that can be used by the

Employee: _____Tim Tall_____

Position: _____file clerk_____

Hours worked: _8:00 AM–4:30 PM_

Use this form to communicate your job duties or daily routine. Use the comments section to document any unusual occurrences.

	Monday	Tuesday	Wednesday	Thursday	Friday
7:30AM					
8:00AM	Locate charts for coders				
8:30AM					
9:00AM					
9:30AM					
10:00AM					
10:30AM	Organize files				
11:00AM	File				
11:30AM					
12:00 noon					
12:30PM					
1:00PM					
1:30PM					
2:00PM					
2:30PM					
3:00PM					
3:30PM					
4:00PM					
4:30PM					
5:00PM					

Comments: _Periodically answer phone calls and bring charts to the floor._

FIGURE 10–7.

Job analysis tool.

employee to analyze his or her job. The employee uses this form to communicate to the manager in detail what the job involves on a daily basis. This is similar to having the employee list the job functions on a sheet of paper, but the employee should also describe the job in his or her own words.

Another management tool that may be initiated to study employee functions is the *productivity report* (Fig. 10–5). Having the employee complete a productivity report can provide the necessary information to analyze his or her job.

Job Description

Once the job analysis is complete, it is possible to organize the employee's tasks into a **job description.** If an old job description needs to be updated, it is appropriate to give the employee a copy of the current job description. Allow the employee to review the job description to determine what has changed in the job. This involvement gives the employee an opportunity to see how the job has changed. The job description is a list of the employee's responsibilities. Each position and employee in the department should have a job description. The job description communicates the expectations of the manager. Job descriptions should be reviewed annually by management and the employee. Employees sign the job description to acknowledge their awareness of their responsibilities and the job functions.

HIT Bit

If you have involved the employee in a job analysis, when the job description is complete the employee should see how the document is a written description of the job's functions and responsibilities.

WRITING A JOB DESCRIPTION

A job description contains several key elements that describe the job specifically. The job description has a heading that briefly describes the position. The heading should include the facility in which the position is located, the title of the position, the supervisor for the position, and the effective date of the job description (Fig. 10–8). The remainder of the job description includes information regarding hours worked, the purpose of the job, the job responsibilities, skills required, and the Americans with Disabilities Act (ADA) requirements.

The job description also contains any numbers or grades used by the human resources department or the organization to describe that position. The job description begins with a statement of the position's duties and responsibilities, explaining who the position reports to or what type of supervision occurs. Following this statement is a list of the job tasks or functions. The job description also includes information describing the environment in which the work is performed and the abilities or skills that the employee must have to perform job duties (this is typically referred to as the ADA information). A complete job description makes it easier to complete performance standards.

PERFORMANCE STANDARDS

The job description should include **performance standards.** Performance standards tell the employee how much work he or she should accomplish within a specific time frame. Additionally, performance standards let the employee know that quality is evaluated in the performance of the job: It is not only important for the employee to complete the job, but the work must be done correctly. Performance standards include requirements for accuracy and quality. Performance standards are used to evaluate the employee following the probationary period, annually, for merit increases, or for promotion.

Performance standards must be related to the job description and the productivity required within the department. Table 10–7 provides a list of performance standards relating to the job description shown in Figure 10–8. The employee's performance standard has a scale that explains how each score is achieved.

Performance standards establish a time frame in which the employee's work is to be completed. For example, the birth certificate clerk is responsible for completing a birth certificate on all newborn admissions according to the facility's policy and state law. Performance standards for this requirement might be stated as follows: "A birth certificate is completed on all newborn admissions according to facility policy and state law prior to the newborn's discharge. If at any time a birth certificate is not completed before the newborn is discharged, the employee has not met the standard, thereby affecting the employee's performance rating."

Employee performance affects the productivity of the entire department. Therefore, the standards are developed specifically for each position to ensure that each employee's performance promotes effective and efficient progress in the HIM department.

Employee Productivity

Now that you understand a typical HIM employee's job responsibility and how the job is evaluated, you can develop a form or tool to collect information that appropriately supports the employee's evaluation. This method involves collecting information about the employee's performance and **productivity.** There are several ways that this information can be collected: manually, by observation, or by using computerized reports from computer applications. The goal is to have an objective tool that reflects the amount of work performed by the employee. Afterward, the accuracy and quality of the employee's work can be followed up by sample review of his or her work.

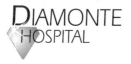

JOB DESCRIPTION

Health Information Management Department
Position Title: Birth Certificate Clerk

Position #: 070530	**Grade:** G2
Reports to: Clerical Supervisor	**Effective:** 01/15/2002

Position Description: Under the general supervision of the Clerical Supervisor, the Birth Certificate Clerk completes a birth certificate, and supporting forms as necessary, for each baby born at Diamonte Hospital. The birth certificates are electronically submitted to the Office of Vital Records, and original certificates with signatures are mailed to the Office of Vital Records in a timely manner. The clerk must maintain a current knowledge of the rules regarding birth certificates. The Birth Certificate Clerk is a member of the Health Information Management department team and maintains knowledge of various other functions in the department to assist as necessary.

Position Qualifications:

Education: High school diploma

Licensure/Certification/Registration: None necessary

Experience: Excellent communication skills. Ability to type 30 WPM. Previous clerical experience preferred. Ability to function in busy office environment with multiple shifting and evolving priorities.

Responsibilities:

1. Monitors Labor and Delivery log and Admission reports to identify all patients requiring a birth certificate.

2. Collects birth certificate information from parent(s) and completes birth certificate accurately. Parent(s) review birth certificate to verify accuracy and sign in appropriate areas.

3. Maintains current knowledge of all birth certificate rules, regulations, and issues. Reviews and implements state laws governing completion of birth certificates.

4. Ensures completion of other forms relating to the birth as necessary, e.g., paternity, social security verification.

5. Maintains current and accurate birth certificate log.

6. Contacts any parents who have left the hospital prior to completion of the birth certificate. Processes new, delayed, or corrected birth certificates.

7. Obtains physician signature on the birth certificate within one week of completion.

8. Submits electronic birth certificates immediately following completion, mailing completed original certificate within 15 days of completion.

9. Maintains electronic birth certificate software in working condition; performs backups regularly.

10. Follows established policies and procedures regarding confidentiality and security of health information, infection control, safety and security management, and emergency preparedness.

FIGURE 10–8.
Job description.

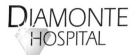

11. Displays a positive and courteous manner toward patients, visitors, customers, and coworkers.

12. Follows all policies and procedures of the facility and HIM department.

13. Completes annual employee in-service and required department training.

Physical Requirements:

Mental and emotional requirements: Employee must be able to manage stress appropriately, work independently, handle multiple priorities.

Working conditions: Employee spends approximately 90% of time inside the health care facility. The work area has adequate lighting, good ventilation, comfortable temperature. Employee work station provided with appropriate access to rest rooms and lunch and break areas.

Physical demands: Employee is responsible for light work—lifting maximum of 20 lb, with frequent lifting or carrying of objects weighing up to 10 lb. Work positions include sitting 50%, standing 20%, walking 20%, lifting/carrying 10%.

Example only

FIGURE 10–8. CONTINUED

TABLE 10–7. Performance Standards*		
Employee/Position	**Standard**	**Performance Rating Scale**
Coder	All health records will be coded within 48–72 hours of patient discharge.	Exceeds expectations: 36 or more records coded daily Meets expectations: 28–35 records coded daily Does not meet expectations: Less than 28 records coded daily *Supervisor uses daily productivity reports to average the coder's performance.*
Coder	Health records will be assigned appropriate and accurate codes according to applicable coding guidelines.	Exceeds expectations: 96–100% of records reviewed are coded appropriately and accurately Meets expectations: 90–95% of records reviewed are coded appropriately and accurately Does not meet expectations: Less than 90% of records reviewed are coded appropriately and accurately *Supervisor will review a representative sample of the coder's work to ensure appropriateness and accuracy of coding.*
Assembly/analysis clerk	All patient health records will be assembled and analyzed within 24 hours of patient discharge.	Exceeds expectations: 95–100% of all records are assembled and analyzed within 24 hours of patient discharge Meets expectations: 85–95% of all records are assembled and analyzed within 24 hours of patient discharge Does not meet expectations: Less than 85% of all records are assembled and analyzed within 24 hours of patient discharge *Supervisor will routinely assess and document the clerks' productivity to determine score.*
File clerk	Accurate filing of all patient health records will be completed daily.	Exceeds expectations: 100% of all health records are filed accurately on a daily basis Meets expectations: 96–99% of all health records are filed accurately on a daily basis Does not meet expectations: Less than 96% of all health records are filed accurately on a daily basis *Supervisor will perform routine checks of filing area to determine accuracy; results will be documented to determine file clerk's score.*

* *Note:* These standards vary in each facility.

Manual Productivity Reports

Manual productivity reports can be designed to obtain information about the employee's performance. Table 10–8 gives a sample form for collection of data on the productivity of a coding employee.

TABLE 10–8. Coding Productivity Sheet																				
Coder: _____ Month/Year: _____																				
	M	Tu	W	Th	F	M	Tu	W	Th	F	M	Tu	W	Th	F	M	Tu	W	Th	F
Date																				
Inpatient																				
Medicare																				
Non-Medicare																				
Outpatient																				
Observation/surgeries																				
Diagnostics																				
Emergency room																				
Hours worked																				
Physician contacts																				
Other (please comment below)																				

Comments:

_____

_____

_____

_____

This form contains information to identify the employee, the time frame in which the information is collected, and specifics about the employee's job. Because the employee in our example is responsible for inpatient coding, Table 10–8 collects information about the number of records coded each day. In addition, the form collects information about activities related to the employee's job, for example, conversations with physicians, problems with chart documentation, and other activities as they occur.

This form can be developed by reviewing the job description and including categories for each responsibility. The employee uses the form to collect statistics regarding his or her job performance. The completed form is turned in to the supervisor. The supervisor is then able to review the employee's productivity against the job's performance standards. This information, collected on a regular basis, provides a picture of the employee's job performance for the entire review period. Routine collection of this information over time provides a larger picture of the employee's performance so that the evaluation is not skewed in one direction toward his or her performance over a limited time period.

Computerized Productivity Reports

Some of the functions in the HIM department are performed in a computer system that produces a productivity report. The report is maintained by the computer system as the employee logs on to the system and completes job tasks. Some computerized reports not only tell the supervisor how much work is performed but they tell the time frame in which the work was done. Referring to our coding example, coders are often expected to code a specific number of records within an hourly time frame, that is, six to eight charts per hour. The software system used by the coders keeps track of this productivity without additional effort from the coder.

Employee Evaluations

Employee evaluations allow management to provide feedback to the employee based on the employee's job performance. This is an important part of management communication with employees. The evaluation is one-on-one communication from the manager about an employee's job performance. Evaluations should be performed at the end of the probationary period and annually thereafter for each employee. Sometimes, the employee's annual evaluation is tied to a merit pay increase. The result of an evaluation can determine whether an employee receives a 1%, 2%, or 5% increase in pay, and occasionally it affects an employee's promotion.

HIT BIT

The employee evaluation is not the first communication the employee receives regarding his or her job performance. Employees are given performance expectations when they receive a copy of their job description and performance standards. Routine communication between the employee and the supervisor should indicate whether the employee's performance is acceptable. The employee evaluation is not the time to let an employee know that he or she is not meeting expectations. Not only is this poor management but it does not effectively improve functions in the HIM department.

Routine feedback to employees about their job performance improves effectiveness if there is a problem and makes the employee performance evaluation smoother because the information necessary has been gathered over the entire evaluation period, that is, 1 year, instead of documenting only the incidents that the manager can recall. The manager may be able to recall only the most recent incidents. If these statistics are not favorable, the manager may not consider the employee's positive performance during the entire evaluation period. In other words, employees should be receiving feedback (positive or negative) from the supervisor on a regular basis. Because they have a job description and understand the productivity expectations, evaluations should not be a surprise to employees.

The employee evaluation should be performed, in person, by the direct supervisor of the employee. It is good for an employee to sit down with his or her manager to discuss the evaluation. It is an excellent opportunity for feedback and communication between the two.

Poor Evaluations

What occurs if the evaluation is not favorable? Is the employee immediately terminated for poor performance? Typically, an employee who has successfully completed a probationary period and then later shows poor performance is put on a performance improvement plan (PIP). The PIP informs the employee of the poor performance and describes the actions that will occur if the employee does not perform according to the acceptable standards, that is, termination of employment.

HIT BIT

The acronym "PIP" stands for various things. For example, HCFA has a program called PIP, for Periodic Interim Payments. "PIP" might also stand for Preferred Internet Provider or Performance Improvement Program. When using acronyms be sure that you understand the meaning in the context in which the acronym is being used.

Hiring Health Information Management Personnel

Hiring the right employee is a very important task performed by the managers and supervisors in a department. When a person is hired to perform a job, an agreement is made between the organization and the employee. The agreement is that the employee will perform the job required for compensation. Sometimes finding the right person for the job is a difficult task.

Advertisement

When a position is vacant, whether because the position is new or because someone has resigned, the process of finding a new employee begins. To locate potential candidates for a job, the organization must let others know that the position is open. There are a number of ways that an open position can be advertised, such as placing an advertisement in local newspapers, professional journals, or community and association newsletters. The advertisement announces the position that is available, qualifications (including the amount of experience and education required for the position), benefits, and how a potential candidate can contact the organization if he or she is interested in applying (Fig. 10–9). Other information that may be included in the advertisement for the position describes the employment status: full-time or part-time, the hours worked per week, responsibilities, and pay scale. Persons who are interested should follow the instructions in the advertisement to apply for the position.

To create the right advertisement, refer to the job description for that position. Be sure to determine all of the qualifications that a candidate should

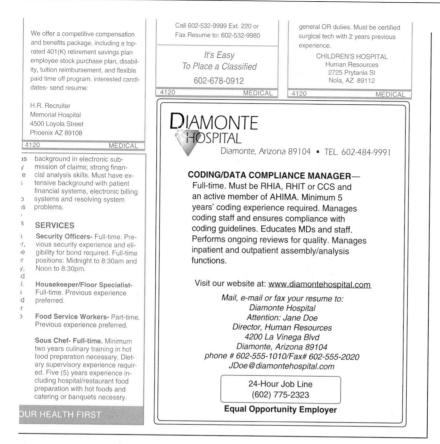

We offer a competitive compensation and benefits package, including a top-rated 401(K) retirement savings plan employee stock purchase plan, disability, tuition reimbursement, and flexible paid time off program. interested candidates- send resume:

H.R. Recruiter
Memorial Hospital
4500 Loyola Street
Phoenix AZ 89108

4120   MEDICAL

background in electronic submission of claims; strong financial analysis skills. Must have extensive background with patient financial systems, electronic billing systems and resolving system problems.

SERVICES

Security Officers- Full-time. Previous security experience and eligibility for bond required. Full-time positions: Midnight to 8:30am and Noon to 8:30pm.

Housekeeper/Floor Specialist- Full-time. Previous experience preferred.

Food Service Workers- Part-time. Previous experience preferred.

Sous Chef- Full-time. Minimum two years culinary training in hot food preparation necessary, Dietary supervisory experience required. Five (5) years experience including hospital/restaurant food preparation with hot foods and catering or banquets necessry.

OUR HEALTH FIRST

Call 602-532-9999 Ext. 220 or
Fax Resume to: 602-532-9980

*It's Easy
To Place a Classified*
602-678-0912

4120   MEDICAL

general OR duties. Must be certified surgical tech with 2 years previous experience.

CHILDREN'S HOSPITAL
Human Resources
2725 Prytania St
Nola, AZ 89112

4120   MEDICAL

DIAMONTE
HOSPITAL

Diamonte, Arizona 89104 • TEL. 602-484-9991

CODING/DATA COMPLIANCE MANAGER—
Full-time. Must be RHIA, RHIT or CCS and an active member of AHIMA. Minimum 5 years' coding experience required. Manages coding staff and ensures compliance with coding guidelines. Educates MDs and staff. Performs ongoing reviews for quality. Manages inpatient and outpatient assembly/analysis functions.

Visit our website at: www.diamontehospital.com

*Mail, e-mail or fax your resume to:
Diamonte Hospital
Attention: Jane Doe
Director, Human Resources
4200 La Vinega Blvd
Diamonte, Arizona 89104
phone # 602-555-1010/Fax# 602-555-2020
JDoe@diamontehospital.com*

24-Hour Job Line
(602) 775-2323

Equal Opportunity Employer

FIGURE 10–9.

Newspaper advertisement for HIM personnel.

possess to apply. Specify how much education is required, for example, college, high school degree or equivalent, and what type of education, such as training in anatomy and physiology, medical terminology, or transcription. It is also important to state the amount of prior experience that a candidate should have. Also specify if the experience needed is specific to a job function or generally related to the HIM field. Then include the way candidates should apply for the position, for example, a résumé sent to your attention via fax or e-mail, or application in person to the human resource department.

HIT BIT

Many HIM positions are advertised by word of mouth. Participation in local HIM associations can put you in touch with large numbers of professionals who are potential candidates for open positions in the department.

Application

Typically, candidates for a position must complete an application for employment in order to be considered for the position. As an applicant, it is important to provide accurate and complete information on this form (Fig. 10–10).

Answer each question on the application. Do not leave spaces blank, even if you think the information is covered on your résumé. Use ink, and write legibly and spell correctly. Read the question or section carefully before completing the information. Think through your answer before writing it on the application, if it involves lengthy communication. Make sure the information is accurate. Do not provide false information. Always provide current and appropriate references; the organization checks the references before making a final decision. Table 10–9 includes a few suggestions for completing employment applications.

SCREENING APPLICANTS

The manager uses the applications to determine who will be interviewed. The applications are carefully reviewed to identify qualified candidates. A legible and complete application is likely to receive a thorough review. Applications that are messy, incomplete, and illegible often receive little attention. Managers review the applications to examine the type of education, training, and experience of each applicant. Those applicants determined to be qualified for the position are contacted for an interview. An applicant can expect that inconsistent, vague, or incomplete information on any part of the application may require further explanation during the interview.

HIT BIT

For those applicants who are screened but not interviewed, at a minimum, some correspondence should be mailed to the applicants to let them know how their application will be handled. The correspondence may thank candidates for the application but explain that their qualifications did not match that of the position; in addition, it can inform them that their application will be kept on file for a specific time period in case any future openings occur.

TABLE 10–9. Do's and Don'ts for Filling Out an Employment Application	
Do	**Don't**
Read the application and question carefully.	Leave sections of the application blank.
Complete the entire application.	Use pencil.
Use ink.	Provide false information.
Write legibly.	
Spell correctly.	

APPLICATION FOR EMPLOYMENT

This application is not a contract. It is intended to provide information for evaluating your suitability for employment. Please read each question carefully and give an honest and complete answer. Qualified applicants receive consideration for employment without unlawful discrimination because of sex, religion, race, color, national origin, age, disability, or other classification protected by law. Applications will remain active for three months.

PLEASE TYPE OR PRINT ALL INFORMATION

Date: _____

Position(s) applying for: _____

How did you learn about us? ☐ Walk-in ☐ Friend ☐ Relative ☐ Job hotline ☐ Employee ☐ Other
☐ Advertisement (Please state name of publication) _____ Referred by: _____

Name: _____
          Last   *First*   *Middle initial*

Mailing address: _____
          City   *State*   *Zip code*

Phone: (_____) _____ (_____) _____ Social Security #: _____
        Home   *Message*

If related to anyone in our employ, state name and department: _____

If you have been employed under another name, please list here: _____

Are you under 18 years of age?... ☐ Yes   ☐ No

Are you currently employed?... ☐ Yes   ☐ No

May we contact your present employer?.. ☐ Yes   ☐ No

Do you have legal rights to work in this country?
  (Proof of legal rights to work in this country will be required upon employment).... ☐ Yes   ☐ No

Have you ever been employed with us before?........................ ☐ Yes   ☐ No   *If "yes," give date(s):* _____

Are you available to work: _____ ☐ Full-time   ☐ Part-time   ☐ Shift work   ☐ Temporary

Are you available to work overtime if required?........................ ☐ Yes   ☐ No

How flexible are you in accepting varying scheduled hours?................... ☐ Very flexible   ☐ Somewhat flexible
                                         ☐ Need set schedule

Minimum salary desired: _____

Have you ever been discharged from a job or forced to resign? .... ☐ Yes   ☐ No
  Explain: _____

Have you ever been convicted of a felony?
  If "yes," please explain: .... ☐ Yes   ☐ No
  Criminal convictions are not an absolute bar to _____
  employment but will be considered with respect _____
  to the specific requirements of the job for which
  you are applying. _____

FIGURE 10–10.

Application for employment.

EDUCATION

High school: _____   High school graduate/GED: ☐ Yes   ☐ No
_____   Date: _____

College: _____   Graduated: ☐ Yes   ☐ No

Major/field(s) of study: _____   Degree: _____

Date: _____

College: _____   Graduated: ☐ Yes   ☐ No

Major/field(s) of study: _____   Degree: _____

Date: _____

Technical, business, or
correspondence school: _____   Graduated: ☐ Yes   ☐ No

Major/field(s) of study: _____   Degree: _____

Date: _____

Describe any specialized training, apprenticeship, and skills such as computer,
office equipment, etc. _____
_____
_____
_____
_____

LICENSES AND CERTIFICATIONS

Type of license(s)/certification(s): _____   Expiration date: _____

Type of license(s)/certification(s): _____   Expiration date: _____

Type of license(s)/certification(s): _____   Expiration date: _____

Verified by: _____

Date: _____

REFERENCES

(Give name, address, and telephone number of three references that you have known for at least one year who are not
related to you.)

Name: _____   Phone: _____   Years acquainted: _____

Address: _____   Business: _____

Name: _____   Phone: _____   Years acquainted: _____

Address: _____   Business: _____

Name: _____   Phone: _____   Years acquainted: _____

Address: _____   Business: _____

FIGURE 10–10. *CONTINUED*   *Figure continued on following page*

EMPLOYMENT EXPERIENCE

(Please list all employment experience, with most recent employment first. If more space is needed, please use the Additional Employment form.)

Employer: _____   Duties and skills performed:_____

Address: _____

Phone number(s) _____

Job title: _____

Supervisor's name/title: _____

Reason for leaving: _____

Salary received: _____ *hourly / weekly / monthly*

Employed from: _____ to _____
               month / year   *month / year*

Employer: _____   Duties and skills performed:_____

Address: _____

Phone number(s) _____

Job title: _____

Supervisor's name/title: _____

Reason for leaving: _____

Salary received: _____ *hourly / weekly / monthly*

Employed from: _____ to _____
               month / year   *month / year*

Employer: _____   Duties and skills performed:_____

Address: _____

Phone number(s) _____

Job title: _____

Supervisor's name/title: _____

Reason for leaving: _____

Salary received: _____ *hourly / weekly / monthly*

Employed from: _____ to _____
               month / year   *month / year*

Do you expect any of the employers listed above to give you a poor reference? ☐ Yes ☐ No

If yes, explain: _____

FIGURE 10–10. *CONTINUED*

Figure continued on following page

APPLICANT'S STATEMENT

I hereby certify that the statements and information provided are true, and I understand that any false statements or omissions are cause for termination. I agree to submit to a drug test and physical following any conditional offer of employment, and I grant permission to Diamonte Hospital to investigate my criminal history, education, prior employment history, and references, and hereby release all persons or agencies from all liability or any damage for issuing this information.

I understand that this application is current for only **three months**. At the end of that time, if I do not hear from Diamonte Hospital and still wish to be considered for employment, it will be necessary to update my application.

_____   _____
Signature of Applicant   *Date*

_____
Print Name

DIAMONTE
HOSPITAL

FIGURE 10–10. *CONTINUED*

Interviewing

The interview is typically a face-to-face meeting between the applicant and the organization's representative. Each organization has a specific process for performing an interview. Some organizations have the applicant interview over the phone or with the human resource department before meeting with the manager in the HIM department. Other organizations perform a group interview, in which the applicant meets with several different members of the organization at the same time. For the applicant, the interview is an opportunity to learn about the organization and the responsibilities of the position. For the organization, the interview is an exploration of the candidate's qualifications for the position. Interviews may be very formal and structured, informal, or somewhere in between. The interviewer should plan ahead, determine an appropriate location, decide on the style, and write down the questions he or she wants to ask.

All interviews begin with some form of a greeting between the candidate and the interviewer. Experienced interviewers say that they can tell a lot about a candidate within these first few moments. Therefore, regardless of your position in the interview process (interviewer or interviewee), be prepared and pay close attention. Greet the other person with a firm handshake, a smile, good posture, and pleasantries. Then take your place in the office, seated at the table or in a chair to begin the interview.

HIT Bit

The handshake is often part of an introduction. The manner in which you participate in the handshake will make an impression on the other party. A good handshake is assertive and has a firm grip. Try out your handshake on a classmate.

During the interview in the HIM department, the manager informs the candidate about the position, discussing requirements, environment, and philosophy of the organization or management style. The manager also asks questions to obtain further information about the candidate's qualifications. This exchange gives the candidate and the organization more information to develop an opinion about the candidate's suitability for the position. The interview is the opportunity to find out if the candidate is appropriate for the job and a good fit for the department. Table 10–10 provides a list of the questions often asked during an interview.

Although the questions asked in an interview are necessary and inform a manager about a candidate's ability and knowledge, in many cases (depending on the position) it is necessary to test the candidate's skills. You must determine whether the candidate can perform the job. For example, if the manager wants to hire a coder who has the skill to code, he or she should give real work to the candidate to determine his or her capability to handle the work in the organization.

TABLE 10–10. Interview Questions
Tell me a little bit about yourself.
Describe your last job. What did you like or dislike about the job?
What expectations do you have of your supervisor? Describe your relationship with your former supervisor.
Explain a stressful situation and how you handled it.
What is the one word that best describes you?
Which of your strengths best suit you for this job?
Which of your weaknesses may cause a problem for you in this job?
Do you have any future education goals?
Where do you see yourself in 5 or 10 years?
Are you available to work weekends, evenings, or some holidays?

Assessment

There are at least two different types of applicant assessments—one for skills and the other for aptitude. A *skills* assessment is designed to identify the applicant's capability for performing the job. The *aptitude* assessment evaluates the applicant's inclination, intelligence, or appropriateness for a position and the likelihood of his or her fitting into a particular organization or position. The assessment is typically a test given during the interview. Some tests are lengthy. Skills assessments should include exercises that the applicant would encounter on the job; for instance, if the position is for outpatient coding, have the applicant code some of your emergency room or outpatient records. It is not fair practice to assess an applicant with a test that is different from the actual work he or she will expected to perform. Health information managers should *always* test the coding skills of an applicant for a coding position and test the typing and terminology skills for a transcription position. Managers and organizations differ in their practices for screening applicants for clerical positions, such as testing filing skills for a file clerk.

Fair Employment Practices

It is extremely important that HIM managers and supervisors comply with appropriate and legal hiring practices. There are a number of laws that regulate the hiring of employees based on age, gender, race, religion, and disability (Table 10–11). Employers must be certain that their hiring practices do not discriminate among candidates. Additionally, employers must be sure that all employees are managed in an appropriate law-abiding manner.

Employers are allowed to require certain standards of their employees; for example, the law allows health care employers to perform a drug screen on candidates before making a job offer. An employee working under the influence of certain substances does not have the ability to provide quality health care. This would be a liability for the employer. Department standards, however, must not contradict the law.

TABLE 10-11. Employment Laws	
Law	**Area of Concern**
Age Discrimination in Employment Act (1967)	Protects employees between the ages of 40 and 70 years
Americans with Disabilities Act (ADA) (1990)	Outlaws discrimination against disabled people and ensures reasonable accommodation for them in the workplace
Civil Rights Act (1964)	Prohibits discrimination on the basis of race, color, religion, sex, or national origin and ensures equal employment opportunity
Fair Labor Standards Act (1938)	Sets minimum wage, overtime pay, equal pay, child labor, and record-keeping requirements for employers. Equal Pay Amendment (1963) forbids sex discrimination in pay practices
Family Medical Leave Act (1993)	Grants unpaid leave and provides job security to employees who must take time off for medical reasons for themselves or family members

Adapted from Abdelhak M, Grostick S, Hanken MA, Jacobs E: Health Information: Management of a Strategic Resource. Philadelphia, WB Saunders, 2001, p 572.

Department Equipment and Supplies

The equipment, or tools, needed to perform the functions in an HIM department vary depending on the size of the facility, the type of health care that the facility provides, and the extent to which the information in that facility has been computerized. The equipment most often recognized in an HIM department includes employee work stations (desks and chairs), filing mechanisms, copiers, fax machines, telephones, computers, and printers. Proper equipment is essential to the functions of the HIM department. Each employee's equipment must be adequate to perform the functions. Old, faulty equipment can have a negative impact on the productivity of an employee, which ultimately affects the entire department. Once an employee has notified the manager of an equipment problem, the manager should be sure to begin the maintenance process in a timely manner.

HIT BIT

Equipment such as computer software programs, copiers, and transcription and dictation equipment is typically purchased with a maintenance contract option. It is important for managers to update and budget for this contract annually. The maintenance contract provides for repair, assistance, and sometimes replacement of certain equipment. The contract option can usually be purchased at minimal cost for maintenance coverage from Monday through Friday, 9 AM to 5 PM, or for the first 90 days. For a higher fee, the contract may cover the equipment 24 hours per day, 7 days per week, including holidays.

Reference material is another necessary tool for any department providing coding and transcription services. Reference materials should be updated periodically. Table 10–12 provides a list of suggested reference materials for these areas. Additional equipment, for example, pens, paper, toner, file folders, envelopes and labels, is commonly referred to as supplies. The HIM department should be appropriately equipped and stocked for the employees to effectively perform their jobs. This includes necessary equipment and supplies for contract employees and those employees who work for the facility from their home.

Supplies

A manager should be sure the amount of each item stocked is adequate to supply the employees. Orders for additional supplies should be placed timely to prevent delay.

FILING

There are a significant number of supplies associated with filing, such as, folders, color-coded labels, and year-band labels. File folders are typically ordered annually; therefore, the manager needs to consider how many folders will be used (annually) before purchasing this item. Remember to account for each

TABLE 10–12. Suggested Reference Materials for the HIM Department

Reference	Updates	Who Needs This Reference Material?
Physicians' Desk Reference (PDR)	Published annually	One copy each for transcription and coding
Medical dictionary	Updated occasionally	One copy each for transcription and coding
Human disease reference		Coding
Specialized word books (e.g., surgical word book, drug book, abbreviation book)		Transcription
ICD-9-CM coding book	Updated annually October 1	Coding must have current codes as of October 1 each year
Coding Clinic for ICD-9-CM	Quarterly newsletter published by AHA	Coding. This tool provides knowledge and advice on implementation of ICD-9-CM coding guidelines
HCFA Common Procedure Coding System (HCPCS)	Updated annually by HCFA	Coding and the person responsible for maintenance of the facility Chargemaster should have access to this reference
Current Procedural Terminology (CPT)	Updated annually	Coding. Outpatient and physician's office coders must have current codes
CPT Assistant	Monthly newsletter published by AHA	Coding. This tool provides examples, explanation, and scenarios for implementation of CPT coding

AHA, American Hospital Association; HCFA, Health Care Financing Administration; HCPCS, Health Care Financing Administration Common Procedural Coding System.

type of patient that will require a folder—inpatient, outpatient, patients in for observation, and newborns. Of course, the number of folders needed depends on the filing system used, whether serial, unit, or serial–unit. In the unit numbering system, the patient uses the same number for all visits; therefore, conceivably one folder could store data for more than one discharge. However, for serial and serial–unit numbering systems each patient will need a new folder. For simplification, we assume that each discharge requires a new folder. The number of discharges for the year should almost equal the number of folders used; the manager should order enough extra folders to allow for errors, mistakes, repair of torn folders, etc. Also, be sure to order sufficient quantities of year-band labels and number labels (see Chapter 5).

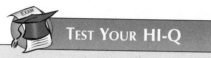

TEST YOUR HI-Q

Using the 2000 statistics for Community Hospital given in Chapter 7 (see Fig. 7–10), determine how many folders you will need for the next year (2001), assuming that you will have a 3% increase in discharges.

COPY MACHINES AND PRINTERS

HIM departments rely on copy machines and printers for many different tasks, but especially to release information to third parties, transfer patient information to a new facility or health care provider, and provide reports as requested by other departments. Copy machines require an adequate supply of paper and toner. Additionally, the department should have a maintenance agreement for the machine so that it can be serviced routinely. Printers also require paper, but their ink comes in the form of cartridges. Managers need to keep a sufficient supply of cartridges on hand so that the department is able to operate efficiently. A good way to stock this supply is to always have one extra ink cartridge (or toner cartridge) for every two printers so that when you run out, you have a replacement. Then you can order a new cartridge before you run out again.

TRANSCRIPTION AND DICTATION EQUIPMENT

Transcription and dictation equipment is important in the communication of patient health information. The dictation equipment is used by the health care professional to record the patient's health information. The transcription equipment is the machine used by the transcriptionist to listen to and type the dictated reports. Transcriptionists access the dictation system to retrieve the recorded voice. They then listen to the voice to type the report. This equipment should have a maintenance agreement, preferably 24-hour, 7-day per week coverage.

SOFTWARE

Many of the operations in the HIM department require the use of computer software. Typical software in a HIM department includes the master patient index, chart locator system, release of information form, electronic birth certificate, and encoders and groupers for coding. This software is critical to the operation of the department. Therefore, each software system should be maintained in an appropriate environment, on computer equipment sufficient to support the applications, with adequate maintenance contracts for upgrades and support.

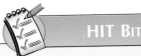

HIT BIT

An *upgrade,* in computer software terminology, refers to a new version of software that is improved in some way.

MISCELLANEOUS SUPPLIES

Remember to coordinate appropriate ordering practices for even routine supplies, such as pencils, ink pens, paper, and flags for analysis. An inadequate supply of these necessary tools may cause unnecessary delays in the processing of health information.

Monitoring Use of Department Resources

HIM department managers must carefully monitor the equipment and supplies so that workflow is not affected. Poor equipment management—whether buying new equipment, maintaining existing equipment, or converting from one system to another—can negatively affect the productivity in the department. It is important to maintain adequate supplies for the employee workforce (on-site, contract, and at home), for example, files, labels, printer or copier paper, and toner or ink cartridges. Minor oversights in department equipment and supplies can cause the workflow to backlog. Backlogs negatively affect employee performance and sometimes affect department budgets. Even such minor details play an important role in the management of health information.

Ergonomics

Ergonomics is the coordination of the work environment with the worker (Random House, 1995). The work environment should be comfortable, allowing the employee to perform the job as necessary, free from injury or harm. Ergonomics is sometimes thought of as proper body positioning of the employee at his or her desk (Fig. 10–11). However, this is not the only office equipment that can be coordinated with employees to keep them free from injury or harm. Other

Anatomy of an Ergonomic Work Station

WORKPLACE ENVIRONMENT

- Most important consideration is working comfortably and efficiently.
- Have sufficient desk area for keyboard, monitor, mouse, document holder, telephone, etc.
- Organize the area so that it reflects the way you use equipment.
- Things you use most often should be within easiest reach.
- Vary your tasks.

- Take frequent breaks.
- If area is shared, be sure all who use it can adjust everything to their needs.
- Document holders should be at the same height and distance from monitor.
- Allow adequate leg room.
- Maintain an unobscured line of sight.

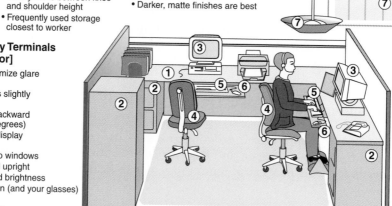

(1) Work Surface
- Proper height and angle
- Neutral postures
- Adjustable
- Standing–prevent slipping, adequate traction
- Sit/stand tools
- Antifatigue floor mats
- Darker, matte finishes are best

(2) Storage Areas
- Good body positions
- Reduce muscular forces
- Avoid excessive reach
- Heavy items between knee and shoulder height
- Frequently used storage closest to worker

(3) Video Display Terminals (VDT) [Monitor]
- Position to minimize glare and reflections
- Top of screen is slightly below eye level
- Tilted slightly backward (less than 15 degrees)
- Distance from display 18–30 inches
- Perpendicular to windows
- Keep your head upright
- Set contrast and brightness
- Clean the screen (and your glasses)
- Antiglare filters
- Adjustable monitor arm

(4) Chairs
- Comfortable (padded seats that swivel)
- Back and seat are adjustable while seated
- Provide good back support (can add additional cushion if necessary)
- Adjustable arm support
- Back straight
- Knees slightly higher than chair bottom
- Thighs horizontal
- Feet flat on the floor (use a footrest if necessary)
- Change positions occasionally

(5) Keyboard
- Back should be lower than front
- Rounded edges
- Wrist rests (sharp edges, neutral position) same height as front of keyboard
- Type properly: don't force your fingers to stretch to incorrect keystrokes

(6) Mouse
- Keep it on the same level as the keyboard or slightly above
- Keep wrist straight
- Do not stretch your arm; keep mouse within immediate reach
- Use the whole arm to move the mouse ... not just the forearm

(7) Lighting
- Less illumination for computer work
- Indirect lighting is best

Avoid:

Awkward posture

Can include reaching behind, twisting, working overhead, kneeling, bending, and squatting. Deviation from ideal working posture can lead to fatigue, muscle tension, and headaches. **Correct working posture** – arms at sides, elbows bent approximately 90 degrees, forearms parallel to floor, wrists straight.

Repetitiveness

Judgment is based on frequency, speed, number of muscle groups used, and required force. Not all people react to the same conditions, so carefully monitor your personal physical response to repetitiveness.

FIGURE 10–11.

Ergonomic environment of an HIM department. (Redrawn from Gaylor L: The Administrative Dental Assistant. Philadelphia, WB Saunders, 2000, p 290.)

ergonomic issues involve lighting, appropriate climate, and the frequency and duration of rest breaks. Because many HIM functions are performed at a computer terminal or desk, appropriate coordination of employees to their work stations is required. Significant time spent in a harmful work environment can compromise employees' health, costing the facility valuable assets when workers' compensation claims are filed.

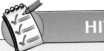

HIT Bit

Workers' compensation is the benefit that pays an employee for time away from the workplace because of a work-related injury.

Areas in the HIM department that require significant ergonomic consideration are the transcription stations and area, employee computer terminal position, chair height in relation to the employee desk or work station, and general office space. The lighting, air conditioning, and heating should also be appropriate. The environment must provide safe and appropriate working conditions. For example, if the employee needs good lighting for reading, then lighting should be adjusted accordingly. But if the employee spends a majority of the day facing a computer screen, dim or indirect lighting may better protect the employee's eyesight.

References

Abdelhak M, Grostick S, Hanken MA, Jacobs E: Health Information: Management of a Strategic Resource. Philadelphia, WB Saunders, 1996.
Random House Webster's School and Office Dictionary. New York, Random House Inc, 1995.

CHAPTER SUMMARY

The management of health information includes the management of the people performing HIM functions. Appropriate organization and management of the department's human resources significantly affects the quality of health information. Quality health information is necessary in the health care environment to provide good patient care. A good place to begin effective management is clear communication of the employee's responsibilities in the job description and performance standards of the position.

HIM supervisors and managers are responsible for the daily operations of the HIM department, as well as future planning in keeping with the facility's mission and vision. In order to guide the department into the future, HIM managers must plan, set goals and objectives, and continually evaluate the services provided within the department.

Knowledge of health information combined with management skills sets the stage for efficient and effective HIM departments.

REVIEW QUESTIONS

1. Explain the difference between unity of command and span of control.

2. Explain how to write a job description.

3. What is the purpose of performance standards?

4. List and describe some of the supplies necessary in an HIM department.

5. Identify some of the issue that must be considered when designing an ergonomic work station.

PROFESSIONAL PROFILE
Health Information Management Director

My name is Mary Catherine and I am the director of the health information management department at Fullmore Hospital, a 250-bed facility that provides acute care, skilled nursing care, rehabilitation, and a geriatric psychiatric service. The medical staff is divided into five sections: Medicine, Surgery, OB/GYN, Pediatrics, and Psychiatric. Our HIM department has 25 employees, 20 FTEs, and 5 part-time employees. I have two supervisors and one assistant director reporting directly to me.

My responsibilities include overseeing the operations of the department and planning and organizing the direction of the health information operations. I attend several meetings each month. I am a member of the Quality Management Committee and the Risk Management Committee. I am also the coordinator for the Health Information Management Committee. As this coordinator, I work closely with the chairman of the committee, a member of the Medical Staff, to organize the meetings, coordinate record reviews, and compile minutes of the meetings.

I also attend a monthly meeting of all the department directors in the facility at which we share important information about our department operations, perform facilitywide strategic planning, and receive communication from administration.

Once a month I hold a department meeting for all HIM employees. During the meeting we discuss department business and quality, and employees receive communication about things that are occurring throughout the facility.

I really enjoy my job. Every day is a new challenge—sometimes from administration, physicians, or employees; at other times, accreditation or federal government requirements present a challenge. Working as a team, we always manage to reach our goals.

APPLICATION

Hiring a Coder

You recently lost a coder at your facility. The department director has asked that you, the coding supervisor, create an advertisement for the local newspaper and participate in the interview for this new position. Using your knowledge of hiring practices and your local newspaper, create an advertisement for this new position.

Before the interview, document at least three questions that you would like to ask the applicant. Be sure to check the list of appropriate interview questions (see Table 10–10).

11

Training and Development

Chapter Outline

Orientation
Organization Orientation
  Personnel Issues
  Customer Service
  Quality
  Building Safety and Security
  Infection Control
  Body Mechanics
  Confidentiality
Health Information Management Department Orientation
Clinical Staff Orientation

Training
Assessment of Education Needs
Audience
Format
Environment
Calendar of Education
  Tracking Employee Education

In-service Education

Educating the Public

Continuing Education

Communication
Employee-to-Employee Communication
Health Information Management Department and Physicians
Health Information Management Department and Outside Agencies or Parties
Written Communication
  Memos
Electronic Communication

Department Meetings
Agenda
Meeting
Minutes
Meeting Records

Web Sites

Chapter Summary

Review Questions

Professional Profile

Application

By the end of this chapter, the students should be able to

- Orient a new employee to the department and his or her job function.

- Orient an employee to a new job procedure.

- Orient medical staff or other facility personnel to the HIM department.

- Identify in-service topics for HIM department personnel.

- Develop an in-service topic for presentation.

- Identify continuing education needs for HIM employees.

- Organize an agenda for HIM department meetings.

- Document minutes from an in-service, or a continuing education session or department meeting.

- Develop appropriate effective written communication.

Vocabulary

agenda	in-service	orientation
continuing education	memorandum (memo)	probation period
credentials	minutes	training

A well-managed health information management (HIM) department spends considerable time on training and development of employees. *Training* involves orientation, education, and practice (practical application) for a particular position or job function. *Development* is the ongoing improvement of staff personally and professionally. The manager of the HIM department is responsible for the hiring, training, developing, and maintaining of employees who perform the department functions. Occasionally, the responsibility is delegated to supervisors as well. Training is a very important part of any department; well-trained employees provide quality service. Training is necessary at many times: in the beginning of employment, as procedures and policies change and processes are improved, and as technology and equipment are improved. Development is equally important because it improves on quality service. A department that develops its employees is making an investment in the future of quality service.

In the previous chapter, we discussed hiring the right candidate for a job. In this chapter, we discuss how a manager trains and develops the employee as an asset to the organization.

Orientation

When an employee begins a job at a new health care facility, he or she needs a few days to learn about the environment and the new job. This is accomplished through **orientation.** The purpose of orientation is to make the employee familiar with the surroundings and assist him or her with the necessary information to function on the job and in the organization. There is an orientation about the organization and another one specific to the employee's job within the department in the organization. Orientation begins with an overall view of the organization and continues with department and job-specific information once the employee reports to the supervisor.

Organization Orientation

Typically before new employees report to their departments, they attend an organization-wide orientation during which they are given information about the organization and have an opportunity to ask questions regarding employment. The typical topics covered in an organization orientation include

- Personnel issues
- Customer service expectations
- Quality
- Building safety and security
- Infection control
- Body mechanics
- Confidentiality
- Tour of the facility

This orientation should take place before employees begin their job activities; however, because these orientations are sometimes offered only once a month, employees may actually begin work before their organization orientation.

PERSONNEL ISSUES

Some of the first information that employees receive during the orientation explains the benefits they are entitled to as employees of the organization. During this part of the orientation, employees learn about special savings plans and will complete necessary forms for income tax and for enrollment in special plans or retirement accounts. Because compensation for the job is important, orientation is an opportunity to ask about pay periods, to learn how to complete payroll forms, or learn how to use the time clock. Employees are also informed of hospital policies and procedures that affect their employment and receive a copy of the employee handbook. Information in the employee handbook includes facility dress code, tardy policy, hours earned for vacation and sick leave, grievance procedures, and holidays.

CUSTOMER SERVICE

During the initial orientation the new employee learns about the organization's expectations of each employee in relation to all customers. Customer service is an important part of health care, and many facilities use this orientation as an opportunity to instill a positive customer focus in all employees. Employees are encouraged to

- Identify all of their customers by name.
- Greet each customer with a smile.
- Provide assistance or find someone who can assist the customer.
- Follow up on a customer's request.

Employees may get an opportunity to role-play a customer encounter and learn how to handle a disgruntled customer.

QUALITY

As we discussed in Chapter 6, quality is critical to all aspects of health care. Because of this, employees are informed about the expectation and methods that the organization uses to ensure quality. The quality improvement method of choice is described. During orientation new employees learn that everyone in the facility is responsible for quality. Employees are encouraged to participate and motivated to identify opportunities to improve quality.

BUILDING SAFETY AND SECURITY

The health care environment should be safe for patients, visitors, and employees. Safety issues are covered in the organization orientation to make the employee aware of the policy and procedures for maintaining a secure environment and for handling situations in the event of an emergency. Two common topics discussed are fire safety and response to "code" emergencies. A common fire response uses the acronym: RACE—rescue, alarm, confine, and extinguish.

Employees learn to *rescue* patients, employees, or visitors from the area of the fire. They should go to the closest fire *alarm* and call the operator with the name, location, and status of the fire. Then they should *confine* the fire by closing all doors in the area. And if possible they should *extinguish* the fire with a fire extinguisher or other appropriate material.

HIT BIT

Each topic in the organization-wide orientation is typically presented by the employee within the organization who is the authority on that issue. For example, the safety topic is presented by the facility's security officer; body mechanics are presented by physical therapy; infection control is presented by the infection control nurse; and confidentiality is presented by an HIM professional.

During a visit to a health care facility you may have heard the operator announce a "code" over the intercom system. Common codes are code blue for cardiac arrest and code red for fire. These codes alert the employees in the facility to an emergency that is occurring in the facility (Table 11–1). These codes may also be announced as code physician names, for example, Dr. Red instead of code red, or Dr. Strong for security. All employees must recognize the codes in the facility and what role they must play in responding to the emergency.

INFECTION CONTROL

Workers in health care can be exposed to the risk of a variety of infections. Because of this, several significant topics are covered under the topic of infection control, for example, hepatitis, acquired immunodeficiency syndrome, and universal precautions for blood and body fluids. During this part of the orientation, new employees will learn how to protect themselves and others from infection. The discussion details information about how these infections are spread and then shares procedures that will help protect employees.

In a discussion about universal precautions for blood and body fluids, employees are informed that one of the best and easiest methods to prevent spread of infection is through washing their hands. Employees are motivated to *always*

TABLE 11–1. Emergency Codes	
Code	**Emergency**
Dr. Strong	Security is requested in a specific area of the facility
Black	Bomb threat
Red	Fire
Orange	Radiation disaster
Pink	Infant abduction
Blue	Cardiac arrest
Yellow	External disaster

wash their hands before and after having contact with a patient, eating, or using the restroom. Universal precautions also include wearing masks and gloves when interacting with potentially infectious material and proper disposal of needles and other contaminated objects.

Because some blood-borne organisms can survive for days outside of the body, health care workers are advised to handle items contaminated with body fluids with care. For example, a paper record contaminated with blood should be filed in a sealed plastic sheath.

BODY MECHANICS

All employees should maintain proper body mechanics. Body mechanics are important while sitting at the work station and when lifting, pushing, pulling, or transporting patients or equipment. This topic is very important to the organization because employees can be injured if they use poor body mechanics. Employee injuries are very costly to the entire organization. An injured employee can miss work or reduce productivity.

CONFIDENTIALITY

Confidentiality is covered during the organization orientation for *all* employees. Typically this topic is presented by an HIM professional. All employees must recognize the sensitivity of the information in a health care facility. The confidentiality policy is reviewed and all employees are asked to sign a confidentiality statement (see Fig. 8–1). Additional information may be covered concerning the policy for release of information and the information management plan.

Health Information Management Department Orientation

Following the organization orientation (optimally), employees report to their supervisor in the new work environment for another orientation specific to their job and the department. During this orientation, employees become familiar with the work station, the environment, other employees, and the policies and procedures regarding their jobs. Each employee is given an opportunity to become acclimated to the work environment, meet the employees that are part of the work group or team, and learn what is expected by management.

During this orientation, the employee is given a copy of the job description, performance standards, rules, and policies and procedures of the HIM department. The employee becomes familiar with the physical layout of the HIM department, including the evacuation route in case of fire, and other related departments within the organization. For example, if the employee is responsible for retrieving information from the emergency room on a daily basis, he or she needs to know where the emergency room is located.

HIT BIT

Employees who change positions within an HIM department also need orientation to their new duties and responsibilities.

One way to orient employees is to have them sit with each section of the department in order to familiarize themselves with everyone's tasks. This helps new employees understand the impact of their role in the department.

Employees also need to understand which holidays they may be required to work or how to request time off. Employees should know the hours they are expected to work. The employee is given a password with access to appropriate computerized information. Once a password is assigned, employees can begin training on the necessary computer system associated with their jobs. An excellent way to keep track of everything that must be covered with a new employee is to complete an orientation checklist (Fig. 11–1). The employee should initial and date each item as it is completed. This form is kept in the employee's file folder as verification of the orientation for future reference.

HIT BIT

The first 90 days of employment for a new employee are called the **probation period.** During the probation period employees are allowed ample time to learn their new tasks and responsibilities.

At the end of this 90-day period, employees who are performing at an acceptable level are considered permanent.

If at any time during this probation period the employer feels that the employee is not performing as expected, the employee can be released from the job.

Clinical Staff Orientation

Department employees are not the only members of the organization who need an orientation. Clinical staff, physicians, and members of other departments should be familiar with the functions and services of the HIM department. A general orientation explaining HIM department operations will assist these members when they interact with the department. HIM customers need to know the requirements for requesting information or records and the procedures for completing or reviewing records.

Physicians require orientation to the HIM department because they will visit the department to complete their health records or perform research. Physician orientation can be by personal appointment or in the form of a letter (Fig. 11–2) introducing or explaining HIM department functions.

DIAMONTE HOSPITAL

Diamonte, Arizona 89104 • TEL. 602-484-9991

EMPLOYEE ORIENTATION CHECKLIST

Employee: _____ Date: _____

Position: _____ Supervisor: _____

The following items have been reviewed with the employee.
(The employee and supervisor should initial and date items as they are reviewed.)

	Employee	Supervisor	Date
Employee identification card policy			
Explanation of payroll procedures, including time clock location			
Absence and tardiness policy			
Employee job description			
Employee performance standards			
Introduction to department employees and physical layout			
Review of department functions			
Review of functions involving related departments			
Departmental Policy and Procedure manual			
Review of specific job-related policies and procedures			
Dress code			
Performance improvement activities			
Security and confidentiality policies			
Review and sign confidentiality statement			
Safety policy, disaster plan, and Safety manual			
Review of break schedule			
Location of restrooms and area to secure belongings			
Password assigned and related policies covered			

Employee signature: _____ Date: _____

Supervisor: _____ Date: _____

Example only. This list is not all-inclusive.

FIGURE 11–1.

Employee orientation checklist.

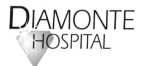

Diamonte, Arizona 89104 • TEL. 602-484-9991

November 30, 2001

Eileen Dombrowski, MD
1101 Medical Center Blvd.
Diamonte, Arizona

Dear Dr. Dombrowski,

On behalf of the Health Information Management department, welcome to Diamonte Hospital. I would like to introduce you to the HIM department staff and the services provided.

Release of information
To obtain copies of health information for a patient under your care, please contact Shelly Pontiac, 565-1411. She will be happy to provide the appropriate forms and process your request.

Coding
Our coding department is supervised by Joanne Davis, CCS. If you have any questions regarding coding, please feel free to contact her.

Request for an old chart for patient care
The unit coordinator will typically request previous records for patients under your care by contacting the Health Information Management department at 565-1400. If you encounter difficulty retrieving a previous patient record, please feel free to contact John Brown, Supervisor.

Medical record completion
In keeping with our policy for timely completion of health records, we will e-mail weekly reminders to your office to notify you of any incomplete records. If you plan to come by our office to complete your records, please call in advance, 565-1455. We will be happy to pull your records and leave them in the physicians' lounge for 48 hours.

I look forward to working with you. If you need any further assistance I can be reached at 565-1416.

Sincerely,

Michelle Parks, RHIA
Director, Health Information Management

FIGURE 11–2.
Orientation letter to physicians.

Department managers need to understand how to request records from the HIM department. Managers often request records for a study or project they are involved in or to obtain information for a meeting. They need to know how much notice the department needs to complete the request. Does the request need to be specific? Does the requestor need to include the patient's name, medical record number, and discharge dates on a request for records? These policies, and others, when covered in an orientation eliminate some confusion and stress in the future.

HIT Bit

Physician orientation is an excellent opportunity to cover information relevant to completion of records, specifically the suspension policy. The suspension policy is typically found in the medical staff bylaws. But even if the orientation is no more than a simple letter of correspondence, it tells the physician how to avoid negative correspondence and unfortunate consequences as a result of delinquent records. Let the physician know who to contact to gain access to incomplete records and how the department can assist the physician in record completion.

Training

Training is an important part of all jobs. Employees need training when they begin a job, but equally important is the training that occurs when processes, procedures, or equipment is changed. Training is education of employees in new techniques and processes within the organization. Training is provided to employees in the health care facility through in-service training sessions and continuing education. Employees require training to ensure the quality of their services. Let's begin by discussing how a training session is organized.

Assessment of Education Needs

The first step in planning a training (in-service or continuing education) session involves an *assessment*. The assessment helps us identify what needs to be taught. Training topics can be identified as the result of

- A management observation from performance standard reviews
- A survey of employees
- Updated or new equipment
- Process improvement

We learned how to create performance standards in Chapter 10. Performance standards tell employees how much and what quality of work they are expected to accomplish. When a manager performs employee evaluations, he or she may determine that additional training is needed in one area due to the employees' low performance.

Occasionally employees may be asked to identify areas in which they would like more expertise. A survey can identify areas of interest to the employees, and training sessions can be developed accordingly. Surveys may also identify ideal areas for cross-training. Cross-training is instructing employees on the procedures for performing other job functions not typical to their job description. Cross-training is a way to prepare a department to handle increased workloads and vacant positions when employees are on a break, are out sick, are on vacation, or leave their position. It can also provide job enrichment for some employees.

With all of the technologic advances that occur in today's health care environment, equipment and computer software are continuously being updated and replaced. These changes typically require training so that employees know how to appropriately use the new technology.

Another opportunity for training is during the "do" and "act" phases of the PDCA (plan, do, check, act) process improvement method. In Chapter 6 we discussed this method for performing and documenting quality improvement efforts. To implement an improved process, all of the employees associated with the process must be trained.

Audience

An important part of planning a training session is learning about the audience. The presenters do not have to know each person individually, but they should know the participants' backgrounds. Their backgrounds with regard to education and work-related experience tell the presenters how to begin the training. When the topic is new to the audience, the presenters begin with an elementary understanding of the topic. If participants are knowledgeable on the topic and have practical experience, the training session can be more advanced. Additionally, knowing the backgrounds of participants affects the organization of the presentation, that is, the vocabulary and knowledge pertinent to the audience. In other words, significantly different vocabulary and examples are used to train physicians as opposed to college students.

Format

The format of a training session explains how the information or topic will be presented. For example, will the training take place as a lecture, or will it be hands-on training? Will the presentation include a video or demonstration? Will there be an instructor, or a self-guided manual? The format is determined by the topic of the presentation and the audience. If the topic involves a procedure and equipment that are new to the audience, a demonstration and hands-on experience would enhance their understanding. However, an in-service training session to describe coding updates to coders may require only a few examples or case studies.

The format of the presentation also determines whether the presenter needs to have audiovisual equipment available. If the training session involves a video, then a TV/VCR monitor must be present in the room. Other audiovisual equipment includes overhead projectors, slide projectors, computer equipment with speakers and video capability, and microphones.

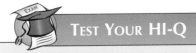

Imagine that you are going to present a training session for new HIM employees. The topic of the training is "How to Organize a Health Record." What format would best suit this presentation?

Environment

The environment or location of the training session is another element that can be determined by the topic of the presentation and the audience. Training sessions can be held in classrooms, auditoriums, via video conference or the Internet, or in the HIM department. If the training requires demonstration of equipment, then the training should happen near the equipment or a demonstration model should be available in the classroom. The location of the training session is also affected by the number of participants. The larger the audience, the more space required. Sometimes multiple sessions can be held to accommodate a large number of participants. However, if the number of participants is small, then the training session may be held in the HIM department. In addition, the audience may need room to take notes, so tables with chairs or desks could be used. If a computer terminal is used for the training, make sure there is adequate seating for one person per computer.

Calendar of Education

How often should employees be trained? At a minimum, *all* employees in the facility should receive annual training regarding customer service, quality, safety, infection control, confidentiality, and body mechanics. Additional training sessions can be organized according to the employee's job function or as the need arises.

In the HIM department there are several positions that require routine training, that is, coding and release of information. Coding employees should participate in quarterly training sessions (coding clinics); for example, inpatient coding changes are effective October 1 of each year. The changes have an impact on all of the coding employees responsible for inpatient coding. A training session should be organized to inform these employees of the upcoming coding changes that will affect their job. Outpatient coding changes (Current Procedural Terminology [CPT]) occur during January. A training session should be organized accordingly to cover these changes. Additionally, other regulations occur at various times during the year, for example, implementation of prospective payment systems (PPSs). A new PPS requires additional training of coders and other clinicians. Release of information employees should receive annual training, and additional sessions should be organized when there are changes in federal or state laws that affect the release of health information.

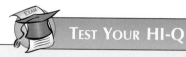

TEST YOUR HI-Q

Create a calendar for education in the HIM department.

TRACKING EMPLOYEE EDUCATION

It is very important to keep a record of employee attendance at training sessions. The record of the employee's attendance supports the communication of a new policy, procedure, or method required as a part of his or her job.

Use a sign-in sheet to record employee participation. This sign-in sheet can be kept in a binder to record employee education, or the information can be transferred to each employee's file. In addition, the information can be transferred to a computer system to track employee education.

Training is an ongoing process. Often it is important to involve other departments so that employees learn the necessary information from the appropriate source. Some topics can be coordinated with members from other departments, such as quality management, nursing, infection control, business office. Also be sure to include *all* of the employees who are affected by the new information, including employees who work at home.

In-service Education

An **in-service** is training for an organization's employees. A training session can be called an in-service when it provides continuing or reinforced education for current employees. An in-service can be part of a monthly department meeting or it can be held separately to cover a new topic, for example, purchase of new equipment. In-services reinforce and develop new skills. In-services can also be used as a method of cross-training staff. Table 11–2 provides a list of in-services for HIM employees. All of the elements of a training session apply to the development of an employee in-service.

TEST YOUR HI-Q

Design an in-service for HIM employees, and discuss all of the elements of a training session.

TABLE 11–2. Examples of In-services
How to use a new copier or printer
How to respond to a fire emergency code, including the use of a fire extinguisher
How to handle a walk-in request for copies of health care records
How to use a clinical pathway
Explanation of a new prospective payment system and how it will affect the organization

Educating the Public

Health care professionals are often called on to educate the public about changes in laws relating to health care or health information as well as health-related topics, such as, cancer awareness, diabetes, infectious disease. Therefore, each of the topics associated with planning a training session for employees can be related to planning a training session for the public.

Continuing Education

Education does not stop simply because a person has completed a program or obtained employment. Professionals recognize that education will continue over the course of their career. As you become an HIM professional, you must recognize that the **credentials** are accompanied by a commitment to lifelong learning. In all health care fields, regulations change, technology advances, and processes improve. Because of this change you must continue your education, as it relates to your job, career, and your special interests.

HIT BIT

The American Health Information Management Association (AHIMA) has a **continuing education** requirement as a part of the certification/registration process. To maintain your credential, you must earn continuing education credits pertinent to the HIM profession. The requirement for the Registered Health Information Technician (RHIT) and Registered Health Information Administrator (RHIA) states that the professional must earn 50% of the required hours in a core content area (Table 11–3). AHIMA has designated the following areas as core content for the HIM profession: Technology, Management Development, Clinical Data Management, Performance Improvement, External Forces, Clinical Foundations, and Other HIM Professional Development.

The RHIA must earn 30 continuing education hours every 2 years. The RHIT must maintain 20 continuing education hours every 2 years. Therefore, the RHIA must have at least 15 (of the 30) hours in any one or multiple core content areas, and the RHIT must have at least 10 of the 20 hours in one or multiple core content areas.

Because certification rules can change, always refer to the AHIMA website for the current requirements.

Continuing education hours can be earned in a variety of ways. Most professionals earn their CE hours by attending local, state, or national HIM association meetings. Some may earn the hours by attending meetings within their facility. Still another method for earning continuing education hours is by reading and responding to the education quizzes found in the *Journal of AHIMA* or visiting the AHIMA Web site.

Additional AHIMA certifications also require a commitment to lifelong learning. The Certified Coding Specialist (CCS) and Certified Coding Specialist—Physician-based (CCS-P) credentials require an annual self-assessment including health record coding scenarios. Depending on the number and nature of coding changes for that year, the number of multiple-choice questions may be as few as 10 or as many as 30.

	TABLE 11–3. RHIT Core Content Areas	
Core Content Area	**Description**	**Example**
Technology	Applications of existing and emerging technologies for collection of clinical data, the transformation of clinical data to useful health information, and the communication and protection of information.	Attending a presentation explaining the process of converting paper records to a virtual file room.
Management Development	Application of organizational management theory and practices as well as human resource management techniques to improve departmental adaptability, innovation service quality, and operational efficiency.	Attending an in-service to learn how to use a new employee evaluation system.
Clinical Data Management	Application of data analysis techniques to clinical databases to evaluate practice patterns, assess clinical outcomes, and assure cost-effectiveness of health care services.	Attending a meeting of the community health information network to learn how to submit information and interpret results.
Performance Improvement	Study of fundamental organizational changes and how they are functionally organized or how they deliver patient care, with special focus on the requisite changes made in health information systems and services.	Attending a meeting to learn how to facilitate quality improvement in your organization.
External Forces	Knowledge of strategies that organizational and HIM professionals in particular have used to effectively address emerging legislative, regulatory, or other external party action that have the potential to significantly impact the collection and use of health data.	Attending a seminar explaining implementation of HIPAA requirements.
Clinical Foundations	Understanding of human anatomy and physiology, the nature of disease processes in humans, and the methods of diagnosis and treatment of acute and chronic medical conditions and diseases.	Attending a conference on breast cancer.

HIPAA, Health Insurance Portability and Accountability Act.
From AHIMA online: Available at www.ahima.org/services/maintenance.rhia-rhit.core.html.

Keeping a record of your continuing education hours is very important. Because continuing education periods vary with each association, you may not remember all of the hours that you earned unless you keep a record of your attendance or completion. The easiest method for keeping track of your continuing education hours is to designate a file folder for material from the meetings you attend, journal article questionnaires submitted, and Web site tutorials completed. If you use a summary form in the file folder, each time you open the folder to file hours you can also write the hours on the summary sheet (Fig. 11–3). This file folder and tracking form are also helpful in the event of an audit of your continuing education hours. Using this file folder and tracking form makes it easier to fill out the continuing education form when your continuing education hours are due. HIM Department managers should also maintain a file of all employees' continuing education in order to document their progress.

Training and education require communication. Communication must occur between staff employees and management, and between management and administration. To educate, we must communicate. Let's discuss communication in the health care environment.

Continuing education for: _____

No. of hours needed: _____

Cycle ends: _____

Date	Topic/Title	Location	Core Content Area	No. of Hours

FIGURE 11–3.

Continuing education tracking form.

Communication

Communication is an important part of management. Employees within an HIM department communicate daily. They use written, verbal, physical, and electronic methods for communicating. The HIM department communicates internally and with other departments in the facility, clinicians and physicians, other health care facilities, insurance companies, attorneys, and patients. Communication should always be clear and appropriate regardless of the parties involved. Let's briefly review a familiar communication scenario (Fig. 11–4).

Communication requires two parties and a message. There must first be a message that needs to be understood by or transmitted to another party. The message can be written, verbal, or electronic or expressed by body language. The first party—called the *sender*—initiates the message. The second party—the *receiver*—is the recipient of the message. This is the basis of all communication.

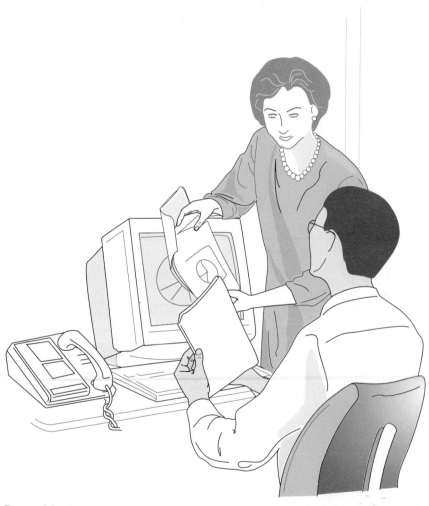

FIGURE 11–4.

Communication.

With this understanding, we can discuss typical communication within the HIM department. We discuss communication between

- Employees within the HIM department
- Employees within the health care organization
- HIM department personnel and physicians
- HIM department personnel and other departments
- HIM department personnel and outside agencies or parties

Employee-to-Employee Communication

Communication occurs between employees within the HIM department and throughout the organization. The type of communication may be verbal, written, or electronic. The communication is job-related and at times personal. Positive appropriate communication between employees enhances productivity.

Most important in a health care facility is that communication about or to patients should be kept confidential. Patient health information should be communicated in an appropriate method to employees as they need to know to perform their job.

Communication between employees and their immediate supervisors is very important. Employees need to know how their performance is perceived by management. They also need to be informed of changes in their work, processes, and functions that affect their daily operations.

Health Information Management Department and Physicians

The HIM department communicates routinely with physicians regarding record completion, release of information, continuity of patient care, and documentation of health information for utilization or reimbursement. Communication with a physician should be respectful. Consider the physician's time and make your communication appropriate. Let it be meaningful, brief if possible, and most important, *clear.*

Health Information Management Department and Outside Agencies or Parties

HIM departments often communicate with agents external to the organization. As discussed in Chapter 8, information should be released only according to applicable policy or state or federal law. Communication should be clear, preferably in writing, and it should provide information so that the recipient can return correspondence as necessary.

Written Communication

Written communication provides documentation of the message intended for the recipient. Therefore, written communication serves two purposes: It conveys a message and records it for later use. A common form of written communication in a health care facility is the memorandum, best known as the memo.

Written communication can be on paper or in electronic form. Written paper communication is typically in the form of a memo or letter. Electronic communication is performed via e-mail.

MEMOS

A **memorandum (memo)** is written or typed communication that informs others. A memo is used to provide clear, concise communication about a new procedure, process, or policy to all those affected by it (Fig. 11–5). The memo is more formal than verbal communication. Memos can be addressed to a group or an individual, but they are not as formal as a letter addressed specifically to an employee.

Memos can also serve as proof of communication to an employee. When a memo is shared with employees in a department, it may be posted in a highly visible and frequented place, for example, near the time clock or in the break room. At other times, memos are copied for each employee and handed to the employee personally by another staff member. Regardless of the means, the management wants to be sure that the message is communicated. One easy method for attaining confirmation of the employee's receipt of the memo is to have the employee initial a master copy of the memo. This method allows management to record employees' verification of their receipt, and preferably review, of the memo.

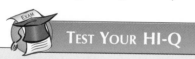

TEST YOUR HI-Q

Write a memo to your instructor to request permission from him or her to miss class because you would like to attend the AHIMA national convention.

Electronic Communication

Today it is extremely common for health care facilities to use a form of electronic communication called e-mail. This communication has changed the way we communicate. E-mail is expeditious if all parties are connected and responding. E-mail allows a message to be typed and sent via electronic means to another party or parties. The message is then kept in the other party's mailbox until he or she opens the message to receive it. E-mail is convenient because messages can easily be returned, forwarded, or saved. Because e-mail is a form of written communication, it is necessary to use appropriate grammar, punctuation, and etiquette when sending a message via e-mail.

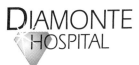

DIAMONTE
HOSPITAL   Diamonte, Arizona 89104 ▪ TEL. 602-484-9991

MEMO

TO: Health Information Management Employees

FROM: Michelle Parks, RHIA
        Director, Health Information Management

DATE: May 8, 2001

RE: Monthly Department Meeting

A Health Information Management department meeting will be held Thursday, May 31, in the hospital auditorium at 2:00 PM.

We will have a brief presentation by the Human Resources department followed by the regular monthly agenda. Please make necessary arrangements to attend this meeting.

Thank you.

FIGURE 11–5.
Memo.

HIT BIT

Do not type an e-mail message in all-capital letters. This is called screaming in e-mail language. Use capital letters sparingly, only to emphasize.

Avoid long messages. Keep the message brief and to the point.

If someone sends you an e-mail message that requires a response, be careful to reply to the sender as appropriate. Include the previous message so that the person knows why you are communicating a specific message.

In a business e-mail, end your message with your name, title, and business address, including phone numbers, as appropriate. You want the person to be able to contact you appropriately.

"Snail mail" is the United States Postal Service.

E-mail is not private. Be careful what you send via e-mail. Messages can be read by others, misdirected, etc. Therefore, send only what you feel comfortable expressing to the whole world.

Use punctuation appropriately.

E-mail is typically faster than snail mail. However, e-mail requires that the intended recipient *read* the message.

Department Meetings

HIM department meetings are another method of face-to-face communication. Department meetings should be held monthly, or more often as the need arises. A good way to schedule the meetings is to set aside one day each month for the meeting, for example, the last Thursday of each month. When this is done, employees and managers know when to expect the next department meeting. The meeting is an opportunity for the department to come together to discuss, learn, communicate, and share information. The department meeting is an ideal place to review policies and procedures (new and old) to make sure everyone understands the appropriate course of action. The department meeting is also a way to make sure everyone in the department hears the same message.

If your department is small to medium-sized, you may need to have only one meeting to communicate necessary information to all employees. However, if your department is larger, you may need to hold more than one meeting during different shifts to reach all employees.

All employees should attend the scheduled monthly HIM department meetings. When employees miss a meeting, they still need to hear the information. Therefore, posting or copying minutes from the meeting serves as notification for these employees. Also, employees should initial the attached transmittal memo indicating that they have read the minutes of the meeting.

Agenda

After the meeting is scheduled, how do you decide what to discuss? Regardless of the style of department meetings (formal or informal), you will need an

TABLE 11–4. HIM Department Meeting Agenda	
I.	Call to order
II.	Review of minutes
III.	Old business
IV.	New business
V.	In-service
VI.	Quality improvement
VII.	Announcements
VIII.	Adjournment

agenda so that you cover all of the necessary topics. Although agendas vary, Table 11–4 provides a typical agenda for a HIM department. A meeting offically begins with the call to order. This is the point at which the events of the meeting begin to be recorded. Employees know that it is time to stop the chatter and begin the meeting. Minutes from the previous meeting can be reviewed, depending on the formality of the meeting. Next any "old business" from the previous meeting is discussed. Occasionally, topics discussed in a meeting cannot be resolved without further investigation or information. Such topics are put under old business to be continued during the next meeting. Topics typically remain under old business until they are resolved, closed, or completed. The next item on the agenda is new business. At this time, new items may be introduced to the meeting. Then some normal course of business as appropriate is conducted during each monthly meeting: reports from sections within the department, quality management activities within the department and relating to the department, safety issues, and special announcements from the administration or about the facility.

HIT BIT

In order to conduct an orderly meeting, many managers have adopted some form of Robert's Rules of Order. These rules explain how business is conducted during the meeting. Employees become accustomed to a typical order. Meetings are formally called to order, the agenda is followed, and the meeting is concluded with adjournment. The rules explain how debate should proceed; and how motions can be made to present new business, make amendments, or vote on issues at hand. Likewise, there is a formal method for keeping track of old business on the agenda until it is resolved to the satisfaction of the meeting members.

Meeting

The HIM department meeting should be held in a place appropriate to the size of the department. A department with many employees will probably have multiple meetings to accommodate all employee schedules and shifts. A department with few employees may have one meeting during business hours in the

Health Information Management
Department Meeting
October 30, 2001

Employees present:

Employees absent:

Topic/Discussion	Recommendation/Action	Follow-up
I. Call to Order The Health Information Management meeting was called to order by Michelle Parks at 2:00 PM.		
II. Review of Old Minutes The minutes from the September Health Information Management department meeting were reviewed and approved as presented.		
III. Old Business **Uniforms** Employees in the department are interested in adopting a uniform as the dress code. During the previous meeting it was decided that the employees would invite three uniform companies to present at the next meeting. M & R Uniforms, Acorn Uniforms, and B & B Direct presented uniforms, pricing, and payment options to the employees.	After review of the information presented by all uniform companies the employees voted for the uniform and options presented by B & B Direct. The uniform company will return in 2 weeks to take orders and the dress code will take effect in 2 months.	11/2001
IV. New Business **HIPAA** Health Insurance Portability and Accountability Act has taken effect. Policies were presented and reviewed with the employees.		
V. Report Intradepartmental quality Interdepartmental quality		
VI. Safety/In-service		
VII. Announcements		
VIII. Adjournment With no further business to discuss the meeting was adjourned at 2:45 PM.		

Michelle Parks, RHIA

Date

FIGURE 11–6.

HIM department meeting minutes.

department. Be sure to consider the time of the meeting in case it is during the normal hours of operation. This may require that one employee miss the meeting or that you have an alternative method for covering the functions within the department while your employees are at the meeting. Be sure to have a sign-in sheet for all of the employees to sign as a record of their attendance at the meeting.

Minutes

Appropriate discussion and decisions from each meeting should be recorded for future reference. This type of documentation is called **minutes.** When preparing minutes, use the agenda as a guide to be sure that you have recorded the content or discussion surrounding each topic presented at the meeting. Review the minutes shown in Figure 11–6; notice how we have recorded the content of the topics discussed as presented at the meeting. Be careful to include only pertinent meeting information and participants' comments without mention of the participants' names in the minutes; do not include slander, slang, or irrelevant comments by the participants.

The minutes should clearly recall the events of the meeting as presented, discussed, and decided. The topics presented are documented under the column marked Topics/Discussion. The decision or action of the meeting members is documented under Recommendation/Action. The final column, Follow-up, identifies whether a topic has been closed, that is, the business for that topic is concluded. Most important, topics that are not finalized should be carried forward to the next meeting until the business is concluded.

Meeting Records

It is important to keep a precise record of each monthly meeting. These records will support any future business, discussion, and accreditation requirements. You can set up a file folder or a binder to organize each month's meeting information. Be sure to keep a copy of the agenda, the sign-in sheet, any attachments or handouts shared with the group, and the final draft of the minutes. The records from these meetings should be kept at least 3 years or as required by legal or regulatory bodies.

Web Sites

www.ahima.org
www.cyberbuzz.gatech.edu/apo/robert.html

CHAPTER SUMMARY

Training and development are critical to the success of an HIM department. New employees in the organization, quality improvement, technology, and policy and procedure changes are continuous reasons for employee training. Development of employees through in-services, continuing education, and communication enhances the HIM workforce.

REVIEW QUESTIONS

1. What is the purpose of orientation?

2. List and briefly explain the issues discussed in the organization orientation.

3. Identify two HIM functions that require annual (at a minimum) training of employees.

4. Explain the importance of the meeting agenda and minutes.

PROFESSIONAL PROFILE
HIM Assistant Director

My name is Michelle, and I am the health information management assistant director in a 220-bed facility, Oakcrest Hospital. This facility provides acute care, emergency services, skilled nursing, and ambulatory services. Our market share is somewhat unique, because we do not provide maternity and pediatric services. Our services are primarily adult and geriatric medicine. We have an HIM department with eight clerical and release of information employees under my responsibility, three coding employees with one coding supervisor, and eight transcription employees with one transcription supervisor.

In our department things are very organized, to the credit of our department director. New employees participate in the organization orientation before reporting to our department for work. During the first few days of employment, employees are oriented to the department. We begin with explaining the employee's job description and expectations (performance standards). Then the new employee goes through the department, sitting with each employee to learn about other HIM functions and how their jobs are related. Finally the employee is oriented to his or her new position. During this process, the employee also obtains a password for our computer systems.

I am responsible for organizing our monthly department meetings and choosing the in-service topic. I set up the agenda, copy and distribute any necessary handouts, and record the minutes. In addition, I coordinate any training required by changes in department policy, procedure, equipment, or federal and state mandates. The employees who report to me are cross-trained in several different functions so that we can cover work for lunch, breaks, vacations, and sick leave.

I really enjoy the training and development aspect of this position. It is rewarding to have a new employee succeed in his or her position, or to have an employee move up into a new position because of appropriate training and development.

APPLICATION

Create a Public Education Information Session

Research the current issues associated with health information. Choose a topic that requires education of the local community (public).

Using the training session information in this chapter, perform an assessment of community education needs, or decide on their educational needs using a new topic. In your preparation consider the audience, format, and environment in which the education will be provided. Prepare a paper presentation of this information for your instructor.

APPENDICES

Managing Personal Workforce Readiness

Jonathan L. Butler*
With an introduction by Nadinia Davis

Introduction

In 1975, microwave ovens were used primarily in professional kitchens. By 1985, they were common in many homes. By 1995, most homes had one, and the food industry had created whole lines of meals and cookware designed to be cooked in them. How did people learn how to use them? How do you know not to put metal utensils in a microwave?

In 1975, PCs had barely been invented. They were a novelty with very little memory, no hard drive, and only rudimentary software. Today, they are in offices, schools, libraries, and homes. Understanding their uses is a necessity in many businesses.

When automated bank cards were developed, many predicted that the average person would not use one. Today, the controversy is not over whether we will use them, but the fees we are being charged to do so!

In several television shows and movies, characters have been depicted as being identified by computer via retinal or fingerprint scan. That technology is actually in use today—how long do you think it will take to become commonplace? How will we learn how to use it?

Have you heard about a new type of computer clothing? Computer circuits are woven into the fabric so that input can be derived at various points on the body, particularly the hands. Data could be collected and downloaded by touch. Wild? Futuristic? Practical? Who knows? But 20 years down the road, it could become the standard in the fashion industry!

Several years ago, electronic books were a dream. Today, they are being advertised in magazines.

How do we keep up with all of this? Do we need to be in school forever? No—but we need to periodically re-evaluate our educational needs and find ways to obtain the knowledge that will help us to achieve our goals.

The purpose of this essay is to convince you that you certainly do need to keep up—that you should want to—and to assist you in figuring out how to do so. It will give you the business perspective: why you need to develop and implement a lifelong learning plan in order to optimize your career strategies. Then, it will explore some practical strategies for keeping yourself up-to-date and even expanding your knowledge in many areas.

We hope that you will find this information useful and practical as you look toward your own future.

*Jonathan Butler is Director of Adult Admissions at Berkeley College, West Paterson, New Jersey. He is a member of New Jersey Association of College Admissions Counselors and a past fellow of the John J. Heldrich Institute for Workforce Development at Bloustein School for Planning and Public Policy, Rutgers University, New Brunswick, New Jersey.

Beginnings

A great beginning! You've made the decision to go back to school. What's next? Where are you going to go? What are you going to study? Do you want a degree, a certificate, or just a class? What about your family, your boss? In fact, how are you going to pay for school? Where are you going to get the time to go to class? Do you still remember how to study, to take tests, or to write papers? What if you fail? Are you going to be the oldest one in class? The only one that doesn't use a computer?

So many questions! I hope I haven't talked you out of returning to school, but there are a few items to consider. In fact, in terms of the problems faced by adult learners returning to higher education, those problems are only the tip of a very large iceberg. Many potential adult learners who really want to return to school either put off their return, sometimes for years, or decide not to return at all. For some, the qualifier is that they cannot find a way to manage all of the obstacles that living in the world present. For others, the reason is their concern about where they will "fit in" within the collegiate community, or how they feel about their ability to handle academic material after years away from the classroom. As an adult learner, you may feel rusty when it comes to such things as your study skills and test-taking prowess, and thus you may have the perception that you are less well prepared than younger students.

Although most of these concerns may be very real for you, you'll be happy to learn that they are balanced against the fact that adult students do exceptionally well in formalized coursework. Adult students' maturity, clear focus and direction, and strong commitment support this phenomenon, as does the fundamental fact that the adult student has never stopped learning. Moreover, despite the once fashionable suggestion that learning is negatively affected as we get older, recent studies have shown exactly the opposite. A growing body of research supports the thinking that the purported adverse affects of aging on learning may be less important to adult students' success than the in-world experience of adult learners, something Sternberg and Wagner (1986) called "practical intelligence."

That being said, you may still feel a fair amount of dissonance surrounding elements of your self-concept that ultimately pit confidence (perception) against competence (reality), the "confidence-competence syndrome." Returning to the classroom can sometimes be framed as a process that includes the setting aside of the fears and anxieties that stem from negative self-perceptions in favor of an adventure that can ultimately be a positive and fulfilling rediscovered self-reality.

Later in the essay I discuss some of the most pressing concerns you may have and strive to help you develop a means to understand how these concerns, left to grow unfettered, become obstacles that can affect your ability to return to school. More importantly, I explore several positive things you can do to manage whatever obstacles life has strewn in your path, and more than that, will challenge you to begin to develop your personal strategy for success. Call it your personal *educational management plan.*

As a beginning, let's acknowledge that returning to school as an adult learner comes only after a change in thinking, a shift in perspective. It is almost an absolute among adult learners returning to campus that a well-designed, step-by-step plan is a prerequisite. Adult learners want information, they want questions answered, and they want no surprises. Adult learners want to see the whole picture right before their eyes, and preferably in living color. Information is the key to the adult learner's ability to schedule something as demanding as schooling into lives already stretched to the point of breaking. Because of that, adults need that information in clear detail. They want it now, not later.

The information exists, although it is sometimes difficult to sift through all the hyperbole to arrive at the fundamental facts you will require in order to clear all the hurdles. A neatly designed educational management plan will be the key to your surviving the process of returning to campus, a tool that can help reduce your anxiety by directing the search for information to those items that are essential for you.

The educational management plan is nothing more than a navigation chart, a step-by-step approach to managing the activities required to reach whatever educational goal you set forth. These activities are directed not only by academic considerations but more fundamentally by the need to manage personal circumstances that may otherwise become a hindrance.

Some important characteristics of an educational management plan are that *you* identify all of the issues that affect you, and *you* begin to gather information that will be of help to you as you work to overcome each of the potential obstacles. It is not something that someone else imposes on you; rather, it is a process of self-knowledge, self-study, and self-direction.

When you set your goals, you will need to develop a plan to achieve those goals, and that planning demands nothing less than a knowledge of self, honesty, and courage. Once you have set your goals, keep in mind that planning is a process refined in the execution and fulfilled in the attainment of the goal.

Organizing all of the variables—your family concerns, the finances, your scheduling—is nothing more than writing an equation, an equation that becomes the framework of your educational management plan. The solution to the equation is this: An educational management plan is a process of self-management.

In the final analysis, the process of self-management—that is, management of your education, your career, or any other aspect of your life—will be successful only to the extent that you are an active participant.

Sighting Your Target

You'll notice that we use the terms "adult learner" and "adult lifelong learning" throughout this essay. These terms have become popular recently as a result of the groundswell of adults returning to formalized education. The need to acquire and maintain skills in the workplace is certainly the primary driver, and rightly so, but actually getting started in an educational program is often a road fraught with peril.

It is difficult for prospective adult learners to see how beginning a program of study can actually become a reality. Some of the many well-founded concerns you may have as a prospective adult student begin with the understanding that your return to school will affect your personal time, your family, your finances, and your job schedule. You may find yourself faced with self-doubt concerning your academic abilities or study skills, particularly if you've been away from formalized education for a number of years. Many successful managers or executives thrive on the pressures of the office but tremble at the thought of a math class. . . .

You may also find yourself at odds with the importance you place on education: do you value education and your participation in educational endeavors, or do you look at it only as a means to an end, something you have to do to get ahead?

Adult learners who have had some success in the marketplace often have concerns about how they will feel as students again. Will they lose their independence, their status, their self-esteem? Consider this from Schlossberg et al (1989): "Older adults . . . are usually colleagues, mentors, or sponsors in their families, jobs, and communities. Suddenly these adults are Bill, Joe, and Anna, and those in charge, sometimes younger and with less experience, are 'Professor,' and 'Doctor'" (p 7). This might be seen as a problem by adult students, particularly if they are used to being nearer to the top of the hierarchy than they will be in a school setting. You may encounter this environment most often in traditionally modeled institutions, whose primary purpose has always been to serve students in earlier transitions, normally right from high school.

Even in those institutions that have acknowledged that separate issues exist for students from different age categories, there are still differences in the way they actually develop and deploy programs and services that support the needs of their nontraditional students. These nontraditional groups are easily differentiated and possess clearly defined needs. The profiles describe working people who need to take a certain amount of continuing education units per year to fulfill job requirements.

1. *Single parents.* Single parents are both male and female, and because they are raising children, they present a wide variety of service needs. These include child care, transportation, and career services that anticipate ongoing child-rearing needs, such as health care or flex scheduling. Don't overlook the basics of family subsistence as the adult, single-parent learner moves through the educational experience. The reality is that women as single parents are much more prevalent than men as single parents. Their needs are pressing and distinct and there is generally much more social program availability to help them through the process of education. Services such as Temporary Assistance to Needy Families (TANF) and other welfare public assistance programs are often available. These programs sometimes include

subsidies for education, transportation, and child care, as well as medical benefits for dependent children. In some instances, benefits extend into the postschooling period of employment so that the transition from school to career is manageable.

2. *Displaced homemakers.* Women returning to the workforce after many years of stay-at-home-mom activities have an impressive list of concerns. Often forced into the work world through the loss of a spouse as a result of death or divorce, these adult learners can require significant counseling. Counseling may address loss and grief, and these adults may need career counseling and academic counseling as well. Additionally, this group of students may have needs for knowledge of other social programs, such as welfare, simply to help them continue to maintain their households.

3. *Unemployed adults.* This segment of the adult learning population has a concern for fast, skills-centered education, followed by aggressive and effective placement services. Their primary need, particularly if they have a background that includes some years in the workforce, is for late-model educational programs that provide a competitive advantage for them in the workplace. Many times they have become disenfranchised workers as the result of organizational downsizing or because a company has chosen to relocate. The trend toward downsizing persists even during a strong employment economy.

4. *Late arrivers.* These are adults for whom school became a priority later in life, after career goals were fashioned. Many students who had not a clue about what they wanted to be when they grew up find that they can only begin to answer that question at age 25, or 30, or 35, or 40 . . . . These students are late arrivers. As more programs are created for adult learners, late arrivers will find more opportunity to chance a return to education.

5. *Skill seekers.* Skill seekers are students for whom competitive skills are a matter of job health. Simply stated, the workplace is changing, and this student is determined to change with it. People currently in a career in which they intend to remain are the backbone of this category and make up a large percentage of those returning to academia.

6. *Career changers.* Arguably, the largest category of adult learner, the career changer, is one for whom education is seen as the bridge to the rest of life. As I discuss later, changes in the marketplace and changes in technology can make career fields that were once viable less attractive in the light of new marketplace trends. Whether disillusioned with a career field or just interested in emerging opportunities, the career changer targets fields that he or she thinks will satisfy the need for achievement and advancement that is not present in the current occupation.

Once you identify your category, it will be important to find an institution that has the type of services you require. Not all institutions will even have considered the basic population characteristics described in the informal typology, which can have significant consequences for you as an adult learner.

As you may sense, there are more questions than answers: hard personal questions, life-stage questions, career orientations, child-care issues, and financial concerns, to name only a few. The process of discovery required to satisfactorily address these questions promises to be arduous. For many adult learners, even finding the time to get the information needed seems to be a daunting task. All too often, prospective adult learners stop right there. Those questions, and many more, hit hard and fast. Most adult learners can't answer them satisfactorily with the information they have at hand. Unanswered, they become obstacles that may seem insurmountable. When that happens, the first, and easiest, response is "Life goes on . . . forget school."

The reality is that life does go on, and so does technology. Technology in the workplace is the number one reason adults are coming back to school. Companies adopt new technologies seemingly every day, racing to compete in an increasingly complex marketplace, and the technologies require workers with new skills. As the global economy becomes more integrated, increased investment in foreign markets underscores the need for workers at every level to develop new perspectives in critical skills. These skills include pronounced abilities in interpersonal relations, forecasting, marketing, organizational development, diversity and cultural issues, and more; and that means a return to school. The staggering truth is that the whole nature of the marketplace has changed so much that it would be virtually unrecognizable to a person who retired only 10 years ago.

It is unsettling to realize that technology is driving change at so rapid a pace that neither business, workers, or educational delivery systems have a hope of catching up with new trends. By the time a college or university can design and implement a training program for a particular technology, it often has been replaced with a new technology.

Yet the need for workplace education, in the face of runaway technologic development, is rapidly reaching critical mass. Employers have an increasingly difficult time finding even entry-level workers with the skills needed to exist in the high-tech, high-skill environment that characterizes business today. On the other end of the spectrum, those who have navigated the workplace successfully for many years often realize that they need new skills simply to maintain their present level.

When we speak of *workplace education* we mean education that provides those skills that *employers* currently demand: hard skills, such as computer and other business machine usage, and soft skills, such as communications skills, team-building and leadership skills, as well as the ability to take responsibility and to be accountable for your work. These skills are not only entry-level skills. They are the critical skills needed by everyone at any stage of a career. As the practice of business continues to change, employers find themselves in need of senior people who can adapt to and manage change; people who can develop and successfully implement new models of business in an economy that demands innovation at every level.

In response to the challenges of the business world, senior-level managers are approaching the concept of adult lifelong learning with the same energy as those who are just beginning to climb the ladder. All are finding a wealth of educational offerings made available from a variety of sources. Without question, returning adult students can find courses in every venue from the traditional classroom, to the Internet, to the corporate training department. No longer are you relegated to endless hours in a classroom for no other reason than that is how education is delivered. (Unless that's what you want.) New educational methodologies are being implemented daily. In many colleges, it is possible for adult learners to design a program that uses a wide variety of the new delivery models, such as Internet-delivered distance education, guided study, contract courses, and telecourses, in addition to the traditional classroom courses. Students are also earning credit through portfolio assessments, vehicles that measure college-level learning that has been gained through life experience. In all, there is more flexibility and more availability of programs and services to the student than ever before. Truly, the nature of educational delivery has begun to change.

Adults are not the only group interested in workplace-targeted education. Our grammar and high schools, in the midst of unprecedented educational reforms and unprecedented pressures on the educational system, are beginning to speak the language of competency-based workplace education. The need for reform is clearly evidenced by the declining entry-level workplace skills of the traditionally schooled high school graduate. Standardized test scores for many years have reflected a need for better computational skills and the need for a stronger grasp of the language.

Our schools' abilities to graduate students with a reasonable chance of integrating into the workforce are severely challenged. The responsibility to make the system work rests not only with those charged with educational leadership but, more critically, in the ability of educators within the system to set aside traditional agendas and to embrace new methodologies and new technologies. Educators, and education, must become more responsive to the changing employment marketplace. Perhaps the foremost means to accomplish the goal of an effective educational system begins by identifying the evolving need for new skills that keep employees competitive, and by developing curricula and services that fulfill that need.

No longer can the primary impetus of education be the maintenance of a status quo long gone; its function can no longer be viewed as "to preserve society as it is, rather than to change it" (Merriam and Caffarella, 1991, p 274). The institution of education must change, dramatically and rapidly, if the hope is to maintain credibility against the revolutionary pace of the technologic world. The only postmodernist constant of the status quo is *change*. Struck with the incongruence of that dichotomy, the question of the sociocultural relevance of entrenched social institutions in an era of remarkable change begs an answer. Are our present social institutions, long recognized as the order-keepers, doomed to incineration in the fire of technologic revolution? or is there hope for institutional responsiveness to a newly articulated social order, a social order driven by the keepers of technology, rather than by those whose mission it is to preserve the traditional values of society as a whole? In the final analysis, our thinking about the mission of education is changing because of the new demands of the workplace.

The demographics of the workforce are interesting to consider as well. With a growing percentage of the workforce at or above middle age, there is the concern that skills learned 15 or 20 years ago have lost some of the punch they once had. Various estimates suggest that adults will have to go back to school at much more than twice the rate of those who are just graduating high school. Nearly three of four workers will revisit education in just the next decade. People at every level will come to realize that their survival within the economy depends on their continued—in fact, continuing—education. The unsettling reality is that your survival is at risk! So, what's your next step?

One of the hardest aspects of returning to school as an adult is choosing the right program of study. Much of the process is simplified if you have a clear understanding of your primary reason for returning to school. Is it for career advancement, or is it to pursue never-learned skills, or refresh aging skills? Your return to school may be for pure enjoyment or to achieve a goal long held but as yet unrealized. More often, adult learners returning to school are seeking a new career. All are great reasons for adults to go back to school. Knowing your particular goals will help you determine what you want to study. Once you make the decision to further your education, the hardest part of going to school still remains. You need a plan.

Planning

You may find some of the earlier comments especially understandable to your life situation, particularly if you are revisiting education because of workplace-based skill issues. How often have you said to yourself, "Someday I'm going to do . . ."? Yet, how often have you found yourself unable to take the first step? How do you change the statement "Someday I'm going to do . . ." to "Today I'm going to do . . ."? With all the difficulties that crop up when you begin to think about going back to school, your best response is probably to create a plan.

Planning is one of the most beneficial steps you can take to support your return to education. Much has been written on the benefits of planning and on all that goes into that activity, yet it is still the area in which I find prospective students to be hesitant. At the most basic level, planning is a first step, an initiative that sets the stage for action. The planning process, done well, not only creates a step-by-step approach to the achievement of your goal but fashions a mindset that is open to the possibility of ultimately achieving that which is set forth in the plan. That open mindset is a critical ingredient for success.

As an example of the need for an open mindset, consider a common experience among adult learners. The vast majority of the adult students that I have dealt with in the past 10 years have had to face their own lack of confidence in their ability to succeed in education. Many, if not most, adult students have experienced the confidence-competence syndrome referred to earlier. In that dynamic, students may actually possess the prerequisite knowledge base to tackle a subject area but at the same time lack the critical confidence in their own knowledge base that would enable them to succeed. Students who have not committed to a plan, who have not decided to take action, might never take a particular course because they suffer from a lack of confidence in their ability. At the same time, they may view *not* taking a course as a means to relieve the anxiety they feel as they contemplate their ability to succeed. Their inaction is negatively reinforced, and a barrier to success is formed.

If you find yourself in this situation you may also feel that it is more comfortable to do nothing, yet by denying yourself the opportunity to take a course you are actually reinforcing your inability to move forward. Fear of failure, founded on lack of confidence, can become a major obstacle to your success by stealing your ability to take action.

Many adults who outwardly profess a desire to return to college can go for years without actually setting foot on a college campus, only because inwardly they haven't faced a simple fear. That fear has become a subconscious wall through which they cannot pass.

Planning takes obstacles such as the confidence-competence syndrome apart by allowing you to set each step on the path in its proper place. It allows you to account for each perceived obstacle, and it allows you to focus on and develop strategies that solve these obstacles. Planning solves problems. Ultimately, as you become aware of the full range of obstacles with which you are faced, you become the driver of your plan. With an understanding of those issues that worked to formulate your worldview, your mindset, you have the knowledge needed to decide how you are going to proceed.

As you think about developing your plan to return to school, remember that your plan needs to speak to all of your issues—all of the things that have kept you from school and all of the reasons you want to return to school. The plan should account for all the issues and concerns in your daily life. Try to highlight the good things, as well as the bad. Take the time to determine all of your goals for education. Make a list of the steps involved to achieving those goals. Begin by taking an inventory of the things you have already done that may support your direction. List, also, those things you still need to complete in order to reach your goal. Don't forget to make a list of all the things that might stand in your way, as well as noting a short response to each of those concerns. Once that step is complete, you will have developed your basic strategy. Your plan may look like the following:

Goal: To gain knowledge of current computer applications so that I can operate the new computer system in the office.

Inventory: I already know basic computer applications.

Needs: I need specific courses in the following subjects:

1. Windows computer program
2. Word processing
3. Spreadsheets

Steps to Reach Goal:

1. Determine what school to choose*
   - Local college or university
   - Company-offered courses
   - Specialized school

   Concerns
   - What courses are offered?
   - How long is the program?
   - Do I get a certificate or college credit?
   - Is there financial aid available, and how do I apply?
   - What kind of class schedule is available?
   - What credentials do the faculty members have?

2. What are the potential obstacles?
   - Schedule around work and family
   - Money
   - Child care
   - Transportation

3. Plans to handle obstacles
   - Get schedule approval from employer.
   - Enlist spouse support for schedule.
   - Contact school's financial aid counselor to develop plan to pay for education.

*It is always a good idea to visit the schools you are thinking of attending. Pay attention to the environment and the equipment used, if appropriate, and ask plenty of questions about the subjects that concern you. If a school will not, or cannot answer your questions, rule it out. Never settle for less than the best.

It's not important that your plan look like the one above; in fact, it will likely be much more detailed than the plan presented in the figure. What is important is that your plan be a format in which you have asked all the questions for which you need answers.

Remember, if it might become a problem someday and you do not address it now, it could very well prove to be unsolvable when it comes up later. Anything that you think *can* come up as an issue, most likely *will* pop up right in the middle of your best laid plans, and at absolutely the worst time. If it seems as if it could be a problem, put it on your plan.

You have heard that terrible but unfortunately true cliché that "the hardest part of the journey is the first step," so don't expect this part of your work to be easy. It's usually not, but planning will help you avoid costly missteps. When you finish, you will have a step-by-step strategy, a clear road to achieving your goals. More importantly, planning helps you identify potential pitfalls.

Be sure that your planning doesn't leave you with just a list of all the obstacles that stand in your way and no answers to help solve them. You will be better served if you talk with professionals in education. A good advisor may be able to provide you with the specific information you need to make a sound decision. You will find that it is easy to talk yourself out of pursuing education if you do not have answers to the specific questions that affect you. When those questions are answered, you will have eliminated all of the reasons that stopped you from going back to school. Let's discuss some of the usual areas that must be visited by prospective adult learners.

Choosing a School

An important aspect of going back to school is choosing the right school for you. Today, there are more opportunities than ever before to further your education, but not all of these opportunities may be appropriate for your needs. Differences in schools are much more than just the superficial measurements of curriculum, price, and location. Some of the more subtle differences lie in areas such as accreditation; the quality of instruction available; the actual course content; the range of student services offered, including advising and tutoring; and laboratory time, if appropriate. Ask if a mechanism for the assessment of prior learning exists, and ask if there are there any hidden charges not detailed up front.

All of these are important considerations as you shop for a school, and they should be thoroughly researched. Schools that are fundamentally different may look very much alike at first, particularly if you are shopping through the newspaper or yellow pages of the telephone book. It is safe to say that every organization that advertises to the public tries to project an image that will attract customers. It should be no surprise that so many competing schools advertise such a tremendous similarity in goods and services. That similarity often ends at the door. Services must be appropriate to your needs if they are to have any value at all for you. Additionally, they must be accessible to you. Great services, well designed in concept and effectively deployed by the institution, can be a tremendous advantage to you, supporting you at critical times in your academic career. More often, great ideas, hampered by too little in the way of deployment, become a source of frustration and disappointment to students who find no realistic approach that actually allows them to take advantage of the promised benefits to be derived from "services." Check with the institutions you are considering so that you can determine whether their programs and services speak to your needs.

The best way to determine the right school for you is to visit the admissions office and ask questions. Get a tour of the area in which your program is offered. Ask about your program of interest, and find out what subject matter is covered to see if it is what you want. Remember that differences often exist in courses from several schools, even if they all have the same course title. Conversely, schools may have differently titled courses that cover the same material. Ask about the faculty and about the credentials they hold. Find out if there is a tutoring service or if there is an extra charge associated with any aspect of their services. Ask about laboratory time and accessibility. Also ask about accreditation and the availability of financial aid. Finally, ask about the admissions process and what steps you need to follow to gain entrance to the institution. Let's touch on several of the more important items you will want to ask about.

Accreditation

Accreditation is much too complex a subject to fully discuss here, but there are general differences that exist even among accredited schools that can make one institution more appropriate than another for you. Basically, accreditation indicates that the institution has been found to maintain certain quality standards. Accreditation says, also, that the institution continually seeks to evaluate and improve its offerings, according to the recommendations of the accrediting body with whom it has elected to be associated.

Young and associates, in *Understanding Accreditation* (1983, pp 17–18), observe that "Accreditation began as a relatively simple idea—a voluntary effort by a small group of educational institutions to agree on standards for distinguishing a college from a secondary school. Over the past seventy years or so, however, accreditation has matured and changed into a much more sophisticated process for evaluating and improving educational quality in colleges, universities and comparable institutions." Not all accreditations are alike, however, and this is an area about which you need to ask questions, particularly if an accreditation may affect the overall value of the courses in which you have an interest.

At a basic level, post–secondary schools may be accredited by a variety of different types of accrediting agencies, depending on their overall mission as well as a host of other factors. Schools can become accredited at a collegiate level or as a career training institution. Institutions may have a specialized accreditation that permits them to offer specialized certificates, degrees, or diplomas. Additionally, some institutions offer courseware accredited by manufacturers, such as many of the current computer certifications that are available.

A simple rule of thumb is that when you need college credit, a professional designation, or a certification, it is important to make certain that the institution you choose has the appropriate accreditation. Ask questions! If you have a doubt about the responses you are getting or feel that you need more information, check with the accrediting body. That will help to determine if the institution and the proposed course complement your needs. There is no sadder student than one who finds out in the 11th hour that the course he or she has been diligently working on, at great expense of money and time, does not fulfill the goals that he or she originally established. Avoid that outcome at all costs, and do so simply by asking questions and making certain that you get the answers.

Financial Aid

Financial aid programs in the United States are excellent and are available for many types of study. You should know that financial aid includes both grants and loans. Grant programs are financial aid vehicles that are awarded usually on a need basis and do not require you to make repayment. Loans, on the other hand, require that you return the money to the lender, just as you would any other type of loan. Obviously, everyone wants grants, but for federal and state aid programs you will have to qualify financially in order to be considered. You should check with your institution regarding any of its grant and scholarship programs for which you may apply. The availability of these programs, as well as the requirements for participation, vary from institution to institution.

There are specific institutional and programmatic requirements that schools must meet to participate in federal and state financial aid programs. Not all schools will have exactly the same financial aid programs. Ask the admissions office what they can offer regarding financial aid, and do not forget to ask if there is institutional aid available for any of their programs. Funding from other sources may be available as well, and information about those sources should be available at your chosen institution.

Just as institutions must meet certain qualifications, you will also have to demonstrate that you qualify for the various financial assistance programs in existence. Your institution's financial aid office often can make a determination of your eligibility very quickly. Keep in mind that not all courses of study will have financial aid eligibility. Ask questions.

Your employer may offer tuition assistance programs as a part of your benefits plan. The company may have specific controls of that benefit, both for the type of program that qualifies and on the grades you must achieve to be considered eligible to participate. If you are not sure, see your company's human resources department for details.

Additionally, recent legislation has passed that provides specific tax credits that may be applicable to you. The Hope Tax Credit and the Adult Lifelong Learning Credit are new tax credits that can help you with the cost of tuition. These credits can be beneficial as you structure your financial plan for school. To find out more about these programs, contact your institutions financial aid office or your accountant, or call the Internal Revenue Service.

A word of encouragement: It is extremely difficult to determine exactly how you are going to afford to go to school until you get all the information from your institution of choice. A school may seem at first to be too expensive for you to consider, but after the financial aid research is done, you may find that it is surprisingly affordable. Don't make decisions without complete information. Get the facts!

At most schools, your process for receiving financial aid will begin with the Free Application for Federal Student Aid (FAFSA). Institutions commonly have an institutional application as well that you will be required to complete. Sometimes you will be required to mail in the FAFSA and wait for a response to determine your eligibility. That can take 8 to 12 weeks, or more. If you are asked to go through a waiting process by your institution, you will need to start the process well before you anticipate going to school. More often, institutions, particularly those specializing in providing services to adult learners, will have developed a streamlined, customer-oriented approach to financial qualification that can reduce your total application process to a matter of minutes.

In very general terms, federal and state financial aid programs normally require that you are either a citizen or a permanent resident as a basic qualification for eligibility. Additionally, males will have had to register for selective service in the United States prior to their 26th birthday. When you meet with the financial aid office, you will be asked to submit various personal records, including your Social Security card, driver's license, birth certificate, or county identification card, as well as your current federal tax filing. Be prepared, as well, to submit information about your personal finances, such as mortgages, bank accounts, and retirement funds, all of which may be required to determine your eligibility. Check with your institution to be sure that you know exactly what documentation it needs you to provide.

Choosing a Course of Study

Do you know what you want to study? If you do, you are more of a rarity than you might realize. The variety of program choices is almost overwhelming, and making a decision about the one that is right for you can be complicated. Often, the choice of subject matter is dictated by the requirements of your job. For example, your company changes to a new computer system. You realize you do not know anything about the capabilities of the system. You decide to take some computer classes. Your problem is solved. If you are in this category, consider yourself lucky. In other circumstances, your choice of a program of study may relate more to a career change.

That's when things can get more complicated.

Marketplace Factors

Can there be anything more difficult than changing your career? It is perhaps the most fear-producing, anxiety-creating, emotionally draining, exasperating process that you can go through. At the same time, it can also be beneficial to your financial and emotional well-being in the long run. The process of career changing requires your total commitment, certainly, but even more importantly, it requires your action.

Career changing is something that the average worker will accomplish several times in his or her working life, sometimes by choice and sometimes by circumstance. In either case, it can be difficult. Whether you make the choice or a choice is made for you, finding your new direction will take concentrated effort. Let's take a look at some of the reasons that career changing has become such a phenomenon.

To begin, you need only look at the same changes in technology and their consequent effect on workers' skills to get a clear understanding of the forces underlying career changing. The rapidity with which skill sets must be upgraded drives both corporations and workers to constantly evaluate their needs. Dramatic evidence of this was presented in the late 1980s and early 1990s as hundreds of thousands of workers were downsized. Many pointed at the recession of 1988 to 1992 as the cause of these downsizings. The recession, particularly in the Northeast, was arguably the deepest and most profound economic downturn since the Great Depression. Although the recession may have contributed to the trend, it was not the cause. What was the cause? The short answer, of course, is technology.

The same technologic progress that continues to create opportunity in today's employment marketplace caused a wholesale slaughter of jobs during that period of time. Almost everyone knows or knew someone who was affected by "re-engineering." In fact, at a recent presentation I gave to a group of workers in a large high-tech company, three of five workers had themselves been downsized in the previous 5 years. Many had been "reorganized" more than once, and a good handful had met that fate as many as five times! It was no surprise that all were eagerly attentive to the subject of adult lifelong learning.

Back to the cause. The last recession was the end of a process that actually had begun many years before. The process developed into a full-blown structural economic shift that changed the makeup of the workforce from largely manufacturing to an economy built around information and services. It was as dramatic a shift as the one that occurred during the Industrial Revolution, and many of us will not see another as profound in our lifetime.

A spinoff result, perhaps even more disturbing, is that a rising angst swept throughout the workforce. People who had grown up believing that they would be able to get a good job and keep it until retirement were faced with the imminent possibility that they would be the next casualty of an economy seemingly in crisis. Whether they actually felt the blade of the axe or not, their confidence and their belief in the workplace was challenged. We will debate for years the extent to which the culture of work, deeply embedded in the psyche of Americans, has been perhaps irreversibly altered. What import that holds for the continuing economic health of the country is certainly a question worth pondering.

The economy, after all, was not in crisis. It was redefining itself in response to the increased demands of globalization and technologic innovation. The United States was shifting from a great industrial and manufacturing giant to one that would be the leader in service and information management. The advent of the knowledge economy, of the imagination-based economy, did not occur without some suffering and uncertainty. As we lost traditional industrial-society manufacturing jobs, we added service and technical jobs. Unfortunately these jobs required skills that a large percentage of downsized workers did not possess. Many workers laid off during that upheaval found that not only was their job gone, but their whole industry had vanished. For those workers, the choice was a simple one: Get new skills . . . fast!

Personal Factors

Workers responding to changes in the economy certainly account for a good percentage of adult learners, but it is not the only arena in which people find a need for retraining.

Large numbers of women, re-entering the workforce after raising a family or after the loss of a spouse through death or divorce, are seeking updated educational credentials.

This group of prospective adult learners presents a host of special needs such as child care and, often, transportation. As students, this group benefits from academic programs such as orientation and advising and from social programs such as peer groups and personal counseling.

More often than not, career changers just "hit the wall" in their career and decide, once and for all, that it's time to do something about getting a good job. There are those, as well, who had decided to take a year off after high school, prior to college, and before they knew it, 5 or 10 years flew by, and in the end, college became just a dream sacrificed to family concerns, bills, and time.

Career Requirements

If you are in the midst of managing your career, you may find that there is a demand for you to add a certain number of continuing education units (CEUs) to your résumé each year. In many industries, CEUs can be obtained through industry-sponsored seminars, normal college courses, or various professional certifications. However they are offered, make it your business to collect at least the minimum number of CEUs. Your position in your industry will be stronger with a more specialized education.

Personal Workforce Readiness

No matter what your circumstances, it is your responsibility to make sure that you are ready for the job market. The new economy demands a skilled workforce, and those with the skills will get the jobs. Those found wanting will become the new poor within a class system defined by knowledge, rather than by race or gender.

The days of companies' displaying loyalty to their workers are all but gone, perhaps for good. In the past, workers right out of high school could, and did, go to work for a company, get educated through the company, and stay on for a long and prosperous career. When the company needed them to know more, the company would train them. In today's economy, that kind of corporate involvement in worker career development is quickly being replaced. The whole issue of worker-company loyalty is being hotly debated, and workers are looking at companies in new ways. Employers in the new economy may tend to value workers only insofar as their skills meet corporate needs for that knowledge base. When the company no longer has that need, the employee may find her- or himself back on the market. Recent headlines bear out the truth of this: The news of a continued low unemployment rate was juxtaposed against a news item relating the restructuring of a pharmaceutical company, along with the downsizing of more than 300 people.

On the other hand, the relationship of the worker to the employer increasingly results from the perceived value of the worker's association with the employer. When that perceived value is diminished, the worker will no longer desire to maintain the relationship. Job-hopping has become prevalent, and in some industries it is used to quickly build a worker's base salary. Loyalty is reduced to the convenience of the moment, rather than being a function of sociocultural belief. It is that shift in behavior and in thinking that most clearly defines what can only be viewed as a fundamental shift in the culture of work.

Today it is the worker's responsibility—your responsibility—to value and protect your personal workforce readiness. No matter your circumstance, you are the driver of your career. You are the one who determines how high you climb. If you have the desire, the drive, and the motivation, there are no barriers to developing a good career today, save one—education. It's simply your choice.

The concept of personal workforce readiness is a valuable weapon that will arm you against the vagaries of the marketplace. It represents your taking control of your circumstances and not your circumstances' being the reason that you fail. It represents your reaching for your highest dream, one step at a time, empowered by your own dreams. There is no secret to building a dynamic career. You just set your goal, find out what is required, put yourself in motion, and go and do it.

Personal workforce readiness says that you understand that you are responsible for your skill level, and that you will do what it takes to gain that knowledge. No one else can do it for you. You must do it for yourself. That is the cold reality of the postmodern economy, but there is more. Once educated is not enough! Once we are educated, we must begin again to make certain that our skills keep pace with the needs of the marketplace. It is truly the age of lifelong learning.

Where do you fit? Downsized; divorced; single mom; career that never got off the ground? Maybe you are academically underprepared? Whatever your circumstances, there are programs that are right for you, choices for you to make. It all comes down to you.

Here are a few real-life examples for you to consider.

Name: Barbara   *Age: 23*

Barbara is a divorced mother of two children who had been collecting welfare. She had attained a high school diploma and married soon afterward. The children came next, but over the years the marriage turned sour. After surviving a few too many beatings, Barbara left the house with her children and moved into a shelter for battered women. In time she qualified for public assistance, but she became desperate to get a career that would allow her the opportunity to raise her family. As soon as she felt able, she decided to investigate the possibilities of college.

Barbara shopped for a college and finally was accepted at a small, private college in the Northeast. Tuition was high, but the financial aid that was available to her because of her circumstances made it possible for her to go to school. Barbara worked hard and was able to graduate with an associate degree and with a high grade point average. The hard work paid off, and Barbara was offered significant scholarships toward her 4-year degree at a prestigious university.

When last we spoke, Barbara was planning to start in the next class toward her 4-year degree. She had begun the process in desperation. Her life had been filled with uncertainty and fear at the prospect of struggling to raise her children. She has become a confident, secure, and engaging person, with bright prospects for a future that will let her care for her children.

For Barbara and for her children, the process of education was a lifesaver. More than that, participating in education was the result of Barbara's overcoming serious obstacles. She overcame not only financial obstacles, but also deep personal obstacles that stemmed from a self-esteem that was dismantled during the years of her marriage. Her success is the result of her inner strength and conviction, and ultimately of her persistence. It was her choice!

Name: Bob   Age: 44

Bob works for a major communications company, with a solid career in the information technology field. Bob has always looked to further his education in order to make himself more marketable, and he has taken several courses over the years. Recently, Bob began a course for professional certification in a computer network administration program. This certificate will further protect his personal workforce readiness. The best thing is, his company paid for the course!

Name: Francine   Age: undisclosed

Francine is a graduate from a local university with a degree in a field that became no longer technically relevant. Although she was still employed, she realized that her days were numbered within the profession, and needed to do something to protect herself. Her choice was between retraining for the field she was already in, or looking for another career where future growth was more ensured. Francine chose to pursue a degree in another field and is working toward an associate degree. Because she is married, there were some scheduling issues that she needed to work out with her spouse. Adults often find that scheduling family time around schooling is difficult, and for some, impossible. Francine was lucky to have a spouse who supported her return to school unconditionally.

Name: George   Age: 46

George has developed a successful career in a dynamic field through hard work and good luck. His problem is that he doesn't have a degree. He feels that he really does need one in order to remain marketable. George looked closely at the various degree programs available to him, and he chose a program that made use of distance learning and guided study, rather than traditional class-room courses. George is looking forward to earning his bachelor's degree soon, and he has talked about pursuing a higher degree in the future. In George's case, having the availability of a course schedule that could be fitted into his schedule was the only way that he ever could have returned to school.

Name: Nina   Age: 37

Nina worked as a secretary for many years, but eventually her company was closed, and Nina became a "displaced worker." More than that, she was having a hard time finding new employment because her skills were not current.

Nina found out from her employment counselor that there was funding for worker retraining available to her through her state unemployment office.* She met with the counselor and soon qualified for the funding. Nina elected to be trained on current computer software and selected a program at a local college. Under the terms of the state retraining program, there was no cost to her. With her newly acquired skills, she had no problem finding new employment. No one will ever say she isn't smart—now she's enrolled in another course that will lead to a college degree. Nina plans to be ready the next time she is downsized.

Name: Patricia   Age: 36

Patricia is a divorced mother of two children. The children, both of whom are learning impaired, require more than the usual care given to other children, and Patricia spends countless hours driving them to various speech and learning therapy appointments. As a result of the divorce, Patricia was forced to add work to her schedule, and she went back to her former business. Patricia always regretted not pursuing her education, particularly in that she had done extremely well in high school. She now began to recognize a pressing need for a career that was more stable, a career that would provide benefits, such as medical insurance and retirement, and an opportunity for her to use her brains.

Her decision to return to school took some time to bear fruit. First she started collecting college catalogs to see what was available. Actually getting started was another story. To begin with, she felt a great deal of anxiety, even fear, at the thought of going back to school. And, of course, there was the matter of the children, her work schedule, and the money.

---

*Most states have programs for worker retraining. If you are down-sized, see your local employment office for information about the training programs available to you.

Finally she decided that it was now or never, and visited a local college, where she was able to get some career counseling. She found a subject major that she thought would work well for her and applied for the program. She had to take an entrance test, and after being away from school for almost 20 years, that test caused her some anxiety. To her surprise, and relief, she scored very high on the test and was accepted to the program.

There was still the matter of the money. How would she be able to pay for the cost of college and still run her household? The counselor had suggested a step-by-step approach to the whole process, so she met with the college financial aid officer. She found that she was eligible for a combination of state and federal grants, as well as a student loan. Much to her surprise, the college found that she was eligible for an institutional grant that covered almost half of the total cost. With the other financial aid programs that she qualified for, her out-of-pocket expenses were reduced to fees and books! That she could handle!

Before she knew it, classes had started—to her surprise (and delight) she had actually made it back to school. When I asked her how she was doing, she said that she was doing great. She had made friends from 18 years old to "whatever" (many years older than she). That solved what had been a source of anxiety because she hadn't known if she would fit in, or if she would wind up to be the oldest one in the class. And although she is sometimes annoyed with younger students, who don't take the opportunity to get an education as seriously as they might, she did say, "You know, I love talking to adults again."

The preceding examples are all taken from real students' accounts, and it is easy to see that they all had different concerns. All were able to overcome whatever obstacles they faced and make a difference in their own lives through their own actions. In the various examples you can see some of the obstacles these adults had to overcome as they came back to school. It was not easy for any of them, and I know that at times many of them thought it was going to be impossible. They all valued and protected their ability to survive in the economy, their personal workforce readiness.

"Great for them," you say, "but how do I choose a career with a future?"

Choosing a New Career

Most of the prospective students I talk with share a common problem when it comes to career changing. "What do I change to?" "What's hot?" "What does the future hold?"

Tough questions for most of us, and tougher still if it's your question and you are faced with maintaining your lifestyle and that of your family. There are several ways that finding out what is available to you can be accomplished.

You can begin by visiting your local library. Ask for a copy of the U.S. Department of Labor's *Occupational Outlook Guide*. That publication can tell you the projected need for workers in a particular field. If there is a good growth projected, you may want to consider the field. Conversely, if the field is dwindling, you might decide not to select it, even if it's something you've been interested in for a time. A great benefit to researching in this way is that you will get to look at career titles with which you have no familiarity, either because they are new fields or because you simply had not known that they existed. More importantly, you are starting outside of yourself, outside your normal frame of reference, with new information that is topical and relevant.

Another great source of information is your local college. Make an appointment with admissions or academic counselors. These are often professionals skilled at identifying your strengths and weaknesses. With you, they may be able to help explore some of the careers you are considering and offer insight into the requirements of those careers.

I recently attended an information technologies career fair. The advertisement said to bring your degree and résumé and interview with hundreds of companies. The advertisement peaked my curiosity, and I had to go and see what the companies were looking for in employees. True to their word, there were hundreds of companies there with literally thousands of positions available. This is a great way to get an inside look at what's hot, and what employers require in order to hire you. Look in your local Sunday newspaper for similar events in your area, and go.

Another very productive area to research is professional trade associations. Once you have selected a small number of possible career choices, get in touch with any applicable trade associations to see exactly what they say is going on within the field. Often they will tell you what educational requirements work well in their field and what trends they are following. You can usually find them on the Internet. Naturally, not all career fields can be referenced to a trade association, but use them when you can for up-to-date information. You can also find out what is available by going online to company Web sites, where specific high-demand positions are sometimes advertised.

Not to be overlooked is your local newspaper. The weekly classified section may not be a great way for you to find a new career, but it will give you an interesting look at what is advertised, and sometimes, what the requirements are for certain fields.

Internet-based job networks provide a database in which to search for jobs in your market area and retrieve complete listings in a matter of seconds. You can post your résumé for reference by employers, and you can often establish contact with the employer.

Lastly, network with everyone you know. That includes "headhunters" who populate the search firms. Employment search firms can give you an insider's look at what careers they represent, what requisites you need to be considered by their clients, and what kind of money you can expect. Talk with friends and acquaintances. When you ask people what they do for a living, also ask them how they chose that career and what education is required. You'll find that most people gladly share information with you, and if you find someone with a career that matches your direction and interests, ask for their help. Most people will offer whatever help they can give as you try to develop your own way.

These are a few examples of ways to search for information on careers. Once you start your research, you will be surprised at how much information about various careers you can find. Use your imagination and have fun with the exploration. When you find something that you like, determine exactly what you need to do in order to participate in that career field, and simply go and do it. In the end, success is just a matter of persistence.

Here is a thought for you to consider:

> Nothing in this world can take the place of persistence. Talent will not; nothing is more common than unsuccessful people with talent. Genius will not; unrewarded genius is almost a proverb. Education will not; the world is full of educated derelicts. Persistence and determination alone are omnipotent. The slogan "press on" has solved, and always will solve the problems of the human race.
>
> Calvin Coolidge

So stated, we leave the topic of career changing with a simple, profound directive: Press on!

Career Building

If you are happy with your field, there are many action steps that you can follow if you want to continue your growth within the field. Almost invariably, education stands right at the top of the list. Many fields today require a certain amount of continuing education units each year. These are usually thought of as the minimum training standards necessary to maintain relevance in the field. If you want to get ahead, though, you may have to do a great deal more than that.

One of the best ways to grow your career is to look at the positions above you on the organizational chart and begin to research the requirements for those jobs. You can call your supervisor or your human resources office for good career planning advice. Ask what is required for certain positions, and don't forget to ask how you can qualify for those positions that interest you. Find out what skills are needed, what credentials, and what experience is preferred. Getting to the end of the road once you have developed that map is not all that difficult. Just go and do the things that these people told you were necessary in order for you to move up.

When more education is recommended, prospective students often feel daunted by the process of continuing their education. Finances and schedule are concerns, as we mentioned earlier, but the most daunting of obstacles might just be the prospect of taking the time required to complete whatever program is indicated. If what you need is an associate degree and you have only a high school diploma, the 2 years required to get the degree may seem like a mountain that is not scalable. If you need a master's degree that requires 42 credits and you're faced with 4 years of part-time matriculation, you may quickly lose your resolve. Sometimes even if you are faced with a short program for a certificate or professional certification, you might fall victim to the "what if's" and not be inclined to continue.

To succeed, you must set aside any thoughts of time and plunge forward! The time required to get your credential is not important. Getting your credential is the prize.

Keep in mind that whether you take the time to get what you need in order to succeed or not, the time will nevertheless go by. As long as you live, you will get to the end of that time, either with credential in hand or not!

Final Thoughts

The pace of change, in our patterns of work, in our economy, in our thinking about institutions that drive our economy, will not slow. It's likely that just the opposite will occur. You will be forced to achieve more, work more, control more, and do it faster and longer with less in the way of resources. You will have to know more. You will need more skills, more weapons, just to survive. It is likely, as well, that those who can't compete will become increasingly disenfranchised. Not a comforting thought.

I have detailed some useful strategies for you to help you through the ongoing process of remaining competitive. The concept of personal workforce readiness can be adopted as a personal philosophy, a self-director of activities that result in your ability to manage your career development and enhancement.

The pace of economic development and technical innovation will rapidly escalate. Change is inevitable and usually uncomfortable. There are several choices that you have as you face continuous change: You can identify yourself as a *leader of change,* welcoming the opportunities that changing circumstances articulate, and leading people through the process of adaptation that results.

Just as easily you can become an *agent of change.* You may not lead the charge perhaps, but you can be comfortable enough in a changing environment to implement new processes and procedures and to facilitate their use by others.

The first two characterizations are of people who are secure, involved, and open-minded, and who are not entrenched in the view that the way things should be is what they used to be. They accept change as inevitable and welcome the prospect of affecting the outcome.

More than that, these active participants prepare themselves to meet unexpected challenges, and because of that, they have the skills necessary to greet change eagerly and effectively.

There also exist those who never seem to be on the right side of the curve. These individuals can't or don't want to see the patterns of change that play out before them. They are invariably underprepared for change and as a result become *victims of change.* Your choice, though not easy, will prepare you to play one of those roles: a leader of change, an agent of change, or a victim of change. Your choices will determine the course of your journey.

What road will be yours?

References

Merriam SB, Caffarella RS: Learning in Adulthood: A Comprehensive Guide. San Francisco, Jossey-Bass, 1991.

Schlossberg NK, Lynch AQ, Chickering AW: Improving Higher Education Environments for Adults. Responsive Programs and Services from Entry to Departure. San Francisco, Jossey-Bass, 1989.

Sternberg RJ, Wagner RK: Practical Intelligence: Nature and Origins of Competence in the Everyday World. Cambridge, England, Cambridge University Press, 1986.

Young KE, Chambers CM, Kells HR, et al: Understanding Accreditation. Contemporary Perspectives on Issues and Practices in Evaluating Educational Quality. San Francisco, Jossey-Bass, 1983.

GLOSSARY

abstract

A summary of the patient record.

abstracting

The extraction of selected fields from a health record to create an informative summary.

access

The ability to learn the contents of a record, by obtaining it and/or having the contents revealed.

accreditation

Voluntary compliance with a set of standards developed by an independent agent, who periodically performs audits to ensure compliance.

activities of daily living

Refers to self-care, such as bathing, as well as cooking, shopping, and other routines requiring thought, planning, and physical motion.

acute care facility

A hospital with an average length of stay less than 30 days, an emergency department, operating suite, and clinical departments to handle a broad range of diagnoses and treatments.

admission record

The demographic, financial, socioeconomic, and clinical data collected about a patient at registration. Also refers to the document in a paper record that contains these data.

agenda

A tool used to organize the topics to be discussed during a meeting.

aggregate data

A group of like data elements compiled to provide information about the group.

allied health professionals

Health care professionals who care for patients or support patient care in a variety of disciplines, including occupational therapy and physical therapy.

ambulatory patient classifications (APCs)

A prospective payment system for ambulatory care, based on medically necessary services.

American College of Surgeons (ACS)

National professional organization of surgeons.

441

analysis	The review of a record to evaluate its completeness, accuracy, compliance with predetermined standards, or other criteria.
assembly	The reorganization of a paper record into a standard order.
assessment	An evaluation. In medical decision-making, the physician's evaluation of the subjective and objective evidence. Also refers to the evaluation of a patient by any clinical discipline.
attending physician	The physician who is primarily responsible for coordinating the care of the patient in the hospital; it is usually the physician who ordered the patient's admission to the hospital.
audit trail	A computer log of computer processing and access activities.
authenticate	To take responsibility for data collection or the activities described by the data collection by signature, mark, code, password, or other means of identification.
average length of stay (ALOS)	The arithmetic mean of the lengths of stay of a group of inpatients.
baseline	A beginning value; the value at which an activity is originally measured, such as the first blood pressure reading at an initial physician's office visit.
bed count	The actual number of beds that a hospital has staffed, equipped, and otherwise available for occupancy by patients.
behavioral health facility	Medical facility that focuses on the treatment of psychiatric conditions.
benchmarking	An improvement technique that compares one facility's process with that of another facility with noted superior performance.
billing	The process of submitting claims or rendering invoices.

brainstorming	A data-gathering quality improvement tool used to generate information related to a topic.
business record rule	An exception to the hearsay rule. Allows health records to be admitted as evidence in legal proceedings because they are kept in the normal course of business, recorded concurrently with the events that they describe, and are recorded by individuals who are in a position to know the facts of the events that are described.
capitation	The reimbursement to a health care provider based on the number of patients, regardless of diagnoses or services rendered.
case management	The coordination of the patient's care and services, including reimbursement considerations.
case mix	Statistical distribution of patients according to their utilization of resources. Also refers to the grouping of patients by clinical department or other meaningful distribution.
census	The actual number of inpatients in a facility at a point in time, usually midnight.
certification	Approval by an outside agency, such as the federal or state government, indicating that the health care facility has met a set of predetermined standards.
character	A single letter, number, or symbol.
charge capture	The systematic collection of specific charges for services rendered to an inpatient.
Chargemaster	The database that contains the detailed description of charges related to all potential services rendered to an inpatient.
charges	Fees or costs.
chart locator system	A system for locating records within a facility.
children's hospital	A specialty facility that focuses on the treatment of children.

claim	The application to an insurance company for reimbursement.
classification	Systematic organization of elements into categories. For example, ICD-9-CM is a classification system that organizes diagnoses and procedures into categories, primarily by body system.
clinical data	All of the medical data that have been recorded about the patient's stay or visit, including diagnoses and procedures.
clinical pathway	A predetermined standard of treatment for a particular disease, diagnosis, or procedure designed to facilitate the patient's progress through the facility.
clinical pertinence	Review of a patient's health record to determine whether the documentation reflects that the care provided to the patient was appropriately related to the diagnosis.
coding	The assignment of alphanumeric values to a word, phrase, or other non-numeric expression. In health care, coding is the assignment of numeric values to diagnosis and procedure descriptions.
coding compliance plan	The development, implementation, and enforcement of policies and procedures to ensure that coding standards are met.
completeness	The data quality of existence. If a required data element is missing, the record is not complete.
compliance	Meeting standards. Also the development, implementation, and enforcement of policies and procedures that ensure that standards are met.
computer-based patient record	Compilation of patient health information in a relational or other computer database.
computerized patient record	A digital form of the patient's paper health record.

concurrent analysis	Any type of analysis (*see* analysis) performed during the patient's stay (after admission but before discharge).
concurrent coding	Any type of coding (*see* coding) performed during the patient's stay (after admission but before discharge). Concurrent coding must be performed in order to obtain the working DRG.
concurrent review	Review occurring during the act or event, i.e., during the patient's stay in the facility.
Conditions of Admission	The legal agreement between a hospital and a patient (or the patient's legal agent) to perform routine services. May also include the statement of the patient's financial responsibility and prospective consent for release of information and examination and disposal of tissue.
confidentiality	Discretion regarding disclosure of information.
consent	An agreement or permission.
consultant	A medical professional who provides clinical expertise in a specialty at the request of the attending physician.
consultation	The formal request by a physician for the professional opinion or services of another health care professional, usually another physician, in caring for a patient. Also refers to the opinion or services themselves as well as the activity of rendering the opinion or services.
continuing education	Education required after attaining a position, credential, or degree intended to keep those persons knowledgeable in their profession.
continuum of care	The broad range of health care services required by a patient during an illness or for an entire lifetime. May also refer to the continuity of care provided by a health care organization.

Cooperating Parties	The four organizations responsible for maintaining the ICD-9-CM: HCFA, NCHS, AHA, and AHIMA.
corrective controls	Procedures, processes, or structures that are designed to fix errors when they are detected. Because errors cannot always be fixed, corrective controls also include the initiation of investigation into future error prevention or detection.
countersignature	*See* countersigned.
countersigned	Evidence of supervision of subordinate personnel, such as physician residents.
CPT-4	Current Procedural Terminology. A nomenclature and coding system developed and maintained by the American Medical Association in order to facilitate billing for physician services.
credentials	An individual's specific professional qualifications. Also refers to the letters that a professionally qualified person is entitled to list after his or her name.
data	The smallest elements or units of knowledge. Also refers to a collection of such elements.
data accuracy	The quality that data are correct.
data collection devices	Paper forms or computer screens designed to capture data elements in a standardized format. Also refers to the physical computer hardware or other tool that facilitates the data collection process.
data dictionary	A list of details about each field in a database.
data entry	The process of recording elements into a collection device. Generally refers to the recording of elements into a computer system.
data set	A group of data elements collected for a specific purpose.

data validity	The quality that data reflect the known or acceptable range of values for the specific data.
database	An organized collection of data.
date-oriented record	*See* integrated record.
decision matrix	A quality improvement tool used to narrow focus or choose between two or more related issues.
deductible	A specified dollar amount for which the patient is personally responsible, before the payer reimburses for any claims.
deemed status	The Medicare provision that an approved accreditation is sufficient to satisfy the compliance audit element of the Conditions of Participation.
defendant	The party or parties against whom the plaintiff has initiated litigation.
deficiencies	Required elements that are missing from a record.
deficiency system	The policies and procedures that form the corrective control of collecting the missing data identified in quantitative analysis. Includes the recording and reporting of deficiencies.
delegate	To give a responsibility, task, or project from a manager to a lower level employee.
delinquent	Status accorded to a record that has not been completed within a specified time frame, such as within 30 days of discharge.
demographic data	Identification: those elements that distinguish one patient from another, such as name, address, and birth date.
detective controls	Procedures, processes, or structures that are designed to find errors after they have been made.
diagnosis	Literally, "complete knowledge"; refers to the name of the patient's condition or illness.

Diagnosis Related Groups (DRGs)	A collection of health care descriptions organized into statistically similar categories.
discharge register (discharge list)	A list of all patients discharged on a specific date or during a specific time period.
discharge summary	The recap of an inpatient stay, usually dictated by the attending physician and transcribed into a formal report.
discounted fee for service	The exchange of cash for professional services rendered, at a rate less than the normal fee for the service.
doctor's orders	*See* physician's orders.
DSM-IV	*Diagnostic and Statistical Manual of Mental Disorders,* Fourth Edition
encounter form	A data collection device that facilitates the accurate capture of ambulatory care diagnoses and services.
epidemiology	The study of morbidity trends and occurrences.
ergonomic	Alignment of the work environment to accommodate the employee's job function.
error report	A list of deficient or erroneous data. Usually a computer-generated document.
ethics	A system of beliefs about acceptable behavior.
etiology	The cause or source of the patient's condition or disease.
exception report	*See* error report.
face sheet	The first page in a paper record. Usually contains at least the demographic data and contains space for the physician to record and authenticate the discharge diagnoses and procedures. In many facilities, the admission record is also used as the face sheet.

family unit numbering	A numeric identification system to identify an entire family's health record using one number and modifiers.
fee for service	The exchange of cash, goods, or services for professional services rendered.
field	A collection or series of related characters. A field may contain a word, a group of words, a number, or a code, for example.
file	Numerous records of different types of related data. Files can be large or small, depending on the number of records they contain.
file folder	The physical container used to store the health record in a paper-based system.
financial data	Elements that describe the payer. For example, the name, address, telephone number, group number, and member number of the patient's insurance company.
fiscal intermediaries	Organizations that administer the claims and reimbursements for the funding agency. Medicare uses fiscal intermediaries to process its claims and reimbursements.
flexible benefit account	A savings account in which health care and certain child-care costs can be set aside and paid using pretax funds.
full-time equivalent (FTE)	An employee who works 32 to 40 hours each week excluding overtime, earning full benefits as offered by the health care facility.
goals	Desired achievements.
graph	An illustration of data.
grouper	The flowchart used to derive the DRG from the ICD-9-CM diagnoses and procedures. Also refers to the computer program that performs this task.

guarantor	The individual or organization that promises to pay for the health care services rendered, after all other sources (such as insurance) are exhausted.
health data	Elements related to a patient's diagnosis and procedures.
health information	Organized data that have been collected about a patient or a group of patients. Sometimes used synonymously with health data.
health information management (HIM)	The profession that manages the sources and uses of health information, including the collection, storage, retrieval, and reporting of health information.
health information technology (HIT)	The area in the field of health information management that focuses on the day-to-day activities of health information management that support the collection, storage, retrieval, and reporting of health information.
health maintenance organization (HMO)	Characterized by the ownership or employer control over the health care providers.
health record	Also called record or medical record. It contains all of the data collected about an individual patient.
hearsay rule	The court rule that prohibits most testimony regarding events by parties who were not directly involved in the event.
history	The physician's record of the patient's chief complaint, history of present illness, pertinent family and social history, and review of systems.
home health care	Health care services rendered in the patient's home. Also refers to organizations that provide such services.
hospice	Palliative health care services rendered to the terminally ill, their families, and their friends. Also refers to organizations that provide such services.

hospital	An organization having permanent facilities that delivers inpatient health care services through 24-hour nursing care, an organized medical staff, and appropriate ancillary departments.
ICD-9-CM	*International Classification of Diseases, Ninth Revision—Clinical Modification.* The United States of America's version of the ICD-9, maintained and updated by the Cooperating Parties.
ICD-10	*International Classification of Diseases, Tenth Revision.*
ICD-O	*International Classification of Diseases—Oncology.* The coding system used to record and track the occurrence of neoplasms (i.e., malignant tumors, cancer).
incidence	Number of occurrences of a particular event, disease, or diagnosis; or the number of new cases of a disease.
incomplete system	*See* deficiency system.
indemnity insurance	Assumption of the payment for all or part of certain, specified services. Characterized by out-of-pocket deductibles and caps on total covered payments.
index	A system to identify or name a file or other item so that it can be located.
indicative data	*See* demographic data.
indices	Collections of patient data (or a database) specific to a diagnosis, procedure, or physician.
information	Processed data; i.e., data that are presented in an appropriate frame of reference.
informed consent	A permission given by a competent individual, of legal age, with full knowledge or understanding of the risks, potential benefits, and potential consequences of the permission.
inpatient	An individual who is admitted to a hospital with the intention of staying overnight.

in-service	Training provided to employees of an organization.
insurer	The party that assumes the risk of paying some or all of the cost of providing health care services in return for the payment of a premium by or on behalf of the insured.
integrated delivery system	A health care organization that provides services through most or all of the continuum of care.
integrated record	A paper record in which the pages are organized sequentially, in the chronologic order in which they were generated; also known as date-oriented record or sequential record.
interdepartmental	Relationship between two or more departments, e.g., HIM and the business office.
intradepartmental	Occurrence or relationship within a department, e.g., assembly and analysis within HIM.
job analysis	Review of a function to determine all of the tasks or components that make up an employee's job.
job description	A list of the employee's responsibilities.
Joint Commission on Accreditation of Health-care Organizations (JCAHO)	The largest and most comprehensive health care accrediting agency.
jurisdiction	The authority of a court to decide certain cases. May be based on geography, money, or type of case.
laboratory	The physical location of the specialists who analyze body fluids.
laboratory tests	Procedures for analysis of body fluids.
length of stay (LOS)	The duration of an inpatient visit, measured in whole days: the number of whole days between the inpatient's admission and discharge.

licensure	The mandatory government approval required for performing specified activities. In health care, the state approval required for providing health care services.
litigation	The term used to indicate that a matter must be settled by the court, and the process of engaging in legal proceedings.
long-term care facility	A hospital that provides services to patients over an extended period of time; an average length of stay is in excess of 30 days. Facilities are characterized by the extent to which nursing care is provided.
loose sheets	In a paper health record, documents that are not present when the patient is discharged. These documents must be accumulated and filed with the record at a later date.
Major Diagnostic Categories (MDCs)	Segments of the DRG assignment flowchart (grouper).
managed care	The blending of the insurance and provider roles.
marketing	Promoting products or services in the hope that the consumer chooses those products or services over the products or services of a competitor.
master patient index	A system containing patient and encounter information, often used to correlate the patient to the file identification.
maximization	The process of determining the highest possible DRG payment.
Medicaid	Joint federal/state program for providing access to health care for the poor and the medically indigent.
medical record	*See* health record; record.
Medicare	Federally funded health care insurance plan for the elderly and for certain categories of chronically ill patients.

medications	Chemical substances used to treat disease.
memorandum (memo)	A communication tool used to inform members of an organization.
mental health facility	*See* behavioral health facility.
microfiche	An alternative storage method for paper records on plastic sheets.
microfilm	An alternative storage method for paper records on plastic film.
middle-digit filing	A modification of terminal-digit filing in which the patient's medical record number is separated into sets for filing and the first set of numbers is called secondary, the second set of numbers is called primary, and the third set is called tertiary.
Minimum Data Set (MDS)	The detailed data collected about long-term care patients. It is collected several times, and it forms the basis for the RUG.
minutes	A tool used to record the events, topics, and discussions of a meeting.
mission	The purpose of the organization documented in a formal statement.
morbidity	Refers to disease.
mortality	Refers to death.
National Center for Health Statistics (NCHS)	One of the ICD-9-CM Cooperating Parties.
nomenclature	A formal system of names that pertain to a profession or discipline.
nurse	A medical professional who has satisfied the academic, professional, and legal requirements to care for patients at state-specified levels. Although usually delivering patient care at the direction of physicians, nurse practitioners may also deliver care independently.
nursing assessment	The nurse's evaluation of the patient.

nursing progress notes	Routine documentation of the nurse's interaction with a patient.
objective	In the SOAP format for medical decision-making, the physician's observations and review of diagnostic tests.
objectives	Directions for achieving a goal.
open access	The physician's office scheduling method that allows for patient visits without an appointment. Some versions of open access focus on group visits for certain types of routine care.
operation	Surgery. An operation consists of one or more surgical procedures.
operative report	The surgeon's formal report of surgical procedure(s) performed.
optical disk	Electronic storage medium.
optimization	The process of determining the most accurate DRG payment.
organization chart	An illustration used to describe the relationship among departments, positions, and functions within an organization.
orientation	Training to familiarize a new employee to the job.
outguide	A physical file guide used to identify another location of a file, in the paper-based health record system.
outpatient	A patient whose health care services are intended to be delivered within 1 calendar day or, in some cases, a 24-hour period.
outsourced	Refers to services that are provided by individuals or organizations that are not employees of the facility for which the services are being provided.

palliative care	Health care services that are intended to soothe, comfort, or reduce symptoms but are not intended to cure.
patient accounts	The department in a health care facility that is responsible for submitting bills or claims for reimbursement.
payer	The individual or organization that is primarily responsible for the reimbursement for a particular health care service. Usually refers to the insurance company or third party.
per diem	Each day, daily. Usually refers to all-inclusive payments for inpatient services.
performance improvement (PI)	Also known as quality improvement (QI) or continuous quality improvement (CQI). Refers to the process by which a facility reviews its services or products to ensure quality.
performance standards	Set guidelines explaining how much work an employee must complete.
physiatrist	A physician who specializes in physical medicine and rehabilitation.
physical examination	The physician's record of examination of the patient.
physician	A medical professional who has satisfied the academic, professional, and legal requirements to diagnose and treat patients at state-specified levels and within a declared specialty.
physician's orders	The physician's directions regarding the patient's care. Also refers to the data collection device on which these elements are captured.
physician-patient privilege	The legal foundation that private communication between a physician and a patient is confidential. Only the patient has the right to give up this privilege.
placebo	A nontherapeutic substance used in clinical drug trials. The patient (and sometimes the physician) does not know whether he/she is receiving the trial drug or the placebo.

plaintiff	The party who initiates litigation.
plan of treatment	In the SOAP format for medical decision-making, the diagnostic, therapeutic, or palliative measures that are taken to investigate or treat the patient's condition or disease.
policy	A statement of something that is done or expected in an organization.
population	An entire group.
postdischarge processing	The procedures designed to prepare a health record for retention.
potentially compensable event (PCE)	An event that could cause the facility a financial loss or could lead to litigation.
Preferred Provider Organization (PPO)	A managed care organization that contracts with a network of health care providers to render services to the PPO's members.
premiums	Periodic payments to an insurance company for coverage (an insurance policy).
prevalence	Rate of incidence of an occurrence, disease, or diagnosis; or the number of existing cases.
preventive controls	Procedures, processes, or structures that are designed to minimize errors at the point of data collection.
primary caregiver	The individual who is principally responsible for the daily care of a patient at home: usually a friend or family member.
primary care physician	A physician who cares for patients.
primary data	Data taken directly from the patient.
probation period	The period of time (grace period) given to a new employee to learn the job and reach the performance standards associated with that job. During this period, the employee is not considered permanent.

problem-oriented record	A paper record with pages organized by diagnosis.
procedure	A process that describes how to comply with a policy. Also, a medical or surgical treatment. Also refers to the processing steps in an administrative function.
productivity	The amount of work produced by an employee in a given time frame.
progress notes	The physician's record of each visit with the patient.
prospective consent	Permission given prior to having knowledge of the event to which the permission applies. For example, a permission to release information before the information is gathered, i.e., before admission.
prospective payment	Reimbursement based on a predetermined amount.
Prospective Payment System (PPS)	The Medicare system for reimbursing acute care facilities based on statistical analysis of health care data.
psychiatrist	A physician who specializes in the diagnosis and treatment of patients with conditions that affect the mind.
qualitative analysis	Review of the actual content of the health record to be certain the information is correct as it pertains to the patient's care.
quality assurance (QA)	A method for reviewing health care functions to determine their compliance to predetermined standards, requiring action to correct noncompliance and then follow-up review to ascertain whether the correction was effective.
quantitative analysis	A detective control designed to identify incomplete data. Usually refers to review of the patient health record for complete content and authentications.

query	To question the database for information or a report.
radiology	Literally, the study of x-rays. In a health care facility, the department responsible for maintaining x-ray and other types of diagnostic and therapeutic equipment as well as analyzing diagnostic films.
radiology tests	The examination of internal body structures using x-rays and other related studies.
reciprocal services	Professional services traded instead of paid for in cash.
record	A collection of related fields. Also refers to all of the data collected about a patient's visit or all of the patient's visits (*see also* health record).
record retention schedule	The length of time that a record must be retained.
referral	The act or documentation of one physician's request for an opinion or services to another health care professional, often another physician, for a specific patient.
registry	A database of health information specific to disease, diagnosis, or implant, used to improve the care provided to patients with that disease, diagnosis, or implant.
rehabilitation facility	A health care facility that delivers services to patients whose activities of daily living are impaired by their illness or condition. May be inpatient, outpatient, or both.
reimbursement	The amount of money that the health care facility receives from the party responsible for paying the bill.
report	The result of a query. A list from a database.
research	The systematic investigation into a matter to find fact.
Resource Utilization Groups (RUGs)	These constitute a prospective payment system for long-term care. Current Medicare application is a per diem rate based on the RUG III grouper.

respite care	Services rendered to individuals who are not independent in their activities of daily living, for the purpose of temporarily relieving the primary caregiver.
retention	The procedures governing the storage of records, including duration, location, security, and access.
retrospective consent	Permission given after the event to which the permission applies. For example, permission to release information after the information is gathered, i.e., after discharge.
retrospective review	Review occurring after the act or event, i.e., after the patient is discharged.
risk	The potential exposure to loss or financial expenditure.
risk management	The coordination of efforts within a facility to prevent and control inadvertent occurrences.
rule out	The process of systematically eliminating potential diagnoses. Also refers to the list of potential diagnoses.
sample	A small group within a population.
scanner	A machine, much like a copier, used to turn paper-based records into digital images for a computerized health record.
secondary data	Data taken from primary data.
sequential record	*See* integrated record.
serial numbering	A numeric patient record identification system in which the patient is given a new number for each visit and each file folder contains separate visit information.
serial–unit numbering	A numeric patient record identification system in which the patient is given a new number for each visit; however, with each new admission, the previous record is retrieved and filed in the folder with the most recent visit.

SOAP format	Subjective, Objective, Assessment, and Plan: the medical decision-making process.
socioeconomic data	Elements that pertain to the patient's personal life and personal habits, such as marital status, religion, and culture.
source-oriented record	A paper record in which the pages are organized by discipline, department, and/or type of form.
span of control	The number of employees that report to one supervisor, manager, or administrator.
standing orders	The predetermined routine orders that have been designated to pertain to specific diagnoses or procedures. For example, the orders to perform specific blood tests, urinalysis, and x-rays prior to admission for certain surgical procedures. Standing orders must be ordered and authenticated by the appropriate physician.
statistics	Analysis, interpretation, and presentation of numbers.
straight numeric filing	Filing folders in numeric order.
subjective	In the SOAP format of medical decision-making, the patient's description of the symptoms or other complaints.
subpoena	A direction from an officer of the court.
subpoena ad testificandum	A direction from an officer of the court to provide testimony.
subpoena duces tecum	A direction from an officer of the court to provide documents.
surgeon	A physician who specializes in diagnosing and treating diseases with invasive procedures.
survey	A data-gathering tool for capturing the responses to queries. May be administered verbally or by written questionnaire. Also refers to the activity of querying, as in "taking a survey."

symptom	The patient's report of physical or other complaints, such as dizziness, headache, and stomach pain.
table	A chart organized in rows and columns to organize data.
Tax Equity and Fiscal Responsibility Act of 1982 (TEFRA)	Established Medicare PPS.
terminal-digit filing	A system in which the patient's medical record number is separated into sets for filing and the first set of numbers is called tertiary, the second set of numbers is called secondary, and the third set of numbers is called primary.
timeliness	The quality of data's being obtained, recorded, and/or reported within a predetermined time frame.
Title XVIII	Amendment to the Social Security Act that established Medicaid.
Title XIX	Amendment to the Social Security Act that established Medicare.
training	Education, instruction, or demonstration of how to perform a job.
treatment	A procedure, medication, or other measure designed to cure or alleviate the symptoms of disease.
Uniform Ambulatory Care Data Set (UACDS)	The mandated data set for ambulatory care patients.
Uniform Hospital Discharge Data Set (UHDDS)	The mandated data set for hospital inpatients.
unit numbering	A numeric patient record identification system in which the patient record is filed under the same number for all visits.
unity of command	Sole management of one employee by one manager.

universal chart order	Pertaining to a paper health record, the maintenance of the same page organization both pre- and postdischarge.
usual and customary fees	Referring to health care provider fees, the rate established by an insurance company, based on the regional charges for the particular service.
utilization management (UM)	The process that ensures appropriate, efficient, and effective health care for patients.
vision	The goal of the organization, above and beyond the mission.
working DRG	The concurrent DRG. The DRG that reflects the patient's current diagnosis and procedures, while still an inpatient.
wraparound policies	Insurance policies that supplement Medicare coverage.

CHAPTER ONE

Q: If a patient is admitted as an inpatient on Monday at 10 AM but dies on Monday at 3 PM, is that patient still considered an inpatient?

A: Yes. Once a patient has been admitted as an inpatient, the status does not change as a result of a same-day discharge. Remember that the physician orders the admission with the *intention* of keeping the patient overnight. The patient is classified as an inpatient regardless of whether the patient actually remains in the hospital.

Q: A patient was admitted on March 14 and discharged on May 3. What was the length of stay?

A: 50 days. 18 days in March; 30 days in April; 2 days in May. Remember that you count the day of admission but not the day of discharge. There are 31 days in March: $31 - 14 = 17$. Add 1 to include the day of admission: $17 + 1 = 18$. May 3 doesn't count, because it is the day of discharge. Therefore, the length of stay is 50 days: $18 + 30 + 2$.

Q: The lines between inpatients and outpatients may become blurred given certain circumstances. An emergency department patient who is treated and released is clearly an outpatient. However, if the patient enters the emergency department at 11 PM and leaves at 4 AM, the patient clearly came on one day and left on the next. Is this patient an inpatient or an outpatient? Why? Additionally, some patients are kept in the hospital for *observation*. This is a special category of patients, neither outpatients nor inpatients, who may stay in the hospital for up to 24 hours without being admitted as an inpatient. Can you think of a reason why this category of patients was created?

A: A patient who is being treated in the emergency room is an outpatient, regardless of the actual time that the patient is admitted or discharged. The *intention* is to treat the patient as an outpatient. Remember that an order from the physician is required to admit the patient as an inpatient.

Students may be able to think of many reasons why the observation category was created. Observation keeps inpatient beds free, reduces paperwork, provides a longer period of time for the physician to decide whether to admit the patient, reduces expensive inpatient admissions, and gives the patient more confidence when returning home that potential life-threatening problems have been investigated.

Q: Deluxe Hospital is a 460-bed facility with an average of 35 discharges per day. The ALOS is 6 days. Deluxe has an emergency department, several operating suites, and a wide variety of ancillary services. The most common reason for admission is childbirth, followed by heart and lung problems. What kind of a facility is Deluxe? What services might it provide?

A: Deluxe Hospital is an acute care facility, sometimes called a short-stay facility. The ALOS is less than 30 days and it maintains an emergency department and operating suites. These are typical of an acute care facility. Deluxe Hospital might provide patient care services ranging from general inpatient care to outpatient clinics and diagnostic services, as well as a variety of community services such as blood pressure screening.

CHAPTER TWO

Q: What other services are provided in an ambulatory care setting? Describe the events that take place in other ambulatory care settings. How does the process differ from the one described earlier? What other personnel are involved?

A: Students may suggest a variety of answers to this question. Diagnostic testing, such as x-rays and blood tests, is performed in an ambulatory care setting, as are certain blood donations and transfusions, physical therapy, dialysis, and dental services. Procedures are very similar in terms of appointments, registration, and payment, although the detail focuses on the service provided. The actual clinical procedures and personnel vary, depending on the service.

Q: Think about a disease with which you are familiar and create a list of all the data elements that you think a physician and allied health personnel in a physician's office would generate for the disease. You can make up the data, but make the list as complete as you can. This exercise will give you an idea of how complex health information is, even at the physician's office level.

A: Answers will vary, depending on student experience. For example, imagine a healthy child visiting a pediatrician for the first time. The doctor will want to know about any childhood illnesses and immunizations as well as any family history of diseases, whether there are any siblings, and the health of the siblings. The doctor will also want to know whether the child is in day care, school, or another setting where he or she is exposed to communicable diseases. The doctor will also want to know about minor health issues, such as colds and fevers, and what medications the caregivers have used to control them. On examination, the physician records all observations, such as vital signs (temperature, pulse, heart rate); condition of the skin, eyes, ears, nose, throat; and response to stimuli. Immunizations are recorded, as well as any discussion with the caregiver about follow-up and continuing care.

Q: Can you give two examples of data and two examples of information from your personal life? Think of two examples of how health data differ from health information.

A: Answers will vary, depending on student experiences. For example, a store receipt that lists the prices and the grand total is data. A store receipt that lists the prices, along with a description of the items, the date, and specific coupons used, as well as the total, is information.

Q: List and describe the four key data categories and what they contain.

A: Demographic data contain data to identify the patient. Socioeconomic data contain specific data about the patient's lifestyle and personal activities. Financial data contain insurance and other payment data. Clinical data refer to the patient-specific data that are collected from and generated about the patient's health.

Q: Create a file of five records that contain name, address, and telephone number. Begin by defining the fields in data dictionary format and then show how you would represent these fields if you were trying to explain them to someone else.

A: See Figure 2–11. The student's definitions may be slightly different.

CHAPTER THREE

Q: The initial data collection for a patient begins to build the hospital's data set on that patient. In Chapter 2, we discussed the Uniform Ambulatory Care Data Set required in a physician's office. Each type of facility has its own particular data set that must be considered when planning data collection strategies. While you are reading this chapter, make a list of the items that you think would be appropriate to include in the data set required in an acute care facility—the Uniform Hospital Discharge Data Set (UHDDS).

A:
1. Patient's identification number
2. Date of birth
3. Sex
4. Race and ethnicity
5. Residence
6. Health care facility identification number
7. Admission date
8. Type of admission
9. Discharge date
10. Attending physician's identification number
11. Surgeon's identification number
12. Principal diagnosis
13. Other diagnoses
14. Qualifier for other diagnoses
15. External cause-of-injury code
16. Birth weight of neonate
17. Other procedures and the date(s) of the procedure(s)
18. Disposition of the patient at discharge
19. Expected source of payment
20. Total charges

Some elements that you may have included in your list are marital status, religion, and past illnesses. Although these data elements are routinely collected in an inpatient record, they are not included in the UHDDS.

Q: Should the "correct" authentication be limited to the attending physician?

A: No. Authentication is performed by any individual who is authorized to record data and must evidence the quality of those data. Also, individuals who share responsibilities, such as medical group partners, may authenticate each other's work, if appropriate.

Q: From our discussion of data in this chapter, can you identify the sources of each of the elements of the UHDDS?

A:

Data Element	Type of Data	Source of Data
Patient's ID number	Demographic	Admission record
Date of birth	Demographic	Admission record
Sex	Demographic	Admission record
Race and ethnicity	Socioeconomic	Admission record Confirmed in history
Residence	Demographic	Admission record
Health care facility's ID	Nonpatient	UB-92
Admission date	Clinical	Admission record
Discharge date	Clinical	Admission record
Attending physician's ID number	Clinical	Identity is part of the admission record Confirmed in history, physician's notes, and discharge summary Actual ID number is administrative data
Surgeon's ID number	Clinical	Identity is part of the operative report and other operative records Actual ID number is administrative data
Principal diagnosis	Clinical	Discharge record Confirmed in physician's notes, pathology reports, operative record, and diagnostic test reports
Other diagnoses	Clinical	Discharge record Confirmed in physician's notes, pathology reports, operative record, and diagnostic test reports
Principal procedure/ date	Clinical	Discharge record Confirmed in physician's notes and operative record

Data Element	Type of Data	Source of Data
Other procedures/ dates	Clinical	Discharge record Confirmed in physician's notes and operative record
Disposition	Clinical	Discharge record Confirmed in discharge summary
Expected source of payment	Financial	Admission record
Total charges	Financial	UB-92

CHAPTER FOUR

Q: When creating a paper form for new patients to complete at registration in a physician's office, what preventive control could be implemented to ensure that the patient lists all significant childhood illnesses?

A: One way to handle this is to list all significant childhood illnesses so that the patient can check them off. In this way, the patient is reminded of illnesses that he or she may have forgotten.

Q: The physician accidentally entered an order into the computer to request a cardiology consultation for the wrong patient. A staff nurse noticed the error. How should the correction be handled?

A: The nurse should call the physician's attention to the error so that the consultation can be ordered for the correct patient. Also, the physician must correct the wrong patient's record. The computer system should enable such corrections by referencing the error and superceding the order with a cancellation.

Q: Answer the following questions after examining the discharge register shown in Table 4–4:

- What is the length of stay for each of these patients?
- What is the average length of stay?
- Why do we want to know the room number if the patient has already been discharged?

A:

| Admission Date | Patient's ID Number | Patient's Name | | D/C 6/5/00 |
		Last	First	LOS
6/2/00	234675	Johnson	Thomas	3 days
6/4/00	234731	Kudovski	Maria	1 day
6/4/00	234565	Kudovski	Vladimir	1 day
5/31/00	156785	Macey	Anna	5 days
6/3/00	234523	Mattingly	Richard	2 days
6/5/00	274568	Ng	Charles	1 day
5/15/00	234465	Rodriguez	Francisco	20 days
6/1/00	198543	Rogers	Danielle	4 days
6/2/00	224678	Young	Rebecca	3 days

Average length of stay for all patients: 4.4 days
(40 days ÷ 9 patients = 4.4 days

The room number helps the HIM department find the record if it has not been delivered to the department. Also, the room number helps quality improvement studies if problems such as an increased infection rate occur on a particular nursing unit.

Q: **What type of control is provided by the first processing step of receiving the records, as previously described?**

A: The first step is to ensure that all records have been received. This can be accomplished by checking the records received against the discharge register. This type of control is a detective control, because it is designed to discover an error: a missing record.

Q: **Because physicians are often not actually employees of the facility at which they have privileges, what incentive do they have to complete their records?**

A: Timely completion of records should be a part of the credentialing process. If a physician does not complete records, he or she could lose the privilege of admitting patients to the facility for treatment.

CHAPTER FIVE

Q: **How many records would this facility have in storage after 5 years?**

A: 19,500 records × 5 years = 97,500 records.

Q: **When you receive a request for an old patient health record, what is the first step to take in locating the record?**

A: 1. Check the master patient index (MPI) to see if the patient has ever been treated in the facility.
   2. If the patient has a history in the MPI, with a prior visit, identify the medical record number.

Q: **What should you do if you are unable to access the computerized MPI? How can you locate a medical record number to find a patient's record?**

A: The facility should maintain a manual method for identifying the patient's medical record number. If a printout exists, access it. However, if a manual system does not exist, ask the clinician if he or she can determine from the patient if he or she has a previous record. If the patient indicates that he or she has been treated in the facility on a previous occasion and can provide an approximate date, you may be able to review the admission, discharge, and transfer logs or the census reports. If a system does not exist, think through the possibilities.

Q: **File the following names in alphabetic order.**

P. B. Josh	Drew B. LaPeu
Hannah Curelle	Cecelia Lower
Ginger Dugas	Wm. Bill Matata
Lauren McIntyre	Amanda Modelle
Beth Katerina Von Amberg	Aubrey Bartolo, III
Sister Gabrielle Brown	Brett Thomasse, Jr.

A: Aubrey Bartolo, III; Sister Gabrielle Brown; Hannah Curelle; Ginger Dugas; P. B. Josh; Drew LaPeu; Cecelia Lower; Wm. Bill Matata; Lauren McIntyre; Amanda Modelle; Brett Thomassee, Jr.; Beth Katerina Von Amberg.

Q: **Using your knowledge of how numbers/identifiers are assigned to patient files in each of the following numbering systems, answer the questions below.**

1. What number will be assigned to Jane for the broken ankle admission?

2. If Green Oaks uses a unit numbering system, what medical record number would be assigned for the broken ankle admission?

A: 1. MR# 23456.

2. Because Green Oaks uses serial numbering each time a patient is treated at the facility, the broken ankle admission would receive a new medical record number.

Q: 1. In a terminal-digit filing system, MR# 658925 would be located in which primary section?

2. In a middle-digit filing system, MR# 658925 would be located in which primary section?

3. Design a filing method for a facility that uses a nine-digit medical record number.

A: 1. 25.

2. 89.

3. Various methods. Could use straight numeric or terminal digit. If terminal digit, decide how many digits will be in each section, that is, 111-222-333, or 111-22-3333, or 11122-33-33.

Q: Marcus counted the number of records in ten 1-foot sections in the file area prior to reorganizing the files. His findings were as follows:

Section #1—12 records, #2—8 records, #3—16 records,
#4—6 records, #5—10 records, #6—24 records, #7—15 records,
#8—14 records, #9—7 records, #10—11 records.

Using this information, calculate the average number of records in a 1-foot section of files.

A: 12.3 records per foot.

Q: Calculate the filing space necessary for a new ambulatory surgery facility. The facility will average 45 surgeries each day, Monday through Friday.

A: Calculate 12 records per inch, 45 surgeries (records) per day, 45 surgeries (records) × 5 days = 225 records each week × 52 weeks in a year = 11,700 records per year. 11,700 records would require 975 inches of filing space (at 12 records per inch). Therefore, 975 inches ÷ 12 inches in a foot = 81.25 linear feet of filing space for 1 year of records.

CHAPTER SIX

Q: Can you think of another use for health information besides those listed above?

A: Determined by the instructor.

Q: What is quality? Take a moment to define quality and then discuss your thoughts with another person. Is that person's perception of quality the same as yours?

A: Review definition found in a dictionary, or use a thesaurus.

Q: Which association was the first to recognize a need for quality in health care and was organized for the purpose of promoting quality health care?

A: The American Medical Association.

Q: What was the name of the first program (set of standards) designed to measure quality in a health care setting?

A: Hospital Standardization Program.

Q: What type of quality monitoring does JCAHO require health care facilities to perform?

A: Quality improvement.

Q: Specify the number of records that would be reviewed at the following facilities using the rule of 5% or 30 discharges (whichever is greater).
Hospital A has 1200 discharges each month.
Hospital B has 400 discharges each month.
Hospital C has 150 discharges each month.

A: Hospital A = 60 charts, because 5% of 1200 = 60 (1200 × .05 = 60); 60 is greater than 30. Hospital B = 30 charts, because 5% of 400 = 20 (400 × .05 = 20); 30 is greater. Hospital C = 30 charts, because 5% of 150 = 7.5 (150 × .05 = 7.5); again, 30 is greater.

Q: Health records contain demographic, socioeconomic, financial, and clinical data. If one of the JCAHO standards requires that the health record contain personal identification information for each patient, where could this information be found in the health record?

A: Face sheet or registration record. Also, each page should contain information to identify the information for a specific patient.

Q: What would you need to do if an employee reports that he or she fell while on a nursing unit, injuring his or her left knee?

A: Complete an incident report.

Q: Which graph would you use to show that the overall percentage of people smoking on campus has remained unchanged?

A: A line graph, because it graphs data (information) over time.

CHAPTER SEVEN

Q: List an example of primary data found in the health record.

A: There are many answers to this question. The following is only a sample: Chief complaint, history & physical (H&P), vital signs.

Q: Is the printed telephone book in your community a data set or a database?

A: Database.

Q: The type of anesthesia used during the surgery is a required data element in the abstract. Using the operative report in Figure 7–5, can you determine what type of anesthesia this patient received?

A: General.

Q: What is the average length of stay (ALOS) for the group of CHF patients described in Figure 7–7?

A: 9.4 days. Total days for all seven patients = 66 (66 ÷ 7 = 9.4).

Q: What other type of report or information could you obtain from the indices?

A: There are many answers to this question. The following are only a sample: a list of patients who have had a particular procedure or diagnosis; patients who were admitted during a particular time period; a list of patients with a specific diagnosis and financial class or age, race, or sex; a list of physicians who perform a specific procedure.

Q: What was the number of average monthly discharges at Community Hospital for the year 2000?

A: 1316 discharges; because 1148 + 1555 + 1430 + 1398 + 1247 + 994 + 1248 + 1148 + 1224 + 1502 + 1598 + 1303 = 15,795 ÷ 12 (months) = 1316.25.

Q: What was the newborn ALOS for 2000?

A: 2 or 2.1; 1974 (total LOS for NB) ÷ 950 (discharges for NB) = 2.07.

CHAPTER EIGHT

Q: Why would an insurance company want a copy of a patient's record?

A: Because the patient's record details the clinical activities related to the patient, the insurance company may want the record in order to confirm that services for which it is paying were actually rendered. Also, the insurance company may want to identify and evaluate those activities for clinical pertinence and efficiency.

Q: In each of the three examples just mentioned, who is the plaintiff and who is the defendant?

A: A patient slips and falls in the grocery store and sues the store: The patient is the plaintiff and the grocery store is the defendant. A physician amputates the wrong foot; the patient sues the physician and the hospital: The patient is the plaintiff and both the physician and the hospital are defendants. A pedestrian is hit by a car and sues the driver: The pedestrian is the plaintiff and the driver of the car is the defendant.

Q: Your facility charges a $5.00 search fee plus $0.75 per page for copying a record. How much will the patient pay for a 125-page record?

A: The patient will pay $98.75 for the record; $125 \times 0.75 = 93.75$; $93.75 + 5 = 98.75$.

Q: If reproduction fees (copying costs) are based on photocopying paper records, how do you think these fees should be affected by reproduction of computer-based records and electronic transmission of information?

A: Answers will vary but should include consideration of personnel time, computer time, and paper costs. Tracking and billing of requests are still needed. Electronic transmission may add an additional follow-up step to ensure correct transmission. In general, it is not safe to assume that costs will go down.

Q: If your state licensure regulations stated that all records in an acute care facility must be completed within 30 days of discharge, or that all requests for records be filled within 30 days of the original requests, how would the health information professional be involved in ensuring compliance with these rules?

A: The HIM professional will identify incomplete records, notify the physicians, and track and report compliance. This process also involves ensuring that the incomplete records are available to the physicians for completion.

CHAPTER NINE

Q: What incentive do physicians have to operate under each of the four methods of reimbursement discussed?

A: Under any method of reimbursement, physician incentive to operate relates to maintaining an efficient and effective method of ensuring optimal reimbursement. The management of the patient may differ slightly as a result of screening requirements and other administrative burdens placed by the insurance company. These administrative burdens may create an environment in which physicians are more likely to become health care delivery system employees or to enter into group partnerships, rather than to operate as solo practitioners.

Q: Based on your knowledge of health records, if an insurance company wanted to check to see whether excessive testing was performed on a patient, where would it look in the chart and why?

A: First, the patient's signs and symptoms would be reviewed, as presented in the history and physical. These data reflect what the physician knew at the time of the initial encounter with the problem. Then the tests results would be reviewed. These would be available on the diagnostic reports pertinent to the tests, for example, the radiology report or the laboratory report related to the radiology examination or the blood test. Finally, the insurance company would review the diagnosis(es), as identified in the physician's notes or the discharge summary. This series of reviews would tell the insurance company what the physician knew, what he or she deduced from that knowledge, and what conclusions were drawn from the evidence. The insurance company would then compare this information with established patterns of practice to determine whether the physician required more or fewer tests than would normally be required.

Q: How do you think a managed care organization controls the utilization of health care resources by all of its subscribers?

A: In general, it controls utilization through the reimbursement process, by defining what it will and will not pay for and by requiring preapproval for certain procedures.

Q: What impact will incorrect coding have on reimbursement by DRG?

A: Incorrect coding may directly result in incorrect reimbursement through incorrect DRGs, APCs, or incorrect HCFA-1500 billing, for example. It may also lead to increased fines or penalties if patterns of abusive overcoding (coding for more services than were actually rendered or coding diseases that did not apply to the current episode of care or that inappropriately increased reimbursement) are detected. In addition, the administrative burden of dealing with insurance audits to validate coding is increased when patterns of overcoding are observed.

CHAPTER TEN

Q: Congratulations! You are the new supervisor in the HIM department at General Hospital. Your facility is licensed for 150 beds. Current census is 90. The facility provides general acute care (130 beds), same-day surgery, a 10-bed skilled nursing facility (SNF) unit, and a 10-bed rehabilatation unit. This facility has a paper-based health record and 10 HIM employees, including the director. Table 10–2 provides a list of employees and their responsibilities, hours worked, and employment status (full-time, part-time, or per diem). Which employees report to the clerical/ROI supervisor?

A: Assembly, analysis, release of information, file, and birth certificate clerks.

Q: Identify the reports required on the health record for a patient who has been in the facility for 24 hours.

A: Face sheet; signed conditions of admission forms; acknowledgments for advance directives and other forms required by law; a history and physical signed by the physician.

Q: Identify another issue that could be addressed in a facility's policy statement.

A: See Table 10–6, an HIM department's Policy and Procedure manual table of contents.

Q: As the new HIM supervisor, how do you know how your predecessor organized HIM functions? Do you rely on what the employees tell you?

A: The Policy and Procedure manual should explain the operations of the department. If the Policy and Procedure manual does not match the practice of department operations, then the policies need to be updated.

Q: Using the 2000 statistics for Community Hospital given in Figure 7–10, determine how many folders you will need for the next year (2001), assuming that you will have a 3% increase in discharges.

A: You will need a minimum of 15,960. You may add more for errors, etc. 2000 discharges (including newborns, who also need folders) = 15,495. 3% of 15,495 = 465. 15,495 + 465 = 15,960.

CHAPTER ELEVEN

Q: Imagine that you are going to present a training session for new HIM employees. The topic of the training is "How to Organize a Health Record." What format would best suit this presentation?

A: Instructor's discretion.

Q: Create a calendar for education in the HIM department.

A: Instructor's discretion.

Q: Design an in-service for HIM employees, and discuss all of the elements of a training session.

A: Instructor's discretion.

Q: Write a memo to your instructor to request permission from him or her to miss class because you would like to attend the AHIMA national convention.

A: Instructor's discretion.

INDEX

Note: Page numbers followed by the letter f refer to figures; those followed by t refer to tables; and those followed by b refer to boxed material.

A

Abbreviations, 21b
Abstracting, 118, 242, 243f–245f, 246, 350, 354. *See also* Database(s).
  coding and, 118, 242, 252
  paper form for, 246b, 247f
  quality of, 208t, 246, 248
Access to records, 106, 106t, 277–285. *See also* Release of information; Security of records.
  by patient, 281, 285
  definition of, 277
  for continuing patient care, 277–278
  for litigation, 279–281, 282f–284f
  for reimbursement, 278
  inappropriate, 277, 297
Accreditation, 28–30, 188–190, 299–300. *See also* Joint Commission on Accreditation of Healthcare Organizations (JCAHO).
  as marketing method, 197
  HIM committee and, 229
  history of, 202
  incomplete records and, 114–115, 189–190, 213
  of HIM education programs, 28b, 428–429
  of managed care organizations, 195
  of medical schools, 201
  organizations providing, 29t, 204
  record review and, 213, 217
Accuracy
  of abstracts, 246, 248
  of coding, 332
  of data, 55, 101t
  of health information, 206b, 213
Acknowledgment form, for advance directive, 210–212, 211f
Acquired immunodeficiency syndrome (AIDS). *See* Human immunodeficiency virus (HIV) infection.
Acquisition of facilities, 10, 11b, 25–26
Acronyms, 21b
ACS (American College of Surgeons), 29, 202, 232

Active records, 165, 165b
Activities of daily living (ADLs), 19, 21
Acute care facility(ies), 10–11. *See also* Health care facility(ies); Hospital(s).
  acquisition of, 10, 11b, 25–26
  average length of stay in, 11, 14, 14f, 15
  clinical flow of data in, 68–71, 69t, 70t, 71t
  licensure of. *See* Licensure of facilities.
  merger of, 10, 11b, 25–26, 123
  prospective payment systems for, 321, 322–324
  services provided by, 18t, 24
    ambulatory, 11, 16
    ancillary, 16–17
  size of, 21–22
ADA (Americans with Disabilities Act), 364, 365, 380t
Addressograph, 138b
Adjunct services, 17
ADLs (activities of daily living), 19, 21
Administration of facility, 190, 344–346, 345f
Admission(s), 11, 68–70. *See also* Census.
  birth as, 256
  by transfer, 259b
  Conditions of Admission form for, 278, 285, 286f, 287
  HIM department notification of, 132
  statistics on, 256, 257t
Admission date, 11
Admission record (face sheet), 69, 69t, 84, 97
  codes on, 252
  sent to HIM department, 132
Admissions department. *See* Patient registration department.
Admitting clerk. *See* Patient registration specialist.
Admitting diagnosis, 117
  data sources for, 252
  working DRG and, 324
Adult day care, 19–20, 30
Advance directive, 210–212, 211b, 211f
Advertising. *See also* Marketing.
  for personnel, 371–372, 372f
  of facility closure, 158, 158f

Against medical advice (AMA), 11, 21b, 258
Age(s)
    calculating average of, 254–255, 255f
    for legal consent, 285
Age discrimination, 379, 380t
Agenda, 410–411, 411t
Aggregate data, 248–249, 249f, 250, 252, 254
AHA (American Hospital Association), 200, 200b, 202, 332
AHIMA. *See* American Health Information Management Association (AHIMA).
AIDS (acquired immunodeficiency syndrome). *See* Human immunodeficiency virus (HIV) infection.
Alcohol abuse records, 274, 287, 292–293, 292f
Alcohol rehabilitation, 19
Allergies, noted on chart, 172–173, 275
Allergist, 6t
Allied health professionals, 8, 9t
  in physician's office, 42, 44, 44f
Allopathic philosophy, 4
ALOS. *See* Average length of stay (ALOS).
Alphabetic field, 51
Alphabetic filing, 142–144, 143f, 144t, 150, 153t
Alphanumeric field, 51, 55b
AMA (American Medical Association), 200, 200b, 201, 202
  CPT codes and, 332
  health insurance and, 316b
AMA (against medical advice), 11, 21b, 258
Ambulatory, definition of, 16b
Ambulatory care facility(ies), 15–17. *See also* Health care facility(ies); Physician's office.
  charge capture in, 328, 329f
  clinical flow in, 45, 70t
  H&P in, 77
  orders in, 78
  progress notes in, 79
  prospective payment systems for, 324
  uniform data sets in, 56–57, 56f, 118, 238
Ambulatory Patient Classifications (APCs), 324
Ambulatory surgery, 16
American Academy of Pediatric Medicine, 5
American Board of Medical Specialties, 4
American College of Surgeons (ACS), 29, 202, 232
American Health Information Management Association (AHIMA), 32
  code of ethics of, 31b, 32, 35, 301
  coding credentials from, 9t, 122, 332, 403b
  coding guidelines and, 332
  continuing education requirement of, 403b

American Health Information Management Association (AHIMA) *(Continued)*
  history of, 204b
  practice briefs of, 301
  record retention guidelines of, 156, 157f
American Hospital Association (AHA), 200, 200b, 202, 332
American Medical Association (AMA), 200, 200b, 201, 202
  CPT codes and, 331
  health insurance and, 316b
American Osteopathic Association (AOA), 188, 204
Americans with Disabilities Act (ADA), 364, 365, 380t
Analysis. *See* Qualitative analysis; Quantitative analysis.
Ancillary services, 17
Anesthesia, consent for, 285
Anesthesia report, 82
Anesthesiologist, 6t
AOA (American Osteopathic Association), 188, 204
APCs (Ambulatory Patient Classifications), 324
Aptitude assessment, 377
Arithmetic mean, 14, 254–255, 255f
Assembly of records, 107f, 109–110, 349
  as priority, 332, 357
  concurrent, 353
  length of stay and, 352
  performance standard for, 368t
  personnel for, 348, 348t
  quality standard for, 207–208, 208t
Assessment, 70, 72, 73t, 77
Assumption of risk, 312–313, 314f
Attending physician, 71
  access to records by, 277
  as data element, 241
  in physician index, 249–250
  UHDDS definition of, 238
Audit trail, 105, 170, 297
Authentication
  by nurse, 78, 111b
  by physician
    of discharge summary, 80
    of H&P, 77
    of operative report, 82
    of orders, 78, 79t, 87, 111b
    of progress notes, 79
    of resident physician's note, 79, 111
    space on form for, 87
  deficiencies in, 111, 112, 112t, 113, 213
  in computer-based record, 90–91, 104
  of corrected data, 105
Authorship, of order, 87, 111, 111b

Average, 254–255, 255f
Average inpatient service days, 265f
Average length of stay (ALOS), 14–15, 14f
    data sources for, 254, 261
    discharge numbers and, 22–23
    in acute care facility, 11, 14, 14f, 15
    in long-term care facility, 17

B

Backup file, 179, 180
Bar graph, 225–226, 225f, 256t
Baseline, 45
Bassinet occupancy ratio formula, 265f
Bassinets, 260b
Batch by days processing, 119
Batch control form, 119
Bed board system, 260b
Bed count, 22
Bed occupancy rate, 265f
Behavioral health facilities, 18–19. *See also* Community mental health services.
Behavioral health records
    classification system for, 116
    release of information in, 287, 292–293, 292f
Benchmarking, 212
Beneficiary, 312t
Benefit(s)
    employee, 342, 343, 393
    in health care services, 312t
Benefit period, 312t
Billing, 326–332. *See also* Insurance; Reimbursement.
    charge capture for, 327–328
    Chargemaster and, 326–327, 327t, 333
    coding and, 117, 187–188, 300, 326, 332–334
    federal enforcement of accuracy in, 300
    for ambulatory care, 327, 328, 329f, 331f, 332
    for physician's services in hospital, 328b
    HCFA-1500 form for, 187, 331f, 332
    patient accounts department and, 326
    UB-92 form for, 187, 240, 328, 330f
Billing services, 327
Binding of health record, 110
Births. *See* Newborns.
Bit, 51b
Blood usage review, 229
Blue Cross, Medicare and, 320
Blue Shield, Medicare and, 320
Board certification, 4–5
Board of directors, 344, 344b
Board of trustees, 344, 344b

Body mechanics, 395, 401. *See also* Ergonomics.
Brainstorming, 223–224
Business record rule, 280
Byte, 51b

C

CAAHEP (Commission on Accreditation of Allied Health Education Programs), 28b, 29t
Capitation, 310–311, 324
Cardiologist, 6t
Care plan, 8–10, 70–71, 72, 77
    case management and, 219–220
    clinical pathway for, 218–219
Career strategies, 418–440. *See also* Continuing education.
    choosing career in, 437–439
    choosing course of study in, 431–433
    choosing school in, 428–429
    distance education in, 424
    financial aid in, 430–432
    for adult learners, 419–423
    for nontraditional students, 422–424
    personal workforce readiness in, 433–437, 440
    planning process in, 425–427
    technology and, 418, 423, 424–425, 433
    workplace education in, 423–424
CARF (Commission on Accreditation of Rehabilitation Facilities), 30, 188, 204
Case management, 219–220
Case mix analysis, 323, 327
Case Mix Groups (CMGs), 322
Case studies, 194
CBC (complete blood count), 82
Census, 259–263, 259f
    bed board system for, 260b
    fiscal year for, 261, 262f
    service days and, 260, 260t, 261t, 262–263, 262b, 263f, 263t
Centers for Disease Control and Prevention (CDC), 26t, 191, 192f, 253
Centralized file area, 168
CEO (chief executive officer), 344–345
Certification, under Medicare COP, 188
Certified Coding Specialist (CCS), 9t, 122, 332, 403b
Certified Coding Specialist–Physician-Office Based (CCS-P), 332, 403b
Certified copy of record, 294–295
Certified nurse technician, 7t
CFR (Code of Federal Regulations), 292
Chain of command, 344, 349b
CHAMPUS (Civilian Health and Medical Program of the Uniformed Services), 319

CHAMPVA (Civilian Health and Medical Program of the Veterans Administration), 319–320

Characters, 50, 51b

Charge capture, 327–328

Chargemaster, 326–327, 327t, 333

Charges, 326–327, 327t, 333. *See also* Billing.

Chart(s). *See* Graphs; Health record(s).

Chart locator systems, 169–173, 171f, 172b, 173f–174f

Chief complaint, 73, 76t

Chief executive officer (CEO), 344–345

Chief of staff, 228, 229

Children's hospital, 23–24

Chronologic order, 62, 63f, 109–110

Civilian Health and Medical Program of the Uniformed Services (CHAMPUS), 319

Civilian Health and Medical Program of the Veterans Administration (CHAMPVA), 319–320

Claim, 312t, 326

Classification systems, 116, 116t, 117t. *See also* Coding.

Clerical employees, 348

Clinic, 16

Clinical data, 73–83, 74f
 definition of, 48
 for consultation, 71, 71t
 from laboratory tests, 74f, 82–83
 from nurses, 74f, 80–81, 81t
 from physicians, 71–80, 73t, 74f, 76t, 77t, 79t
  in office visit, 48–49, 49f
 from radiology tests, 74f, 83
 in operative records, 82

Clinical flow of data
 in acute care facility, 68–71, 69t, 70t, 71t
 in physician's office, 44–45, 70t

Clinical pathways, 218–219

Clinical pertinence, 215, 216f, 217

Clinical professional, definition of, 8

Clinical trials, 195b

Closed chart review. *See* Record review.

Closure of facilities, 156–158, 158f

CM (Clinical Modification). *See* ICD-9–CM (International Classification of Diseases) codes.

CMGs (Case Mix Groups), 321

Code of ethics, of AHIMA, 31b, 32, 35, 301

Code of Federal Regulations (CFR), 292

Coder(s), 122
 certification of, 9t, 122, 332, 403b
 performance standards for, 368t
 productivity reports on, 368–369, 369t, 370
 supervisor of, 268
 targeted review of, 333

Codes, emergency, 393, 394, 394t

Coding, 115–118, 116t, 117t, 350. *See also* Coder(s); Current Procedural Terminology (CPT) codes; International Classification of Diseases (ICD) codes.
 abstracting and, 118, 242, 252
 auditing of, 333–334, 336
 guidelines and rules for, 332–333
 in-service training in, 334, 399, 400
 order of processing and, 107f, 120
 outpatient, 115–116, 116t, 117t, 334
 quality of, 208, 208t, 300, 333–334
 reimbursement and, 117, 187–188, 300, 326, 332–334

Coding Clinic, 332, 333, 381t

Coding compliance plan, 300, 333

Collection of records, 108, 109b, 349

Color coding, 139, 140, 142

Commission on Accreditation of Allied Health Education Programs (CAAHEP), 28b, 29t

Commission on Accreditation of Rehabilitation Facilities (CARF), 30, 188, 204

Committees, 228–231, 230f
 JCAHO steering committee as, 300
 Medical Executive Committee as, 209, 229

Communication, 404–409, 405f
 by e-mail, 407, 409b
 by memo, 407, 408f
 patient data for, 129

Community awareness, health information for, 193

Community mental health services, 325

Competency, of patient, 285

Complaint, legal, 280

Complete blood count (CBC), 82

Completeness. *See also* Quantitative analysis.
 of data, 100–101, 101t
 of health record, 206b

Completion of records, 104, 113–115, 350
 physician orientation about, 396, 398f, 399b

Compliance, 298–301, 333. *See also* Accreditation; Licensure of facilities; Professional standards.

Compressible shelves, 160, 161f, 163t

Computer files
 backups of, 179, 180
 indexing of, 137–138, 155
 Computer interface, 133, 134b

Computer software, 178, 383, 383b

Computer-assisted function
 definition of, 105b
 example of, 113

Computer-based patient record, 65–67, 67f, 137. *See also* Computerized patient record.
 abstract of, 242

Computer-based patient record *(Continued)*
  assembly of, 110
  audit trail of, 105, 170, 297
  authentication in, 90–91, 104
  completeness of, 115, 295
  confidentiality of, 275, 277, 297
  correction of errors in, 105–106
  database created from. *See* Database(s).
  definition of, 105b
  design of screens for, 88–89, 90–91, 90t,
    92, 240
  HIM department workflow and, 353
  paper printouts and, 97
  prospective payment systems and, 321, 321b
  quantitative and qualitative analysis of, 218,
    353
  security of, 175b
  standardization of, 202b
  validity of data in, 90, 90t, 101–102
Computerized chart locator systems, 172–
    173, 172b, 173f–174f
Computerized document
  definition of, 105b
  policies and procedures manual as, 361,
    361t
  productivity report as, 369–370
Computerized master patient index, 133–
    136, 134f–135f, 136b
Computerized patient record, 137–138,
    155–156. *See also* Computer-based pa-
    tient record.
  audit trail of, 170
  imaging manager and, 182
  security of, 178, 179, 180
Concurrent analysis, 112–113, 352–353, 353t
  of computer-based patient record, 218
  planning for, 354–355
Concurrent coding, 117, 352, 353t, 354
Concurrent review, 187, 217
Conditions of Admission, 278, 285, 286f, 287
Conditions of Participation (COP), 27, 30, 188
Confidentiality, 274–277. *See also* Access to
    records; Security of records.
  definition of, 274
  employee orientation to, 395, 401
  employee's signed agreement on, 275, 276f
  hypothetical application of, 304
  of computer-based record, 275, 277, 297
  of released health record, 295–296, 296f
  within family, 149
Confidentiality Statement, 275, 276f
Consent
  definition of, 285
  for medical procedures, 285, 287, 288f
  for release of information, 287, 289–290,
    289f

Consent *(Continued)*
    special, 287, 292–293, 292f
    to payer, 278
    validation of, 293–294
  informed, 285, 287, 293
  on admission to facility, 278, 285, 286f, 287
  prospective, 278, 287, 293
  retrospective, 278, 287
Consultant, 71
Consultation, 6, 71, 71t, 80
  missing report of, 113
  physician's order for, 78
Continuing education, 194, 399, 403–404,
    404t, 405f, 433, 439
  AHIMA requirement for, 403b
Continuous quality improvement (CQI). *See*
    Quality improvement (QI).
Continuum of care, 24–26
Contracts
  managed care, 195
  of facility with vendors, 190
Cooperating Parties, 332
COP (Conditions of Participation), 27, 30, 188
Co-payment, 312t, 316
Copy machines, 382
Copy services, 303
Coronary care unit, 92
Corporate compliance, 300–301, 333
Corrective controls, 104–105, 113–115, 114f,
    198. *See also* Completion of records.
Correspondence, 118, 281. *See also* Release of
    information.
Cost basis, 327, 327t
Countersigned note, 79, 111
Court order, 281, 284f
Coverage, definition of, 312t
CPT Assistant, 381t
CPT codes. *See* Current Procedural Terminol-
    ogy (CPT) codes.
CQI (continuous quality improvement). *See*
    Quality improvement (QI).
Credentialing, of physicians, 34
Credentials, of HIM professional, 403
Critical care units, 92
Crosby, Philip, 199, 200
Cross-training, 400, 401
Current Procedural Terminology (CPT)
    codes, 115–116, 116t, 117t, 187, 332–
    333, 334
  Chargemaster field for, 327t, 333
  employee training about, 401
  in outpatient prospective payment, 324–325
  on encounter form, 328
  reference materials on, 381t
Customer service, 392, 400
Customers, 197, 197b–198b

D

Data. *See also* Health record(s).
 accuracy of, 55, 101t
 aggregate, 248–249, 249f, 250, 252, 254
 as plural form, 42b
 categories of, 45–49, 46f–49f
 clinical. *See* Clinical data.
 clinical flow of
  in acute care facility, 68–71, 69t, 70t, 71t
  in physician's office, 44–45, 70t
 definition of, 38, 39f, 236b
 description of, 50–53, 51f–52f, 54f
 health data as, 39–40, 41f
 interpretation of, 254
 optimum source of, 252–253
 primary, 236, 236f
 quality of, 54–55, 100–101, 101t
  controls over, 90–91, 90t, 101–106, 102t, 103f
 reporting of, 190–191, 253–254, 268
 retrieval of, 248–253, 249f–251f
 secondary, 236, 236f
 statistical analysis of, 254–256, 255f, 256t
 validity of, 55, 101t, 206b, 213
  preventive controls over, 90–91, 90t, 101–102, 103f
 visual presentation tools for, 224–228, 225f–227f, 227t, 256t
Data collection devices, 83. *See also* Forms.
 control of, 91–92
 design of
  for computer screen, 88–89, 90–91, 90t, 92
  for paper forms, 84–88, 86f, 88f, 90t
Data dictionary, 51, 51f, 90, 90t, 240, 241t, 252
 development of, 59, 92
Data entry
 in abstracting data, 118
 in recording data, 100
Data flow. *See* Clinical flow of data.
Data sets, 55–57, 56f, 93, 238–240, 238t, 239t
 codes in, 118
 for patient's gender, 239–240, 239f, 240b
Data transfer, to electronic medium, 118
Database(s), 240–241. *See also* Abstracting.
 federal requirements for, 240b
 quality check of, 246, 248, 248b
 querying of, 241, 241b, 242, 246
  identifying population for, 251–252
  information needed for, 249
  strategies for, 253
  to create indices, 249–250, 250f–251f
 relational, 65–66, 105b
 reporting of data from, 253–254, 268
 statistical analysis of, 254–256, 255f, 256t

Data-gathering tools, 223–224, 224t
Date-oriented record, 62, 63f–64f, 66
Datum, 42b
Day of discharge, 11
DD (date dictated), 190, 190b
Death(s)
 as discharge from facility, 11, 257f, 258
 statistics on, 191, 257f, 258
Death certificate, 254
Death rate, 200b
Decentralized file area, 168
Decision making, medical, 73, 75f
 computerized support for, 218
 payers' involvement in, 219
Decision matrix, 226–228, 227t, 256t
Decision support, computerized, 218, 218b
Deductible, 314–315, 316
 definition of, 312t
Deemed status, 30, 188
Defendant, 279
Deficiencies in record, 111–115, 112t, 114f
Deficiency sheet, 113, 114f
Deficiency system, 113–115, 114f. *See also* Completion of records.
Delegation of responsibility, 342
Delinquent records, 114–115, 357
 medical staff bylaws and, 399b
Deming, Edward, 199
Demographic data, 46, 46f, 69, 84
Department heads, 346
Department of Health and Human Services (DHHS), 26t, 191
 HIPAA regulations of, 301
 Office of the Inspector General in, 300
Dermatologist, 6t
Destruction of records, 179–180, 281
Detective controls, 103, 110–112, 112t, 114f, 198. *See also* Quantitative analysis.
Detoxification, 19
Development, of employees, 392
Diagnosis, 8b
 admitting, 117, 252, 324
 at discharge, 80
 coding of, 116–118, 116t, 117t, 187. *See also* International Classification of Diseases (ICD) codes.
 development of, 70, 71–73, 73t
Diagnosis index, 250–251, 250f–251f
Diagnosis Related Groups (DRGs), 321, 322–324, 326
 auditing of records and, 336
 optimal reimbursement and, 332
Diagnostic and Statistical Manual of Mental Disorders (DSM-IV), 116, 116t
Dictation equipment, 382
Dietician, registered, 9t

Digital imaging, 153. *See also* Optical disk.

Disaster planning, 175–176

Discharge(s), 11. *See also* Census; Postdischarge processing.
  by transfer to other facility, 258, 259b
  facility size and, 22–23
  HIM department workflow and, 351–352
  length of stay and, 12–13, 12f–13f, 20f, 22–23
  statistics on, 256, 257f, 258

Discharge register, 107–108, 108t, 109

Discharge summary, 80, 113, 206

Discharged no final bill (DNFB) list, 326

Discounted fee for service, 309, 310, 324, 328
  in ambulatory health care, 324
  UB-92 form for, 328

Discovery, in lawsuit, 279, 280t

Discrimination, in employment, 379, 380t

Disease(s). *See also* Diagnosis.
  definition of, 38
  federal monitoring of, 191
  incidence of, 191
  prevalence of, 191

Disposition of patient, 242

DNFB (discharged no final bill) list, 326

Doctor(s). *See* Physician(s).

Doctor of Medicine (MD), 4

Doctor of Osteopathy (DO), 4

Doctor's order(s). *See* Order(s).

Document imaging manager, 182

Documentation, importance of, 201b

DRGs (Diagnosis Related Groups), 321, 322–324, 326
  auditing of records and, 336
  optimal reimbursement and, 332

Dropping a bill, 326, 332

Drug and alcohol abuse records, 274, 287, 292–293, 292f

Drug and alcohol rehabilitation, 19

Drug screen, on job candidate, 379

DSM-IV (Diagnostic and Statistical Manual of Mental Disorders), 116, 116t

DT (date transcribed), 190, 190b

Durable medical power of attorney, 211b

E

Education. *See also* Career strategies; Training.
  continuing, 194, 399, 403–404, 404t, 405f, 433, 439
    AHIMA requirement for, 403b
  for public, 416
  health information for, 194
  medical, history of, 201
  of public, 403

Electronic communication, 408, 410b

Electronic data
  abstracted from paper record, 118
  definition of, 104b

Electronic patient record, 53. *See also* Computer-based patient record.

Electronic signatures, 91

E-mail, 408, 410b
  for sending records, 296

Emergencies
  chart locator system and, 170, 172–173
  release of information in, 290–292, 291f

Emergency codes, 393, 394, 394t

Emergency department, 10
  admission to hospital from, 70
  outpatient in, 17b

Employee(s)
  classification of, 342–343, 343t
  confidentiality agreement signed by, 275, 276f
  evaluations of, 370–371, 370b
  health record of, 297
  HIM staff positions of, 347–349, 347f, 348t
  hiring of. *See* Hiring.
  inappropriate access to records by, 277, 297
  insurance premiums paid by, 312
  job analysis of, 362, 363f, 364
  job description of, 364–365, 366f–367f
  performance improvement and, 208–209, 210
  probation period of, 365, 370, 371, 396b
  productivity of
    equipment and supplies for, 383
    measurement of, 352, 352f, 358, 364, 365, 368, 369t, 370
      performance standards for, 365, 368t, 399
  supervisors of, 343, 346, 348, 350
    communication by, 407
    monitoring of operations by, 358

Employee handbook, 393

Employer
  HMOs offered by, 317
  insurance provided by, 311, 312, 313, 315

Employment laws, 379, 380t

Encounter, 15

Encounter form, 328, 329f, 333

Epidemiology, 40

Equipment, for HIM department, 380, 380b, 381

Ergonomics, 383, 384f, 385. *See also* Body mechanics.

Error report, 103, 112

Errors. *See* Corrective controls; Data, quality of.

Ethics, AHIMA Code of, 31b, 32, 35, 301
Etiologies, 78
Examination, 72, 76–77, 77t. *See also* History & physical (H&P).
Exception report, 103, 112
Exclusion, definition of, 312t
Exempt employees, 348b
Expert testimony, 193, 194

F

Face sheet (admission record), 69, 69t, 84, 97
    codes on, 252
    sent to HIM department, 132
Facilitator, 223
Facilities. *See* Health care facility(ies).
Facsimile (fax) transmissions
    to release records, 296, 296f
    to request release of records, 291–292
Fair employment practices, 379, 380t
Family Medical Leave Act, 380t
Family practitioner, 4, 5–6, 6t
Family unit numbering system, 146–147, 149, 149t
Federal government, 26–27, 26t
    corporate compliance and, 300
    database requirements of, 240b
    health policies of, 191–192, 193f
    reimbursement by, 319–322. *See also* Medicaid; Medicare.
    special consent regulations of, 292–293, 292f
Fee for service, 308–309, 310, 324, 327
    in ambulatory health care, 324
    UB-92 form for, 328
Fees. *See* Charges; Reimbursement.
Fields, 51, 51f, 55b
File(s)
    of data, 53, 54f
    on computer
        backups of, 179, 180
        indexing of, 141, 153–156
File cabinets, 158–159, 159f, 163, 163t
File clerk, 368t
File folder(s), 110, 349
    identification of, 141–142
        alphabetic, 142–144, 143f, 144t
        family unit numbering for, 146–147, 149, 149t
        serial numbering for, 146, 147f, 149t
        serial–unit numbering for, 146, 148f, 149t
        unit numbering for, 144–145, 145f, 149t
    labeling of forms in, 138
    multiple for single patient, 139

File folder(s) (*Continued*)
    recommended features of, 138–140, 140f–141f, 141b
    recommended quantities of, 381–382
File rooms, 162–164
Filing. *See also* Storage of records.
    performance standard for, 368t
    personnel for, 348, 348t, 368t
    quality standard for, 208t
Filing furniture, 158–162, 163, 163t, 164
Filing methods, 150–156
    advantages and disadvantages of, 153t
    alphabetic, 142–144, 143f, 144t, 150, 153t
    conversion between, 183
    middle-digit, 152, 152t, 153t
    straight numeric, 150–151, 153t
    terminal-digit, 151–152, 151t, 153f, 153t
Financial data, 47–48, 48f, 69, 84
Fire security, 176–177, 393, 394
Fiscal intermediaries, 312t, 320
Fiscal year, 261, 262f
Flagging, by analyst, 112
Flexible benefit account, 319
Flexner Report, 201, 202
Flowchart, 228
Forms
    control of, 91–92
    design of
        for computer screen, 88–89, 90–91, 90t, 92
        for paper, 84–88, 86f, 88f, 90t
    for billing, 187, 240, 328, 329f–331f, 332
    for clinical evaluations, 73
    for record review, 213, 214f
    in prospective payment systems, 321b
    master file of, 91, 92
    patient identification on, 137
Forms committee, 84, 87, 91–92, 229
Formulary, 229
For-profit organization, 23, 196, 327, 344b
Fraud, 188, 188b, 332, 333
Full-time equivalent (FTE), 342, 343b, 343t
Furniture, for filing, 158–162, 163, 163t, 164

G

Gastroenterologist, 4, 5, 6t
General ledger code, 327t
General practitioner, 4, 5–6
Geriatric aide, 7t
Goals, of HIM department, 356–357, 356t, 358
Governing board, 229, 344, 344b, 345
Government, in health care, 26–28, 26t. *See also* Federal government; State governments.

Graphs
  of clinical data, 39, 40f, 73, 81
    in critical care unit, 92
  types of, 225–226, 225f–227f, 256, 256t
Group practice, 15–16
Grouper, 323, 325
Guarantor, 48
Guardian, 285
Gynecologist, 6t

H

H&P. *See* History & physical (H&P).
Hand washing, 393–394
Handshake, 378b
HCFA. *See* Health Care Financing Administration (HCFA).
HCFA-1500 form, 187, 331f, 332
HCPCS (HCFA Common Procedure Coding System), 115–116, 116t, 327
Health, definition of, 38
Health care costs, 315–316
Health care facility(ies), 10–32
  accreditation of. *See* Accreditation.
  acute care. *See* Acute care facility(ies).
  administration of, 190, 344–346, 345f
  admission to. *See* Admission(s).
  adult day care as, 19–20, 30
  ambulatory. *See* Ambulatory care facility (ies).
  behavioral health, 18–19
  closure of, 156–158, 158f
  committees in, 228–231, 230f
    JCAHO steering committee as, 300
    Medical Executive Committee as, 209, 229
  comparison of, 20f, 21–24
  continuum of care and, 24–26
  discharge from. *See* Discharge(s).
  financial status of, 23, 196, 344b
  hospice as, 20–21
  legal and regulatory environment of, 26–28, 26t
  length of stay in. *See* Length of stay (LOS).
  long-term care, 17, 18t
    H&P in, 77
    prospective payment system for, 325
    state regulation of, 28
  marketing by, 196–197
  organization chart of, 344–346, 345f
  ownership of, 23
  patient population of, 23–24
  physician's office as. *See* Physician's office.
  professional standards in, 31–32, 301
  rehabilitation, 18t, 19

Health care facility(ies) *(Continued)*
  accreditation of, 30
  care plans in, 71
  prospective payment system for, 326
  services provided by, 18t, 24
  size of, 21–23
  statistics of. *See* Statistics, of facility.
  transfers between, 258, 259b
  transfers within, 258, 258f, 259b
Health Care Financing Administration (HCFA), 27, 30, 188, 320
  Ambulatory Patient Classifications of, 323–324
  billing form of (HCFA-1500), 187, 331f, 332
  coding guidelines and, 332, 333
  DRGs published by, 323
  HCPCS coding system of, 115–116, 116t, 327t, 381t
  record retention requirement of, 156
  Uniform Hospital Discharge Data Set and, 238, 240
Health care professionals, 4–8, 6t, 7t, 9t
  standards for, 31–32, 301
Health care providers, in managed care, 195
Health data, 39–40, 41f. *See also* Data.
Health information, 40, 41f, 42
  quality of, 205, 205b–206b. *See also* Quality improvement (QI).
  uses of, 186, 196t. *See also specific uses.*
Health information administrator. *See* Registered Health Information Administrator (RHIA).
Health information analyst, 110
Health information management, 53–54
Health information management (HIM) department
  alternative names for, 347
  assistant director of, 233, 347
  collection of records for, 108, 109b, 349
  communication in, 405–410, 406f
    by e-mail, 408, 410b
    by memo, 408, 409f
  compliance with regulations in, 298–299
  director of, 347, 388b
    certification of records by, 294–295
    compliance with regulations and, 298
    human resources and, 342
    on HIM committee, 229
    on JCAHO steering committee, 300
    sequestered records and, 220b
  equipment for, 380, 380b, 383
  ergonomics in, 383, 384f, 385. *See also* Body mechanics.
  functions of, 205, 349–350, 351f
    standards for, 352–353, 353t

Health information management (HIM) department *(Continued)*
  goals and objectives of, 356–357, 356t, 358
  meetings of. *See* Meetings.
  monitoring operations in, 358
  organization chart of, 347–349, 347f
  orientation to
    for clinical staff, 396, 398f, 399, 399b
    for HIM employees, 395–396, 396b, 397f
  planning in, 354–357, 356t
  policies and procedures of, 298, 300, 358, 359f, 360–362, 360t–361t
  prioritization in, 357
  quality in. *See* Quality improvement (QI).
  reference materials for, 381, 381t
  retention policy of, 156
  sequestered file in, 220b, 297
  staff positions in, 347–349, 347f, 348t. *See also* Employee(s).
  standards in, 352–353, 353t, 357
    for concurrent processing, 354, 354t
  supplies for, 381–383
  workflow in, 349–354, 351f–352f, 353t, 354t, 357
Health information specialist, 110
Health information technician, 348, 348t. *See also* Registered Health Information Technician (RHIT).
Health information technology, 54
Health insurance. *See* Insurance.
Health Insurance Portability and Accountability Act (HIPAA), 191, 240, 300, 301
Health Level Seven (HL-7) standards, 240
Health maintenance organizations (HMOs), 191, 317–318, 320
Health record(s), 53. *See also* Data.
  access to. *See* Access to records.
  active vs. inactive, 165, 165b
  assembly of. *See* Assembly of records.
  binding of, 110
  certified copy of, 294–295
  clinical data in. *See* Clinical data.
  clinical flow and
    in acute care facility, 68–71, 69t, 70t, 71t
    in physician's office, 44–45, 70t
  collection of, 108, 109b, 349
  completion of, 104, 113–115, 350
    physician orientation about, 396, 398f, 399b
  compliance with regulations for, 298–299
  computer-based. *See* Computer-based patient record.
  computerized. *See* Computerized patient record.
  confidentiality of. *See* Confidentiality.
  contaminated with blood, 395

Health record(s) *(Continued)*
  demographic data in, 46, 46f, 69, 84
  destruction of, 179–180, 281
  duplicate copies of, 180
  filing of. *See* File folder(s); Filing; Filing methods.
  financial data in, 47–48, 48f, 69, 84
  HIM department processing of, 205, 349–350, 351f. *See also* Postdischarge processing.
  identification of, 129, 130, 130f, 141–142
    alphabetic, 142–144, 143f, 144t
    numeric. *See* Medical record number (MR#).
  in physician's office, 45
  location of. *See* Master patient index (MPI).
  Medicare reviews of, 204–205
  minimum content of, 202, 203f
  of employee patient, 297
  of potentially compensable events, 220, 220b
  of transferred patient, 259b
  organization of, 62–67, 63f–68f. *See also* Assembly of records.
  photocopying of, 294–295, 303
  qualitative analysis of, 212–213, 214f, 215, 216f, 217–218
  release of. *See* Release of information.
  retention of, 106, 106t, 118, 155–158, 157f–158f, 179
  retrieval of. *See* Retrieval of records.
  security of, 106, 106t, 175–180, 175b
    in computer environment, 175b, 240b
  sensitive, 220b, 297
  socioeconomic data in, 46–47, 47f, 69, 84
  storage of. *See* Storage of records.
  tracking of, 119–120
Health unit coordinator, 9t
Health-related professionals, 8, 9t
  in physician's office, 42, 44, 44f
Hearsay rule, 280
HIM committee, 229, 230f, 233
HIM department. *See* Health information management (HIM) department.
HIM Tech I and II, 348, 348t
HIPAA (Health Insurance Portability and Accountability Act), 191, 240, 300, 301
Hiring, 371
  advertisement for, 371–372, 372f
  application form for, 373, 373t, 374f–377f
  assessment for, 379
  interviewing for, 378, 379t
  legal restrictions in, 379, 380t
  screening applicants for, 373, 373b
History, 73, 75, 76t

History & physical (H&P), 77. *See also* Physical examination.
  deficiencies in, 111, 113, 115
  JCAHO standards for, 77, 213
  timeliness of, 205b, 213
HL-7 (Health Level Seven) standards, 240
HMOs (health maintenance organizations), 191, 317–318, 320
Home health care, 21, 326
Home health care assistant, 7t
Hospice, 20–21
Hospital(s). *See also* Acute care facility(ies).
  definition of, 10
  historical development of, 200, 202
Hospital privileges, 34
Hospital Standardization Program, 202
Human immunodeficiency virus (HIV) infection
  consent to testing for, 285, 287
  release of records about, 292–293, 292f
Human resources, 342–343, 343t. *See also* Employee(s).

I

ICD-9-CM (International Classification of Diseases) codes, 116, 117t, 187, 332
  DRGs derived from, 322, 323
  in ambulatory care, 325
  in long-term care, 325
  on encounter form, 328
  reference materials for, 381t
ICD-10 (International Classification of Diseases) codes, 116, 337
ICD-O (International Classification of Diseases–Oncology), 116, 117t
IDSs (integrated delivery systems), 26
Impression, 77. *See also* Assessment.
Inactive records, 165, 165b
Inadvertent occurrence, 220, 221f–222f
Incidence, 191
Incident report, 220, 221f, 231
Incomplete records
  completion of, 104, 113–115, 350
  physician orientation about, 396, 398f, 399b
  release of, 294
Incomplete system, 113–115, 114f. *See also* Completion of records.
Indemnity insurance, 313–316
Independent practice association (IPA), 318
Indexing. *See also* Indices; Master patient index (MPI).
  of computerized record, 137, 155, 167, 182
Indicative data, 46, 46f
Indices, 249–250, 250f–251f

Infection control
  annual training about, 401, 402
  orientation to, 394–396
Infection control committee, 229–230
Infectious disease statistics, 190–191
Information, 38–39, 39f–41f, 40, 42. *See also* Health information.
Informed consent, 285, 287, 293. *See also* Consent.
Initial assessment, 70
Inpatient
  definition of, 10, 17b
  in long-term care facility, 17
Inpatient service days (IPSD), 260, 260t, 261t, 262–263, 262b, 263f, 263t
  average, 265f
In-service training, 399, 400, 402, 402t
Insurance, 310–318. *See also* Billing; Medicaid; Medicare; Reimbursement.
  access to records and, 278
  AMA position on, 316b
  assumption of risk and, 312–313, 314f
  cost control and, 315–316, 317
  definition of, 312t
  history of, 311–312
  legislative impacts on, 191
  managed care and, 195, 316–318
  preapproval of procedures and, 219, 316, 317
  prospective payment systems and, 309, 326
  release of information and, 287
  terminology of, 312t
  types of, 313–319, 319t
Integrated delivery systems (IDSs), 26
Integrated record, 62, 63f–64f, 66
Intensive care unit, 92
Interdepartmental performance improvement, 209b, 210
Interface, computer, 133, 134b
Interhospital transfer, 258, 259b
Internal medicine, 4
International Classification of Diseases (ICD) codes
  Ninth Revision (ICD-9-CM), 116, 117t, 187, 331
    DRGs derived from, 322, 323
    in ambulatory care, 325
    in long-term care, 325
    on encounter form, 328
    reference materials for, 381t
  Tenth Revision (ICD-10), 116, 337
International Classification of Diseases–Oncology (ICD-O), 116, 117t
Internet, records sent by, 296
Internist
  in behavioral health facility, 18

Internist *(Continued)*
  in rehabilitation facility, 19
Interpretation of data, 254
Interviewing, of job applicant, 378, 379t
Intradepartmental performance improvement, 209b, 210
Intrahospital transfer, 258f, 259b
Invoice, for copies of record, 295, 303
IPA (independent practice association), 318
IPSD (inpatient service days), 260, 260t, 261t, 262–263, 262b, 263f, 263t
  average, 265f

J

JCAHO steering committee, 300
Job analysis, 362, 363f, 364
Job application form, 373, 373t, 374f–377f
Job description, 364–365, 366f–367f
Joint Commission on Accreditation of Healthcare Organizations (JCAHO), 29–30, 188, 204, 299–300
  accreditation manuals of, 202, 203t
  blood usage review and, 229
  completion of records and, 77, 112, 114, 189, 213
  disaster planning and, 176
  filing systems and, 142
  founding of, 202
  medication usage review and, 229
  quality improvement standards of, 206–208, 207t, 208t, 209b
  record review and, 215, 217
  safety requirements of, 230
  surgical case review and, 229
  surveys by, 252–253, 299–300
Juran, Joseph M., 199–200
Jurisdiction, of court, 280

L

Laboratory services, 16–17, 24
Laboratory tests, 82–83
  orders for, 78
Laundry companies, 190
Lawsuits. *See* Litigation.
Length of stay (LOS), 12–15, 12f–14f, 13b, 20f
  aggregate data on, 248, 249f, 254
  assembly of records and, 352
  average. *See* Average length of stay (ALOS).
  diagnosis coding and, 117
  discharge statistics and, 22–23
  for obstetric patients, 191

Length of stay (LOS) *(Continued)*
  in acute care facility, 11, 14, 14f, 15
  in long-term care facility, 17
  prospective payment systems and, 321, 323
Licensed beds, 22
Licensed practical nurse (LPN), 7, 7t
Licensed vocational nurse (LVN), 7, 7t
Licensing of health care professionals, 4, 6, 31–32
Licensure of facilities, 10, 27–28, 30, 188–190, 298–299
Line graph, 225–226, 226f, 256t
Litigation, 193–194, 279, 280t
  against HMOs, 191
  health records for, 193
    access to, 279–281, 282f–284f
    certified copy of, 294–295
    potentially compensable events and, 220, 220b
    security of, 220b, 297
Living will, 211b
Long-term care facilities, 17, 18t. *See also* Health care facility(ies).
  H&P in, 77
  prospective payment system for, 325
  state regulation of, 28
Loose sheets, 119
LOS. *See* Length of stay (LOS).
LPN (licensed practical nurse), 7, 7t
LVN (licensed vocational nurse), 7, 7t

M

Maintenance contract
  for equipment, 380b, 382
  for software, 383
Major Diagnostic Categories (MDC), 322–323
Malpractice claims. *See* Litigation.
Managed care, 195, 316–318
Managers, 343, 346, 358. *See also* Supervisors.
Manipulative approach, 4
Marketing, 196–197
Master forms file, 91, 92
Master patient index (MPI), 129–136
  computerized, 133–136, 134f–135f, 136b
  contents of, 130–131, 131f
    in manual system, 132b
  duplication of patient in, 131, 133b
  in serial–unit numbering system, 146
  manual, 129, 132–133, 132b, 133b, 133f
    conversion of, 136, 137b
  medical record number in, 129, 130, 130f
  on-site storage and, 168
  removal of cards from, 133b
  retention of, 136, 138b

Maximization of reimbursement, 332
MD (Doctor of Medicine), 4
MDC (Major Diagnostic Categories), 322–323
MDS (Minimum Data Set), 325
Mean, 14, 254–255, 255f
Median, 255
Medicaid, 188, 192, 204, 319, 320, 321
Medical assistant, 42, 45, 327
Medical decision making, 73, 75f
  computerized support for, 218
  payers' involvement in, 219
Medical education, history of, 201
Medical evaluation process, 71–73, 73t, 77
Medical Executive Committee, 209, 229
Medical record(s). *See* Health record(s).
Medical record analyst, 110
Medical record committee, 229, 230f
Medical record department. *See* Health information management (HIM) department.
Medical record librarian, 204
Medical record number (MR#)
  assignment of, 129
  filing methods and
    middle-digit, 152, 152t, 153t, 154f
    straight numeric, 150–151, 153t
    terminal-digit, 151–152, 151t, 153f, 153t,
  for each separate facility, 142b
  in master patient index, 129, 130, 130f, 136
  numbering systems and
    family unit, 146–147, 149, 149t
    serial, 146, 147f, 149t
    serial–unit, 146, 148f, 149t
    unit, 144–145, 145f, 149t
  on each form, 138
  on file folder label, 139, 141f
Medical secretary, 42
Medical specialties, 4–6, 6t. *See also* Consultation.
Medical staff. *See also* Physician(s).
  board of directors and, 344
  committees of, 228–229
  organizational structure of, 344, 345f
Medical terminology, 5b
Medicare, 27, 188, 192, 319, 320
  accreditation and, 30
  Conditions of Participation (COP), 27, 30, 188
  long-term care reimbursement by, 325
  peer review organizations and, 321
  prospective payment systems of, 321, 322, 324, 325, 326
  reviews of health records by, 204–205
  UB-92 form used by, 328, 330f
  Uniform Hospital Discharge Data Set and, 238

Medicare HMO plans, 320
Medication(s)
  nurse's administration of, 81
  physician's order for, 78, 84–85, 87, 89
  research on, 194, 195b
  usage review of, 229
Meetings, 410–413
  agenda for, 410–411, 411t
  in quality improvement process, 222–223
  minutes of, 223b, 412f, 413
  Robert's Rules of Order in, 411b
Memorandum (memo), 408, 409f
Mental health facilities, 18–19
Mental health records. *See* Behavioral health records.
Mental health services, ambulatory, 324
Merger of facilities, 10, 11b, 25–26, 123
Microfiche, 165, 166f, 167
Microfilm, 165–167, 166f, 169, 179
Middle-digit filing, 152, 152t, 153t, 154f
Midnight census. *See* Census.
Minimum Data Set (MDS), 325
Minimum data sets. *See* Data sets.
Minutes, of meeting, 223b, 412f, 413
Misfile, 155–156
Mission statement, 355–356
Mode, 255
Modified terminal-digit filing, 152, 152t, 153f, 153t
Morbidity statistics, 191
Mortality statistics, 191
MPI. *See* Master patient index (MPI).
MR#. *See* Medical record number (MR#).
Multispecialty group, 15, 16

N

National Center for Health Statistics (NCHS), 332
National Committee for Quality Assurance (NCQA), 195, 195b
Neonatologist, 6t
New patient, 132b, 134
Newborns
  census of, 260b
  health records on, 84, 92
  reporting to state on, 254
  statistics on, 256, 257f, 265f
Nomenclature, 115. *See also* Current Procedural Terminology (CPT) codes.
Nonclinical professionals, 8
Nonexempt employees, 348b
Nosocomial infections, 82, 230b, 264
Notarization, of consent form, 293–294

Not-for-profit organization, 23, 196, 344b
NP (nurse practitioner), 7–8, 7t, 42, 44
Numbering systems
  advantages and disadvantages of, 149, 149t
  family unit numbering as, 146–147, 149, 149t
  serial numbering as, 146, 147f
  serial–unit numbering as, 146, 148f
  unit numbering as, 144–145, 145f
Numeric field, 51
Nurse(s)
  data elements contributed by, 73, 80–81, 81t
  execution of physician's order by, 78, 87
  in physician's office, 42, 45
  levels of practice of, 6–8, 7t
  on performance improvement team, 212
  on record review team, 217
Nurse anesthetist, 7
Nurse assistant, 7t
Nurse midwife, 7
Nurse practitioner (NP), 7–8, 7t, 42, 44
Nursery, 260b
Nursing assessment, 80
Nursing homes. *See* Long-term care facilities.
Nursing progress notes, 81, 81t

O

Objective data, 72, 73t, 77
Objectives, of HIM department, 356–357, 356t, 358
Observation, stay in hospital for, 17b
Obstetric patients, 84, 92, 191
Obstetrician, 6t
Occupancy rate, 22, 262, 263, 265f
Occupational Safety and Health Administration (OSHA), 26t, 230
  filing area requirements of, 162–163
Occupational therapist (OC), 9t, 19
Occurrence report, 220, 221f
Office of the Inspector General (OIG), 300
Off-site storage, 168–169
Old patient, 132b
Oncologist, 5, 6t
Oncology classification system, 116, 117t
On-site storage, 168
Open access
  to emergency department, 70
  to physician's office, 44b
Open shelves, 159–160, 160f, 163t
Operation, 82. *See also* Surgery.
Operative note, 82, 189
Operative report, 82
  abstracting from, 245f
  completion of, 113, 115, 189–190, 189f
  for same-day surgery, 92
  in patient's personal files, 281

Ophthalmologist, 6t
Optical disk, 153, 154–155, 166f, 167, 169, 179
Optimization of reimbursement, 331
Order(s), 70, 78, 79t, 111b
  computer-based, 89, 97
  paper form for, 84–85, 87, 88f
Organization charts, 343–344
  for health care facility, 344–346, 345f
  for HIM department, 347–349, 347f
Organization of records, 62–67, 63f–68f, 349. *See also* Assembly of records.
Orientation
  of clinical staff to HIM, 396, 398f, 399, 399b
  of employees, 392–399
    to HIM department, 395–396, 397f
    to new position in HIM, 396b
    to organization, 391–395, 394b, 394t
Orthopedist, 6t
OSHA (Occupational Safety and Health Administration), 26t, 230
  filing area requirements of, 162–163
Osteopathic doctor, 4
Osteopathic facilities, 204
Outguide, 146, 170–171, 171f
Out-of-pocket costs
  definition of, 312t
  under managed care, 317
Outpatient. *See also* Ambulatory care facility(ies).
  definition of, 15, 17b
Outpatient coding, 115–116, 116t, 117t, 334. *See also* Current Procedural Terminology (CPT) codes.
Outpatient surgery, 16
Outsourcing, of release of information, 285, 303

P

P&T (pharmacy and therapeutics) committee, 229
Paid time off (PTO), 342
Palliative care, 20
Paper forms. *See* Forms.
Paperless environment, 97
Part-time (PT) employee, 342, 343, 343t
Password, 178. *See also* Authentication.
  for HIM employee, 396
  for physician, 77
Pathologist, 6t
Patient
  access to record by, 281, 285
  competency of, 285
  disposition of, 242
  name of
    as identifier, 287

Patient *(Continued)*
    in alphabetic filing, 142–144, 143f, 144t
    new vs. old, 132b
    on quality improvement team, 211, 212
Patient accounts department, 326
Patient care. *See* Quality, of patient care.
Patient care plan, 8–10, 70–71, 72, 77
    case management and, 219–220
    clinical pathway for, 218–219
Patient registration department, 68–69. *See also* Admission(s).
    admitting diagnosis and, 117
    master patient index and, 129, 134, 136
Patient registration specialist, 59, 68
Patients' rights, 211b, 212
Pay-back period, 169
Payer, 47–48, 187b. *See also* Reimbursement.
    definition of, 312t
    in medical decision making, 219
    release of information to, 278, 287
PCEs (potentially compensable events), 220, 220b
PCP (primary care physician), 6, 318
PDCA method, 209, 210f, 400
Pediatrician, 5, 6t
Peer review organizations (PROs), 321
Per diem employee, 342, 343, 343t
Per diem reimbursement rates, 309
    for long-term care, 325
Percentages, 264–265, 264f–265f
Performance improvement (PI). *See* Quality improvement (QI).
Performance improvement plan (PIP), 371, 371b
Performance standards, 365, 368t, 399
Personal workforce readiness. *See* Career strategies.
Personnel. *See* Employee(s).
Pertinence, clinical, 215, 216f, 217
Pharmaceutical research, 195b
Pharmacy and therapeutics (P&T) committee, 229
Phlebotomist, 9t
Phonetic searching, 136
Photocopying, 294–295, 303
Physiatrist, 19
Physical examination, 72, 76–77, 77t. *See also* History & physical (H&P).
Physical files. *See* File folder(s).
Physical medicine, 19
Physical therapist (PT), 9t, 19, 21
Physician(s), 4–6, 6t
    after-hours access to records by, 178
    billing for hospital services by, 328b
    communication with, 407
    data elements contributed by, 71–80, 73t, 74f, 76t, 77t, 79t

Physician(s) *(Continued)*
    in office visit, 48–49, 49f
    education of, 201
    hospital privileges of, 34
    in managed care, 316–317, 318
    orders by, 70, 78, 79t, 111b
        computer-based, 89, 97
        forms for, 84–85, 87, 88f
    orientation to HIM for, 396, 398f, 399
    plan of care and, 70–71, 72
Physician assistant, 42
Physician index, 241, 249–250
Physician office liaison, 34–35
Physician-patient privilege, 274
Physician's office, 15. *See also* Ambulatory care facility(ies).
    billing in, 327, 328, 329f, 331f, 332
    certified coding specialist for, 332, 403b
    clinical flow of data in, 42, 43f, 44–45
    closure of, 157–158, 158f
    compared to inpatient stay, 70t
    personnel in, 42, 44, 44f
    services provided in, 18t
PI (performance improvement). *See* Quality improvement (QI).
Pie chart, 225–226, 227f, 256t
PIP (performance improvement plan), 371, 371b
Placebo, 195b
Plaintiff, 279
Plan of care, 8–10, 70–71, 72, 77
    case management and, 219–220
    clinical pathway for, 218–219
Planning, in HIM department, 354–357, 356t
Pneumatic tube systems, 108, 109b
Policies and procedures, 298, 300, 358, 359f, 360–362, 360t–361t
Policy
    insurance, 312t
    of facility, 358
Pool employee, 342, 343t
Population, retrieval of data on, 251–252
Postdischarge analysis, 113. *See also* Quantitative analysis.
Postdischarge processing, 106–120, 350–353
    abstracting in. *See* Abstracting.
    analysis in. *See* Quantitative analysis.
    assembly for. *See* Assembly of records.
    billing and, 332
    coding in. *See* Coding.
    identification of records for, 107–109, 108t
    personnel involved in, 106
    processing flow in, 107f, 120, 351f
    retention of records and, 106, 106t, 118
    tracking of records in, 119–120
Potentially compensable events (PCEs), 220, 220b

PPO (preferred provider organization), 318
PPSs. *See* Prospective payment systems (PPSs).
Preapproval
for out-of-plan care, 318
for procedures, 219, 316, 317
Preexisting condition, 312t
Preferred provider organization (PPO), 318
Premium(s)
definition of, 312t
historical increases in, 312, 313
President. *See* Chief executive officer (CEO).
Prevalence, 191
Preventive care, 195, 317
Preventive controls, 101–102, 102t, 103f,
198
Primary care physician (PCP), 6, 318
Primary data, 236, 236f
Primary digits, 151, 151t, 152, 152t, 154f–155f
Primary payer, 47–48
Printers, 382
Privileges, hospital, 34
PRN employees, 342, 343t
PRO (peer review organization), 321
Probation period, 365, 370, 371, 396b
Problem list, 67, 68f
Problem-oriented record, 64–65, 66, 66f,
67
Procedure(s), 8b. *See also* Policies and proce-
dures.
coding of, 115–116, 116t, 117–118, 117t,
187–188. *See also* Coding.
consent for, 285, 287, 288f
physician's order for, 70. *See also* Order(s).
preapproval for, 219, 316, 317
Procedure index, 250
Productivity of employees
equipment and supplies for, 383
measurement of, 352, 352f, 358, 364, 365,
368–370, 369t
performance standards for, 365, 368t
Productivity report, 352, 352f, 358, 364,
368–369, 369t
computerized, 369–371
Professional standards, 31–32, 301
Professional standards review organizations
(PSROs), 372
Progress notes, 78–79
anesthesia note in, 82
by nurse, 81, 81t
computerization and, 115
operative note in, 82
timeliness of, 206
Prospective consent, 278, 287, 293
Prospective payment systems (PPSs), 309–310,
321–322
advantages and disadvantages of, 326

Prospective payment systems (PPSs) *(Continued)*
comparison of, 326t
DRGs for, 321, 322–324, 326
auditing of records and, 336
optimal reimbursement and, 332
employee training about, 401
for ambulatory care, 324–325
for home health care, 326
for long-term care, 325
for rehabilitation, 326
PSROs (professional standards review organizations), 321
Psychiatric facilities, 18–19. *See also* Behavioral health records; Community mental
health services.
Psychiatrists, 6t, 18, 19
Psychologists, 18, 19
PT (physical therapist), 9t, 19, 21
PT (part-time) employee, 342, 343, 343t
PTO (paid time off), 342

Q

Qualitative analysis, 212–213, 214f, 215, 216f,
217–218
Quality
of coding, 208, 208t, 300, 333–334
of data, 54–55, 100–101, 101t
controls over, 90–91, 90t, 101–106, 102t,
103f
of database, 246, 248, 248b
of health information, 205, 205b–206b
of patient care
customer perspectives on, 197, 197b–
198b
historical development of, 200–205,
201f, 203f
record review and, 186–187, 215, 216f,
217
Quality assurance (QA), 206–208, 208t, 358
Quality improvement (QI), 206–207, 207t,
208–210, 210f
data audits and, 248b
data-gathering tools in, 223–224, 224t
employee orientation to, 393
for advance directives, 210–212, 211f
HIM committee and, 229
models of, 209, 209b, 210f
JCAHO 10-step method as, 206–207,
207t, 209b
team meetings on, 222–223, 223b
visual presentation tools in, 224–228, 224t,
225f–227f, 227t
Quality management, theories of, 198–200

Quality management (QM) department, 198
  signing out records to, 173
Quality standards, 207–208, 208t
Quantitative analysis, 110–115, 112t, 114f,
    206b, 212–213, 349–350
  as priority, 357
  in record review, 215
  performance standard for, 368t
  quality standard for, 207, 208t
Quarters, of year, 261, 262f
Querying a database, 241, 241b, 242, 246
  identifying population for, 251–252
  information needed for, 249
  strategies for, 253
  to create indices, 249–250, 250f–251f

R

RACE acronym, for fire response, 393–394
Radiologist, 5, 6t
Radiology services, 16, 18t, 24
Radiology tests
  data elements derived from, 83
  orders for, 78
RAI (Resident Assessment Instrument), 325
Rates, calculation of, 264–265, 264f–265f
Receipt, for health record, 296
Receiver of message, 406
Receiving hospital, 259b
Receptionist, 44, 45
Reciprocal services, 309
Record, 52, 52f, 53. *See also* Health record(s).
Record retention schedule, 155–156, 157f
Record review, 212–213, 214f, 215, 216f,
    217–218
  frequency of, 213
  HIM assistant director and, 233
  HIM committee and, 229
Record review form, 213, 214f
Record review team, 217
Reference materials, 381, 381t
Referral, 6. *See also* Consultation.
Registered dietician, 9t
Registered Health Information Administrator
    (RHIA), 9t, 204
  continuing education for, 403b, 404t
Registered Health Information Technician
    (RHIT), 9t, 204, 354
  continuing education for, 403b, 404t
Registered nurse (RN), 7, 7t
  orders dictated to, 78, 111b
Registrar. *See* Patient registration specialist.
Registries, 116, 253

Rehabilitation facilities, 18t, 19
  accreditation of, 30
  care plans in, 71
  prospective payment system for, 326
Reimbursement, 187–188. *See also* Billing; In-
    surance.
  access to records for, 278
  by government, 319–321. *See also* Medic-
    aid; Medicare.
  coding and, 117, 187–188, 300, 326,
    332–334
  definition of, 308, 312t
  false claims for, 188, 188b, 332, 333
  fiscal intermediaries in, 312t, 320
  maximization of, 332
  optimization of, 332
  types of, 308–311, 309t. *See also specific
    types.*
    facility profit and, 327
Relational database, 65–66, 105b. *See also*
    Database(s).
Release of information, 118, 281
  confidentiality in, 295–296, 296f
  consent for, 287, 289–290, 289f
    in release to payer, 278
    special, 287, 292–293, 292f
    validation of, 293–294
  employee training about, 401
  fees for, 295
  in emergencies, 290–292, 291f
  in incomplete record, 294
  log of, 294, 294t
  outsourcing of, 285, 303
  preparing record for, 293–296, 294t, 295t
  quality standard for, 208, 208t, 357
  steps in, 295t
  to department managers, 399
  to facility personnel, 296–297
  without consent, 290
Reporting of data, 190–191, 253–254, 268.
    See also Database(s).
Research, 118, 194
  as evidence in trial, 193, 194
  on medications, 194, 195b
Resident, in long-term care facility, 17
Resident Assessment Instrument (RAI), 325
Resident physician, 4
  countersigned notes by, 79, 111
Resource utilization, 323, 324, 332
Resource Utilization Groups (RUGs), 325
Respiratory therapist, 9t
Respite care, 20
Retention of master patient index, 136, 137b
Retention of records, 106, 106t, 118,
    155–158, 157f–158f, 179. *See also* Stor-
    age of records

Retrieval of data, 248–253, 249f–251f

Retrieval of records, 118, 205, 294, 350. *See also* Chart locator systems; Release of information.
fee for, 295
in computerized system, 141
on optical disk, 154–155
purposes of, 129, 129b

Retrospective analysis, 113. *See also* Quantitative analysis.

Retrospective consent, 278, 287

Retrospective processing. *See* Postdischarge processing.

Retrospective review, 187

Reverse chronologic order, 62, 64f, 110

Review of systems, 76t

Revolving file system, 161–162, 162f, 163t

RHIA (Registered Health Information Administrator), 9t, 204
continuing education for, 403b, 404t

RHIT (Registered Health Information Technician), 9t, 204, 354
continuing education for, 403b, 404t

Rider, definition of, 312t

Risk, assumption of, 312–313, 314f

Risk management, 220, 221f–222f

RN (registered nurse), 7, 7t
orders dictated to, 78

Robert's Rules of Order, 411b

ROI. *See* Release of information.

RUGs (Resource Utilization Groups), 325

Ruling out a diagnosis, 72

S

Safety. *See also* Security of records.
annual training about, 401
orientation to, 393–394

Safety committee, 230–231

Safety officer, 230, 231b

Same-day surgery, 92

Sample, from population, 252

Scanning of records
into computer system, 141, 153, 167, 182
onto microfilm, 165, 167
onto optical disk, 167

Scheduling appointments, 44, 44b

Search fee, 295

Second opinion, 317

Secondary data, 236, 236f, 242

Secondary digits, 151, 151t, 152, 152t, 153f–154f

Secondary payer, 48

Secretary, medical, 42

Security of records, 106, 106t, 175–180, 175b. *See also* Confidentiality.
in computer environment, 175b, 240b
litigation-related, 220b, 297

Self-insurance, 318–319

Sender of message, 406

Sequential record, 62, 63f–64f, 66

Serial numbering system, 146, 147f, 149t, 382

Serial–unit numbering system, 146, 148f, 149t, 382

Service days, 260, 260t, 261t, 262–263, 262b, 263f, 263t
average, 265f

Shareholders, 344b

Shelves, 159–160, 160f–161f, 163, 163t, 164

Shewhart, Walter, 209

Signature, 111b. *See also* Authentication.
electronic, 91
for release of information, 293–294

Skilled nursing facilities (SNFs), 325. *See also* Long-term care facilities.

Skills assessment, 379

Snail mail, 410b

SOAP format
for medical evaluation, 72–73, 73t, 77
for progress notes, 79

Social Security Act, 319, 320. *See also* Medicare.

Social Security number
as identifier for ROI, 287
data field for, 55b, 90
for terminal-digit filing, 152

Social services personnel, 18, 19

Socioeconomic data, 46–47, 47f, 69, 84

Software, 178, 383, 383b

Source-oriented record, 63–64, 65f, 66, 110

Span of control, 346

Special consents, 287, 292–293, 292f

Specialist physician, 4–6, 6t. *See also* Consultation.

Speech therapist, 19

Staff employees, 343, 346

Standards of care, 193–194

Standing order, 78

State governments
advance directives and, 212
confidentiality regulations of, 274, 287
health care legislation of, 191
licensure of facilities by, 27–28, 30, 188, 298–299
Medicaid and, 204, 320
prospective payment systems and, 321
record retention laws of, 155–156
reporting by facilities to, 28, 253, 290

Statistical analysis, 254–256, 255f, 256t

Statistics, of facility, 256–265, 257f. *See also* Census; Database(s).
 ALOS calculated from, 261
 fiscal year for, 261, 262f
 on admissions, 256, 257f
 on discharges, 256, 257f, 258
 on transfers, 258, 258f, 259b
 percentages in, 264–265, 264f–265f
 rate calculations with, 264–265, 264f–265f
 reporting of, 190–191
Statute, definition of, 274
Storage of records, 106, 106t, 107, 118, 205, 348. *See also* File folder(s); Filing; Filing methods; Retention of records.
 alternative methods of, 165–169, 166f, 179
 importance of, 128, 129
 locations in. *See* Master patient index (MPI).
 number of records in, 128b
 security for, 106, 106t, 175–180, 175b
Straight numeric filing, 150–151, 153t
Strategic planning, 355
Subjective data, 72, 73t, 77
Subpoena, 281, 282f–284f
Subscriber, definition of, 312t
Supervisors, 341, 346, 348, 350
 communication by, 407
 monitoring of operations by, 358
Supplies, for HIM department, 381–383
Surgeon, 82
Surgeon General, 192, 193f
Surgery
 consent for, 285, 287, 288f
 second opinion for, 317
Surgical case review, 229, 252
Surgical facilities, 10, 18t, 24
 ambulatory, 16
Surgical supply companies, 190
Surgical technologist, 7t
Survey
 by JCAHO, 252–253, 299–300
 for information gathering, 224, 224t
Suspension policy, 399b
Symptoms, 49, 72

T

Tampering with records, 177–178
Targeted reviews, of coding, 333–334
Tax Equity and Fiscal Responsibility Act (TEFRA), 321
TD order. *See* Terminal-digit filing.
Technical employees, 348, 348t
Telephone orders, 78
Temporary employee, 342, 343, 343t

Terminal-digit filing, 151–152, 151t, 153f, 153t
Terminology, medical, 5b
Tertiary digits, 151, 151t, 152, 152t, 153f–154f
Theft of records, 177–178
Therapeutic procedure, 8b, 70
Third party payer, 187b. *See also* Insurance.
 accreditation and, 188
 definition of, 312t
 preapproval of procedure by, 219
Time studies, 352
Timeliness, 100, 101t, 205b–206b
 of coding, 332
 qualitative analysis of, 213
Title XVIII of Social Security Act, 319, 320
Title XIX of Social Security Act, 319, 320
Tracking records, 119–120
Training, of employees, 392, 399–402, 402t
Transcription, 348, 350
 equipment for, 382
 quality improvement in, 207t
 standards for, 353t, 354t, 357
Transcriptionist, 96, 348t
 of operative report, 190b
Transfer form, 259b
Transfers
 interhospital, 258, 259b
 intrahospital, 258f, 259b
Treatment. *See* Order(s); Plan of care.
Trial, of lawsuit, 279, 280t
TRICARE, 319, 320
Tumor registry, 116, 253

U

UA (urinalysis), 82
UM (utilization management). *See* Utilization review (UR).
Unbilled list, 326
Uniform Ambulatory Care Data Set (UACDS), 56–57, 56f, 118, 238
Uniform Bill (UB-92), 187, 240, 328, 330f
Uniform Hospital Discharge Data Set (UHDDS), 93, 118, 238, 239t
Unique patient identification number (UPIN), 289
Unit numbering system, 144–145, 145f, 149t, 382
Unity of command, 346
Universal chart order, 110
Universal precautions, for blood and body fluids, 394–395
Upgrade, software, 178, 383
Urinalysis (UA), 82
Urologist, 5

Usual and customary fees, 309
Utilization management (UM). *See* Utilization review (UR).
Utilization of resources, 323, 324, 332
Utilization review (UR), 219, 248, 252, 254

V

Validation of consent, 293–294
Validity of data, 55, 101t, 206b
    preventive controls on, 90–91, 90t, 101–102, 103f
    qualitative analysis of, 213
Verbal orders, 78, 79t, 111b
Vice presidents, of facility, 345
Vision statement, 356
Visit, 15
Vital signs, 81
    in critical care unit, 92
Vital statistics, 254
Volume reduction, 118

W

Water damage
    to computers, 179
    to paper records, 175b, 176, 177
Workers' compensation, 385b
Workflow, in HIM department, 349–354, 351f–352f, 353t, 354t, 357
Working DRG, 324
Wraparound policies, 319
Written communication, 408, 409f

X

X-ray tests. *See* Radiology tests.

Z

Zero defects, 200
Zip-code field, 55b